OXFORD MEDICAL PUBLICATIONS

Oxford Handbook of
Clinical Pharmacy

Published and forthcoming Oxford Handbooks

Oxford Handbook of Clinical Medicine 6/e (also available for PDAs and
    in a Mini Edition)
Oxford Handbook of Clinical Specialties 7/e
Oxford Handbook of Acute Medicine 2/e
Oxford Handbook of Anaesthesia 2/e
Oxford Handbook of Applied Dental Sciences
Oxford Handbook of Cardiology
Oxford Handbook of Clinical Dentistry 4/e
Oxford Handbook of Clinical and Laboratory Investigation 2/e
Oxford Handbook of Clinical Diagnosis
Oxford Handbook of Clinical Haematology 2/e
Oxford Handbook of Clinical Immunology and Allergy 2/e
Oxford Handbook of Clinical Pharmacy
Oxford Handbook of Clinical Surgery 2/e
Oxford Handbook of Critical Care 2/e
Oxford Handbook of Dental Patient Care 2/e
Oxford Handbook of Dialysis 2/e
Oxford Handbook of Emergency Medicine 3/e
Oxford Handbook of Endocrinology and Diabetes
Oxford Handbook of ENT and Head and Neck Surgery
Oxford Handbook for the Foundation Programme
Oxford Handbook of Gastroenterology and Hepatology
Oxford Handbook of General Practice 2/e
Oxford Handbook of Genitourinary Medicine, HIV and AIDS
Oxford Handbook of Geriatric Medicine
Oxford Handbook of Medical Sciences
Oxford Handbook of Nephrology and Hypertension
Oxford Handbook of Nutrition and Dietetics
Oxford Handbook of Neurology
Oxford Handbook of Obstetrics and Gynaecology
Oxford Handbook of Oncology 2/e
Oxford Handbook of Ophthalmology
Oxford Handbook of Palliative Care
Oxford Handbook of Practical Drug Therapy
Oxford Handbook of Psychiatry
Oxford Handbook of Public Health Practice 2/e
Oxford Handbook of Rehabilitation Medicine
Oxford Handbook of Respiratory Medicine
Oxford Handbook of Rheumatology 2/e
Oxford Handbook of Tropical Medicine 2/e
Oxford Handbook of Urology

UKMI specialist information centres

Specialist topic	Centre
Prescribing in pregnancy	Newcastle Regional MI
Drugs in breast milk	Sutton Coldfield and Leicester Regional MI
Complementary medicine	Cardiff Regional MI
Medicines in children	Alder Hey Children's Hospital MI
Drugs in liver impairment	Leeds Regional MI
Drugs in renal impairment	Bristol Regional MI
Oncology	Royal Marsden Hospital MI
Ophthalmic drugs	Moorfields Hosiptal MI
HIV/AIDS	St Marys Hospital (London) MI
	Chelsea and Westminster Hospital MI

Phone numbers are in the British National Formulary and on the UKMI website (www.ukmi.nhs.uk).

UK National Poisons Information Service

NPIS is comprised of six Poison Centres (Belfast, Birmingham, Cardiff, Edinburgh, London, and Newcastle) with a single national telephone number: 0870 600 6266

Oxford Handbook of
Clinical
Pharmacy

Philip Wiffen

Director of Training UK Cochrane Centre
and Co-ordinating Editor Cochrane Pain,
Palliative and Supportive Care Group
Pain Research Unit, Churchill Hospital
Oxford, UK

Marc Mitchell

Divisional Pharmacist
Surgery, Cancer, Neurosciences
& Critical Care, Oxford Radcliffe Trust, UK

Mel Snelling

Lead Pharmacist
HIV and Infectious Diseases
Oxford Radcliffe Hospitals NHS Trust, UK

Nicola Stoner

Lead Cancer Pharmacist
Cancer Directorate and Cancer Research UK
Oxford Radcliffe Hospitals NHS Trust;
and Principal Visiting Fellow
School of Pharmacy
The University of Reading, UK

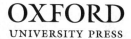

OXFORD
UNIVERSITY PRESS

OXFORD
UNIVERSITY PRESS

Great Clarendon Street, Oxford OX2 6DP

Oxford University Press is a department of the University of Oxford.
It furthers the University's objective of excellence in research, scholarship,
and education by publishing worldwide in

Oxford New York

Auckland Cape Town Dar es Salaam Hong Kong Karachi
Kuala Lumpur Madrid Melbourne Mexico City Nairobi
New Delhi Shanghai Taipei Toronto

With offices in

Argentina Austria Brazil Chile Czech Republic France Greece
Guatemala Hungary Italy Japan Poland Portugal Singapore
South Korea Switzerland Thailand Turkey Ukraine Vietnam

Oxford is a registered trade mark of Oxford University Press
in the UK and in certain other countries

Published in the United States
by Oxford University Press Inc., New York

© Oxford University Press 2007

The moral rights of the authors have been asserted
Database right Oxford University Press (maker)

First published 2007

British Library Cataloguing in Publication Data

Data available

Library of Congress Cataloging in Publication Data

Data available

Typeset by Newgen Imaging Systems (P) Ltd., Chennai, India
Printed in Italy
on acid-free paper by
Legoprint S.p.A.

ISBN 0–19–856710–3 (flexicover: alk.paper) 978–0–19–856710–3 (flexicover: alk.paper)

10 9 8 7 6 5 4 3 2 1

Foreword

The world we live and work in has changed, and continues to change rapidly. Clinical pharmacy is one area where change is at its most rapid, and the extent and speed of change poses a major challenge. Although this book covers a huge amount of ground, perhaps three main areas stand out to a non-pharmacist looking over the pharmacist's shoulder.

The first is the interpretation of clinical evidence about efficacy (or effectiveness) and harm of medicines. The number of new medicines, and studies of existing medicines, is exploding, producing more information than we can handle. The key to handling it is often to have good systematic reviews of good randomized trials, when the results will be secure.

The second is to reassess how we look at harm. Adverse events that are rare, but serious, will hardly ever be uncovered in randomized trials because of insufficient numbers. The trend is to perform large observational database studies of clinical practice, often with millions of participants; some of these will make us think again about medicines we have always considered safe.

The third is the translation of knowledge into clinical practice. There are any number of different ways this can affect clinical pharmacists–from use of expert computer systems to halve the rates of adverse drug reactions, to the generation of care pathways to deliver better outcomes for patients, with less hassle and at lower cost. This requires real management skills–not bureaucracy, let me emphasize, which is what most of us see badged as management.

All three of these demand that clinical pharmacists have a range of skills, and the key is that they know and understand the tools of evidence-based healthcare. This includes management as well as knowledge of clinical trials in order to convert efficacy into effectiveness.

The use of evidence is massively misunderstood. The most often used definition of evidence-based medicine is the *'conscientious, explicit and judicious use of current best evidence in making decisions about the care of individual patients*.[1] It is interesting that this was in response to a critic of evidence-based medicine, John Grimley Evans, who made a very similar point: *'Managers and trialists may be happy for treatments to work on average; patients expect their doctos to do better than that'.*[2]

Both of these emphasize the point that each of us is an individual, and that we have to treat average results from trials or reviews with a degree of caution, both for efficacy and harm. Robert Temple, a thoughtful FDA researcher, has recently commented that *'whether accomplished by sophisticated genetic or receptor analyses or by empirical observation of response to treatment, there is growing recognition that people are not all the same in the way that they respond to treatment and that groups that might*

1 Sackett DL, Rosenberg WM, Gray JA, Haynes RB, Richardson WS (1996). Evidence based medicine: what it is and what it isn't. *BMJ*, **312**, 71–72.
2 Grimley Evans J (1995). Evidence-based and evidence-biased medicine. *Age Ageing*, **24**, 461–463.

respond differently should be studied, a change from the established wisdom of conducting trials with broad entry criteria while eschewing subset analyses.[3]

There are some intriguing results out there, relating differences in efficacy to genetic polymorphisms affecting drug absorption and metabolism, the way drugs pass the blood–brain barrier, as well as changes in receptors. Keeping up, and coping with these changes is by no means going to be easy, let alone incorporating them into clinical pharmacy. All we can be sure of is that more change is on the way.

Andrew Moore
Chief Editor, *Bandolier*
October 2006

3 Temple RJ (2005). Enrichment designs: efficiency in development of cancer treatments. *J Clin Oncol*, **23**, 4838–4839.

Preface

One of the authors began their clinical pharmacy career at a time when pharmacists entered a ward with trepidation and more than once was shouted at by a feisty ward sister protecting her territory. Since then, things have moved on a long way such that an internationally renowned surgeon stated recently that clinical pharmacy (provided by his capable clinical pharmacist) was one of the best things anyone had provided for him in his professional career.

This illustrates, perhaps, that clinical pharmacy services are only as good as the pharmacists who provide them and there are still battles to be fought and won. It remains a disappointment that clinical pharmacy in the UK has not embraced the academic rigor seen in some countries and that the research culture inbred into junior doctors has yet to infect pharmacists in the same way.

This book is the distillation of 60–70 years of combined experience between the authors with the hope that it will contribute to assisting clinical pharmacists fulfil their potential. The book is organized into chapters that follow, we hope, a logical layout with additional information organized into chapters designed to provide additional know-how. This handbook was never perceived as a formulary, but hopefully it will provide wisdom that can be used at the bedside, in the department, or for on-call.

The Oxford Handbook series is well established and although pharmacists have used many of the volumes, this is the first is written specifically for pharmacists. We hope that it will prove useful to clinical pharmacy practitioners and teachers.

PW
MM
MS
NS
2006

Contents

Contributor

Mark Borthwick
Lead Pharmacist, Critical Care Oxford Radcliffe Hospitals NHS Trust,
UK, wrote six monographs on critical care.

Acknowledgements

We are grateful to the following people who provided comments and help: John Beale, Sarah Cripps, Mrudula Patel, Rhoda Welsh, and Rebecca White.

We are also grateful to the following reviewers: Jon Hayhurst, Phil Rogers, and Nicola Walker.

Detailed contents

Symbols and abbreviations

↑	increased
↓	decreased
>	greater than
<	less than
♂	male
♀	female
°	degrees
28d	one-stop supply
A&E	accident and emergency
A&W	alive and well
AAA	abdominal aortic aneurism
ABC	airway, breathing, and circulation
abdo	abdominal
ABPI	Association of the British Pharmaceutical Industry
ACE	angiotensin-converting enzyme
ACV	assist control ventilation
ADR	adverse drug reaction
AF	atrial fibrillation
AFB	acid-fast bacilli
APPT	activated partial thrombin time
AUC	area under the plasma concentration curve
AV	arteriovenous
BiPAP	bilevel positive airway pressure
BMI	body mass index
BMR	basal metabolic rate
BNF	British National Formulary
BP	blood pressure
BPH	benign prostatic hyperplasia
C/O	complaining of
CAPD	continuous ambulatory peritoneal dialysis

CAVD	continuous arteriovenous haemodialysis
CAVH	continuous arteriovenous haemofiltration
CD	controlled drug
CFTR	cystic fibrosis transmembrane conductance regulator
CHM	Commission on Human Medicines
C-MRSA	community-acquired MRSA
CMV	continuous mandatory ventilation
CNS	central nervous system
CO_2	carbon dioxide
COC	combined oral contraception
COPD	chronic obstructive pulmonary disease
COREC	central office for research ethics committees
COSHH	Committee on Substances Hazardous to Health
CPAP	continuous positive airway pressure
CTC	common toxicity criteria
CVC	central venous catheter
CVS	cardiovascular system
CVVHDF	continuous venovenous haemodiafiltration
CXR	chest X-ray
CYP450	cytochrome P450
DDx, $\Delta\Delta$	differential diagnosis
DHx	drug history
DIC	disseminated intravascular coagulation
DOE	disease-orientated evidence
DoH	Department of Health
DTI	direct thrombin inhibitor
DUE	drug-use evaluation
DVT	deep vein thrombosis
Dx, Δ	diagnosis
E/C	enteric-coated
EBM	evidence-based medicine
ECF	extracellular fluid
ECG	electrocardiogram
ESBL	extended-spectrum beta-lactamases
EU	European Union
FH	family history
G6PD	glucose 6-phosphate dehydrogenase

GABA	γ-aminobutyric acid
GAfREC	governance arrangements for research ethics committees
GCP	good clinical practice
GFR	glomerular filtration rate
GI	gastro-intestinal system
GIT	gastrointestinal tract
GMP	good manufacturing practice
GOR	glucose oxidation rate
GP	general practitioner
GSL	general sales list
GTAC	gene therapy advisory committee
GTN	glyceryl trinitrate
HbA_{1c}	glycosylated haemoglobin
HD	haemodialysis
HDF	haemodiafiltration
HF	haemofiltration
HIV	human immunodeficiency virus
HPA	Health Protection Agency
HPC	history of presenting complaint
HRS	hepatorenal syndrome
ICF	intracellular fluid
IM	intramuscular
IMP	investigational medicinal product
IMV	intermittent mandatory ventilation
INR	international normalized ratio
IPS	Institute of Purchasing Supply
ITU	intensive therapy unit
IV	intravenous
Ix	investigations
K^+	potassium
KCCT	kaolin cephalin clotting time
LFT	liver function test
LREC	local research ethics committee
M/R	modified-release
MARS	molecular absorbent recirculating system
MDA	Medical Devices Agency
MDI	metered-dose inhaler

MDS	monitored dose system
MEMS	medicines event monitoring system
MHRA	Medicines and Healthcare Products Regulatory Agency
MHV	mechanical prosthetic heart valve
MI	myocardial infarction
MIC	minimum inhibitory concentration
MREC	Multicentre research ethics committee
MRSA	Methicillin-resistant Staphylococcus aureus
MSSA	methicillin-susceptible Staphylococcus aureus
NHS	National Health Service
NICE	National Institute of Clinical Excellence
NNH	number needed to harm
NNT	number needed to treat
NPSA	National Patient Safety Agency
NSAID	nonsteroidal anti-inflammatory drug
NSF	National Service Framework
NSTEMI	non-ST-segment elevation myocardial infarction
O/E	on examination
O_2	oxygen
ortho	bones and joints
PABA	para-amino benzoic acid
$PaCO_2$	partial pressure of carbon dioxide in arterial blood
PaO_2	partial pressure of oxygen in arterial blood
PAS	patient addresso-graph sticker
pc	percutaneously
PC	presenting complaint
PCI	percutaneous coronary intervention
PEEP	Positive end-expiratory pressure
PEG	percutaneous endoscopic gastroscopy
PGD	patient group direction
PICC	peripherally inserted central catheter
PMCPA	prescription medicines code of practice authority
PMH	past medical history
PMR	prescription medication records
PMS	pre-menstrual syndrome
PNS	peripheral nervous system
po	per os (by mouth)

POD	patient's own drugs
POEM	patient orientated evidence that matters
POM	prescription only medication
PONV	postoperative nausea and vomiting
ppm	parts per million
pr	per rectum (by the rectum)
prn	pro re nata (as required)
PSV	pressure support ventilation
PT	prothrombin time
QP	qualified person
Resp	respiratory system
RPSGB	Royal Pharmaceutical Society of Great Britain
S	stock
SC	subcutaneous/ly
S/R	systems review
SH	social history
SIMV	synchronous intermittent mandatory ventilation
SOB	short of breath
SR	sinus rhythm
SSA	site-specific assessment
Stat	once only
STEMI	ST-segment elevation myocardial infarction
TB	tuberculosis
TBC	to be confirmed/awaiting confirmation
TDM	therapeutic drug monitoring
TENS	transcutaneous electronic nerve stimulation
TIA	transient ischaemic attack
T_{max}	time to maximum drug concentration
t-PA	tissue plasminogen activator
U&E	urea and electrolytes
UFH	unfractionated heparin
UKMI	UK Medicines Information
v/v	volume in volume
v/w	volume in weight
VAC	vacuum assisted closure
VAS	visual analogue scale
VAT	value added tax

VLCD	very-low-calorie diet
VRE	vancomycin resistant enterococci
VRSA	vancomycin resistant MRSA
VTE	venous thromboembolism
VV	venovenous
w/v	weight in volume
w/w	weight in weight
WHO	World Health Organization

Adherence

Introduction

What is adherence?

'To be taken as directed' is an instruction that frequently appears on medicine labels. It suggests that a patient will obey the doctor's 'orders' without question. However, as most pharmacists are well aware, patients frequently choose not to 'take as directed'.

'Compliance' is a term used to describe whether or not a patient takes their medicines as directed. It implies a paternalistic relationship between the doctor (or other healthcare professional) and the patient, with little, if any, discussion or negotiation.

'Concordance' is a two-way exchange between healthcare professional and patient. The patient participates in both the consultation and the decision-making process, and the patient's preferences and beliefs are taken into account (see www.medicinespartnership.org/about-us/concordance). However, this rarely happens in full in a busy general practitioner's (GP's) surgery, hospital ward, or out-patient clinic.

'Adherence' is somewhere between compliance and concordance. The healthcare professional accepts that the patient's beliefs, preferences and prior knowledge influence medicine taking and attempts to address this. However, adherence interventions are frequently made after the prescription is written and the patient might not have had much influence on the choice of drug. Consequently, pharmacists and specialist nurses tend to have a bigger role in facilitating adherence than doctors.

Concordance requires a high level of resources and a multidisciplinary effort. Although less than ideal, adherence support can be carried out by pharmacists to some extent in their everyday practice. Thus this discussion will concentrate on adherence.

Why is adherence important?

It is estimated that, on average, 50% of patients on long-term therapy do not take their medicines 'as directed'. The costs of this are potentially significant on both personal and public levels. It is estimated that up to 30% of drug-related hospital admissions result from nonadherence. In one study, 91% of non-adherent renal-transplant patients experienced organ rejection or death compared with 18% of adherent patients[1]. The cost of wasted medicines and ↑ health expenditure to treat uncontrolled disease represent a significant public cost.

Why do patients not take their medicines?

Numerous studies have attempted to identify the causes of nonadherence and many factors have been identified (Table 1.1). Different factors are relevant to different diseases or settings, for example cost is an issue in the USA (because patients have to pay for medicines/health insurance) but rarely in the UK. The reasons for nonadherence generally fall into two categories:

- Involuntary or behavioural—eg simply forgetting.
- Voluntary or cognitive—eg concerns about side effects.

---

1 De Geest S et al. (1995). Incidence, determinants, and consequences of subclinical noncompliance with immunosuppressive therapy in renal transplant patients. *Transplantation*, **59**(3):340–7.

Pharmaceutical manufacturers tend to concentrate on behavioural factors—producing combination tablets or once daily versions of their medicines, which are supposedly easier to take. There is evidence to suggest that adherence is reduced if the dose frequency is more than three times daily, but no data are available to support once daily over twice daily dosing. Patients might prefer combination products or once daily dosing, but preference does not necessarily relate to adherence. Once daily dosing could, in fact, lead to a worse therapeutic outcome because missing one dose means missing a whole day's therapy.

Many adherence strategies focus on cognitive issues. Intuitively it seems right that if patients do not adhere because of fears or misconceptions about their medicines, addressing these issues should improve adherence. However, it is not clear whether nonadherent patients lack knowledge and understanding or whether these are the patients who fail to seek advice.

Ultimately, it is the patient's, not the healthcare professional's, agenda that influences whether or not they take their medicines.

Table 1.1 Factors reported to affect adherence

Ability to attend appointments
Age
Beliefs about medicines
Chaotic lifestyle
Complexity of regimen
Concerns about confidentiality
Cost
Cultural practices or beliefs
Depression
Educational status
Frequency of doses
Gender
Health beliefs and attitudes (towards self and others)
Impact on daily life
Language (if the patient's first language is different to that of healthcare professional's)
Literacy
Manual dexterity
Past or current experience of side effects
Satisfaction with health care
Self-esteem
Side effects
Socioeconomic status

Assessing adherence

Various methods of measuring adherence have been developed, but none of them is entirely satisfactory:

- Treatment response—the most clinically relevant method of assessing adherence. If the patient has been taking their medicines, logically their health should improve (assuming the choice of therapy was appropriate). A reasonably noninvasive and simple marker of treatment success is necessary (eg measuring blood pressure [BP] or cholesterol levels). However, some markers might only show recent adherence (eg blood glucose levels).
- Therapeutic drug monitoring (TDM)—has limited use for assessing adherence. If serum levels are within the therapeutic range, recent, but not long-term, adherence can be assumed. Subtherapeutic levels can be an indicator of erratic or recent nonadherence but could also reflect malabsorption of the drug or a drug interaction.
- Medicines event monitoring systems (MEMSs)—these are special bottle caps that record each time the bottle is opened. The information can be downloaded so that each time and date the bottle was opened can be read. However, MEMS caps can only record whether the bottle has been opened, not whether any drug (or how much) was taken out of the bottle. Ideally, they should be used in conjunction with some form of patient diary so that if the bottle is opened or not opened for some reason (eg taking out two doses at once), this can be recorded. MEMS caps are expensive and are usually only used in clinical trials. Blister-packed medicines have to be popped into a suitable container, which can be time consuming and inconvenient.
- Pharmacy records (refills)—can be used to check whether the patient collects the correct quantity of tablets each time, so they do not run out if they have been taking their drugs correctly. However, this system cannot determine whether the patient actually takes the tablets.
- Patient self-report—the patient should be asked (in a nonjudgemental way) whether they have missed or delayed any doses, and if so, how many. Patients tend to overestimate their level of adherence and could give the answer they feel the enquirer wants to hear rather than a true picture. However, patient self-report correlates well to other measures and is relatively cheap and easy to do.

Strategies to improve adherence

Numerous strategies have been used to attempt to improve adherence, but there is little evidence that any of these strategies are effective in the long term. Interventions to support adherence are discussed here.

Monitored dose systems (MDSs)

MDSs ('dosette boxes') are useful for patients who might have difficulty understanding or following instructions—because of language, learning or memory problems. Different types of box are available and it is important to ensure that the patient has the dexterity required to use them. There is no guarantee that the patient will actually take their tablets, but MDSs provide a useful check for whether or not a dose has been taken—if the tablets are still there, clearly the dose has been missed, but an absence of tablets doesn't necessarily mean the tablets have been swallowed.

MDSs are time consuming to fill and pharmacists must ensure that if a patient starts to use an MDS in hospital, a continuing supply of filled MDSs can be ensured in the community. MDSs can only be used for solid-dose formulations and are not suitable for hygroscopic tablets (eg sodium valproate), 'as required' drugs (eg analgesics) or variable-dose medicines (eg warfarin).

Alarms

Alarms, bleeps and phone calls have all been used to remind patients to take their medicines. Many patients find it useful to set the alarm on their mobile phone because this is less obvious than a special alarm. Text messaging has also been used to remind patients to take their tablets but requires a system to be set up to send the messages and should only be done with the patient's consent.

Refill/follow-up reminders

Patients who attend follow-up clinics and collect refill or repeat prescriptions are more likely to adhere to their medication regimen. Adherence support should not just concentrate on medicine taking, but also ensure the patient adheres to other therapies, out-patient appointments etc. Keeping the patient engaged with the whole of their care could be the most important adherence intervention.

Regimen simplification

Patients who have to take their medicines more than three times daily are less likely to adhere fully to their regimen. Further complications, such as having to take medicines with food or on an empty stomach, make adherence even harder. Ideally, the regimen should be simplified to three times daily or less, with times that fit in with the patient's lifestyle.

Written and oral patient information

Bombarding the patient with drug information can be counterproductive, but well thought out advice is important. Much of this can be done when handing out the medicine. A simple explanation of the dosage schedule and probable side effects should be given with every prescription handover. Remember that patients might not understand terms that seem obvious to a healthcare professional. For example, 'take two tablets twice daily' could be interpreted as 'take one tablet morning and evening' (ie two tablets in 24h). Clearly stating that the patient should 'take two tablets in the morning and two tablets in the evening' helps to clarify exactly what is expected.

Manufacturers' patient information leaflets are frequently complex and beyond the reading ability of many patients. A list of side effects can scare patients and confirm the belief that the medicine could do more harm than good. A brief explanation of common side effects and what to do about them, in addition to reassurance that the patient is unlikely to experience other less common side effects listed, can be of considerable benefit.

For more complex or problematic therapies, it might be necessary to spend a substantial amount of time discussing treatment with the patient. This is often a task for specialist pharmacists (where available) in hospitals or GP's surgeries. The patient should be given time to express their fears and beliefs and to ask questions about therapy. Two-way communication between patient and healthcare professional has the following benefits:

- Improves patient satisfaction with care.
- Improves patients' knowledge of their condition and treatment.
- Increases the level of adherence.
- Improves health outcomes.
- Leads to fewer medication related problems.

Verbal information should be backed up with written information. For many chronic diseases, there is a wealth of literature available from the Pharmaceutical Industry or self-help organizations (eg the British Diabetic Association). It might be appropriate to write tailor made patient information for certain drugs or therapies.

Comprehensive management

This involves a multidisciplinary approach, which encompasses all the above strategies. It is potentially complex, labour intensive (with associated costs) and not feasible or necessary in many situations. However, it is appropriate for some diseases and treatments (eg diabetes mellitus and antiretrovirals). Some schemes can be quite intensive and care must be taken that patients do not lose autonomy as a result of the scheme. Expert patient schemes are a good example of comprehensive disease self-management (alongside conventional care), whereby patients are taught by their peers. See www.expertpatients.nhs.uk. These schemes deal with complete management of the disease, not just drug therapy.

Adherence counselling

Pharmacists involved in adherence counselling should ideally employ the communication skills discussed in Chapter 4 (p.84).

When discussing treatment with the patient for the first time, it is important to establish what they already know and any beliefs they hold. Possible questions to ask the patient include the following:
- Tell me anything you already know about the disease/treatment.
- What have the doctors already told you?
- Have you read/found any information about the disease/treatment (eg on the internet)?

Having established baseline knowledge, the pharmacist can then proceed to fill in gaps and attempt to correct any misconceptions. The latter must be done tactfully, in order not to undermine patient self-confidence and their confidence in others (bear in mind that the most cited sources of medicines information are family and friends). A checklist of information that could be provided is shown in the table on p.9 but this should be tailored according to the setting and patient's needs.

Sometimes it is useful to provide written information (to complement verbal information) at the beginning of the session so that you can go through the information with the patient, but sometimes it is better to supply written information at the end so that the patient is not distracted by what they have in their hand. Suggest other sources of information, such as self-help organizations and suitable websites and provide your contact details for further questions.

When questioning the patient about the in level of adherence, it is important to do so in a non-judgemental way. A reasonably accurate picture of adherence, and whether the patient's lifestyle affects it, can be obtained if the patient is asked how many doses they have missed or delayed:
- In the past month.
- In the past week.
- Over a weekend.

This method tends to give a more realistic idea of adherence, but patients tend to underestimate how many doses they have missed. It is also important to confirm that the correct dose (eg number of tablets) has been taken and that any food restrictions have also been adhered to.

If the patient has been nonadherent, ask them why they think they missed doses and if they can think of ways to overcome this. Work together with the patient to find strategies to overcome nonadherence. Ask the patient to tell you in their own words why adherence is important and reflect this back, correcting any inaccuracies as you do so. Verify that the patient understands the regimen—eg ask the patient 'tell me exactly how you take your medicines'. Try to find something positive to say about their adherence, even if this is saying something along the lines of 'I'm glad you've told me about these problems with taking your tablets…'.

Give positive reinforcement to patients who are fully adherent and encourage any improvements. Be careful not to be patronizing! If you have access to any results that could reflect adherence (eg BP readings and glycosylated haemoglobin [HbA1c]), show the patient these results and explain how they reflect improvement in control of the disease.

Checklist of medication information for patients

Basic information
- Drug name (generic and trade name), strength and formulation
- How it works—nontechnical explanation
- Why it is important to keep taking the treatment correctly

Using the treatment
- How much to use—eg number of tablets
- How often to use—eg twice daily, about 12h apart
- Special information—eg with food or drink plenty of water
- Storage—eg in the original container, in the fridge or expiry date

Side effects
- Common side effects—eg when they might occur and what to do about them
- Managing side effects—eg taking drugs with food might reduce nausea or over-the-counter drug treatments
- Serious side effects—eg what to do and whether to contact the clinic (provide a phone number, if appropriate), local doctor or hospital

Drug interactions
Any drugs that the patient should avoid/be cautious with—in particular, mention over-the-counter medicines, herbal and traditional medicines and recreational drugs

Other
- Availability
- Cost (per month/per year)
- Monitoring—eg frequency of tests and costs of tests

Patient preferences for tone and style of written information

Likes
- Positive tone
- Friendly
- Encouraging
- Reassuring
- Non-alarmist
- Honest
- Practical
- Understanding
- Not condescending
- Talking to you personally
- Using 'you' a lot
- Warm

Dislikes
- Negative tone
- Stress on what could go wrong
- Unrealistic
- Over optimistic
- Misleading
- Patronizing
- Childish
- Cold

Writing patient information leaflets

Written information is an important supplement to the verbal information on medicines and disease that pharmacists provide. Patient information leaflets help patients retain the information discussed and provide a source of information for future reference. In the European Union, pharmacists are required to distribute the patient information leaflets supplied by the pharmaceutical industry with each drug when it is dispensed, but additional information might also be required.

Pharmacy-generated patient information leaflets can be used to describe the following:

- The disease and how it could affect the patient's daily life.
- Disease prevention—eg stopping smoking.
- Treatment or treatment options if there is more than one.
- Details of drug therapy, including:
  - Dose and regimen.
  - The importance of continuing chronic therapy even if the patient feels well.
  - Side effects—eg risks and benefits, and what to do if they occur.
  - Drug interactions—eg over-the-counter and herbal medicines, food, alcohol and, recreational drugs.
  - Other special considerations—eg use in pregnancy and lactation.
  - Further sources of information and support—eg pharmacy contact details, self-help organizations and websites.

Before you start

- Discuss with patients:
  - Do they feel they need additional information? What information would they like?
  - What are they worried about?
  - What type of leaflet design do they prefer?
- Don't reinvent the wheel! Check whether a leaflet covering the topic you intend to write about is already available—useful sources are the pharmaceutical industry and patient organizations.
- Look at other leaflets and see how they have been written:
  - Does the style and layout fit what you want to do?
  - Do you find it easy to read and understand?
  - What good/bad aspects of design and content can you learn from these?
- Check whether your hospital or primary care trust has guidelines on writing patient information leaflets. Some organizations require leaflets to be written in a standard format and the final version to be approved by a senior manager.
- Check what facilities there are for printing and distribution and what funding is available. There is no point spending hours producing a full-colour leaflet that requires professional printing if the funds will only stretch to a black and white photocopy.
- Talk to your organization's information technology adviser/medical illustration department—they might have access to computer programmes that will make designing the leaflet much easier.

Content

- State the aim of the leaflet at the beginning—eg 'This leaflet is for people starting treatment for….'.
- Be relevant—decide on the scope of the information you are providing and stick to that, don't get sidetracked into providing information that is not directly relevant to the aim. The leaflet should provide sufficient detail so that the reader can understand the main points but not so much that it becomes confusing and the main points are lost.
- Be accurate—the leaflet must include the most up to date information available and should also address the following points:
  - Be consistent with current guidelines or best practice.
  - Give an honest description of risks and benefits.
  - Where there is a lack of clear evidence, explain that this is the case.
  - Be updated as new information becomes available or guidelines are updated.
- Be understandable, acceptable and accessible to the audience:
  - Apply the rules for clear writing discussed in Chapter 4, p.72.
  - Consider the target group—are there any religious or cultural issues that could influence the content? How can you make the leaflet accessible to patients with visual impairment or who do not speak English? Be careful about getting leaflets translated bcause sometimes the meaning can be inadvertently changed.
  - Get patient's opinions on the content—check that they understand/interpret the information correctly, tone and style are acceptable (see lower box on p.9), layout and presentation are easy to follow, and they think it covers all the relevant issues.

Design and layout

Once you have drafted the text, think about how best it can be presented. Use the guidance on p.73 on font type and basic layout.

Large amounts of type on an A4-size sheet of paper is hard work for anyone to read. A5 size (ideally a single side) is the maximum size that should be used. If you have a lot of information to present, use an A5 or smaller booklet format or a three fold A4 leaflet.

Graphics can be helpful to break up the text and 'signpost' new ideas, but be careful not to overdo it so that the graphics overwhelm the text. Graphics must be relevant to the text. Ensure graphics are culturally acceptable and bear in mind that some stylized pictures or icons could be interpreted differently by people of different cultures (eg a crescent moon to indicate night time would be interpreted as a religious symbol).

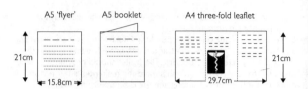

Fig. 1.1 Writing reports: design and layout

Review and update regularly

The leaflet should state the author's name and job title, the date of production and a future review date. Depending on what new information becomes available, it might be necessary to update the leaflet sooner than the review date. If the information is significantly out of date, the leaflet should be withdrawn from use until an updated version is available.

Adverse drug reactions and drug interactions

Introduction

Adverse drug reactions (ADRs; also known as 'side effects', 'adverse drug events' or 'drug misadventures') are a frequent cause of morbidity in hospital and the community. They have a significant cost both financially and in terms of quality of life. Few studies of ADRs have been carried out in the community so the effect on primary care is harder to assess, but studies in the hospital environment have shown the following

- ADRs occur in 10–20% of patients in hospital.
- ADRs are responsible for 5% of admissions to hospital.
- ADRs might be responsible for 1 in 1000 deaths in medical wards.
- ADRs are the most common cause of iatrogenic injury in hospital patients.

The World Health Organization defines an ADR as the following:
'a drug-related event that is noxious and unintended and occurs at doses used in humans for prophylaxis, diagnosis or therapy of disease or for the modification of physiological function.'

However, this definition does not take into account the following scenarios, all of which can also cause ADRs:

- Overdose (including prescribing or administration errors).
- Therapeutic failure.
- Drug interactions.
- Drug withdrawal.

Pharmacists have an important role in identifying, reporting and preventing ADRs.

Classification of ADRs

A number of classification systems exist but the most widely accepted is to group ADRs as either type A (predictable) or type B (unpredictable) reactions. This system is not ideal because some types of reaction (eg teratogenic effects) do not easily fit into either category. However, it is a useful system in most cases because immediate management of the ADR and future drug choices can be guided by the ADR type.

Type A reactions

An exaggerated, but otherwise normal, pharmacological action. Type A reactions have the following characteristics:
- Largely predictable.
- Usually dose-dependent.
- Incidence and morbidity high.
- Mortality low.

Examples of type A reactions include respiratory depression with opioid analgesia, cough with angiotensin-coverting enzyme (ACE) inhibitors and withdrawal effects with benzodiazepines or alcohol.

Type B reactions

Idiosyncratic, aberrant or bizarre drug effects that are unrelated to the pharmacology of the drug. Type B reactions have the following characteristics:
- Usually unpredictable.
- Might not be picked up by toxicological screening.
- Not necessarily dose-related.
- Incidence and morbidity low.
- Mortality high.

Type B reactions are most commonly immunological (eg penicillin allergy).

Adverse reactions: drug or disease?

Determining whether or not a symptom is an ADR can be difficult, especially if the patient has multiple pathologies. Experience has shown that pharmacists tend to blame the drug and doctors to blame the disease. Questions to ask are as follows:

• Is there another explanation for the symptom (eg disease-related)?
• Is this a previously reported side effect of this drug? How common is it? This is harder to assess for new drugs because there is less information available.
• Is the timing right? Most ADRs occur soon after starting a drug, although some ADRs (eg hepatotoxicity) might be delayed. The onset of some hypersensitivity reactions (eg penicillin rash) can be delayed for up to 10 days after starting the drug. This can cause confusion, especially if the antibiotic course has been completed before the rash appears.
• Is the dose excessive? Check serum levels if available. Check renal function—was the dose too high if renal function is impaired? If the symptom can be explained as a type A reaction and the dose is high for whatever reason, it is more probable that the reaction is drug-induced.
• Does the symptom resolve on stopping the drug or reducing the dose (de-challenge)? Type A reactions are usually dose-dependent and so will worsen on dose increase but rapidly resolve or improve on dose reduction or drug withdrawal. Type B reactions are dose-independent and will rarely resolve with dose reduction. Drug withdrawal is necessary but if symptoms are caused by immunological effects (rather than direct drug action) it could take some days or weeks for symptoms to resolve.
• Does the symptom recur on restarting the drug (re-challenge)? Remember that re-challenge can be especially hazardous for type B reactions and is usually not advised.

If the answer to the first question above is 'no' and the answer to (most of) the other questions is 'yes', it is highly probable that the event is an ADR.

Factors predisposing to ADRs

Factors that predispose to ADRs are many and varied and some are related only to specific disease/drug interactions, such as rash with amoxicillin in patients with glandular fever. However, the following factors are generally considered to ↑ patient risk:

• Age
• Renal impairment
• Hepatic impairment
• 'Frailty'
• Polypharmacy
• ♀
• Previous history of ADRs
• Genetics.

The first four factors predispose to type A reactions because they are determinants of drug toxicity, but the remaining factors predispose to type A or type B reactions.

Helping patients understand the risk of ADRs

Terms such as 'common' and 'uncommon' are used to describe levels of risk of ADRs in patient information leaflets and summaries of product characteristics. The terms are standardized by the European Union according to the reported frequency found in clinical trials, for example, (Table 2.1) but patients routinely overestimate the level of risk that these terms are intended to imply.

The following strategies should help in communicating risk to patients:
- Avoid using verbal descriptors such as 'common'.
- Use frequencies rather than percentages—eg 1 person in every 1000 rather than 0.1%.
- Use the same denominator throughout—ie 1 in 1000 and 10 in 1000 rather than 1 in 1000 and 1 in 100.
- Give both positive and negative information—eg 95 out 100 patients did not get the side effect and 5 patients did.
- Give information about baseline risk eg
  - The risk of deep vein thrombosis (DVT) in nonpregnant women who are not taking the combined oral contraceptive (COC) is 5 cases per 100 000 women per year.
  - The risk of DVT in pregnancy is 60 cases per 100 000 pregnancies.
  - The risk of DVT in women taking the COC is 15–25 cases per 100 000 per year.

Table 2.1 Terminology as standardized by the European Union according to reported frequency in clinical trials.

EU terminology	Level of risk
Very common	>10%
Common	1–10%
Uncommon	0.1–1%
Rare	0.01–0.1%
Very rare	<0.015

Reporting ADRs

Most ADRs are not reported and this can lead to delays in identifying important reactions. The reasons for failure to report ADRs have been called the 'seven deadly sins' (Table 2.2). Pharmacists should attempt to address these and encourage their medical and nursing colleagues to report ADRs, in addition to sending in their own reports.

The regulatory authorities in many countries have systems for reporting ADRs and it is important to find out how ADRs are reported and whether pharmacists can submit reports. In the UK doctors, dentists, pharmacists, nurses and patients can report ADRs to the Commission on Human Medicines (CHM) through the yellow card scheme. New drugs are labelled with a black inverted triangle in the British National Formulary (BNF) and the CHM requests that all ADRs to these drugs are reported. For established drugs, unusual or significant reactions should be reported. Yellow card data can be accessed online.[1]

Table 2.2 Failure to report ADRs: the 'seven deadly sins'

1 **Complacency**—a mistaken belief that only safe drugs are allowed onto the market and that these will not cause serious ADRs
2 **Fear** of involvement in litigation, or of a loss of patient confidence
3 **Guilt** that a patient has been harmed by a prescribed treatment
4 **Ambition**—to collect and publish a personal series of cases
5 **Ignorance** of what should be reported or how to make a report
6 **Diffidence**—a reluctance to report an effect for which there is only a suspicion that it is drug related
7 **Lethargy**—this may include a lack of time or interest, inability to find a report card etc.

Drug interactions

Drug interactions occur when the effect of a drug is altered by the co-administration of any of the following:
● Another drug.
● Food.
● Drink.

The outcome of this is as follows:
● Frequently clinically insignificant.
● Sometimes beneficial.
● Occasionally potentially harmful.

Mechanisms of drug interactions

Interactions can be caused by pharmacokinetic (ie the handling of the drug in the body is affected) or pharmacodynamic (ie related to the pharmacology of the drug) mechanisms. Sometimes the interaction can be caused by more than one mechanism, although usually one mechanism is more significant. The majority of interactions are caused by the mechanisms listed below.

Pharmacokinetic mechanisms

Absorption

One drug will ↑ or ↓ the absorption of another. This is most frequently owing to one drug or compound interacting with another—by adsorption, chelation or complexing—to form a product that is poorly absorbed. This can be beneficial (eg activated charcoal adsorbs certain poisons) or problematic (eg antacids and tetracyclines).

Changes in gastric pH affect the absorption of certain drugs—eg ketoconazole and itraconazole require an acidic environment to be absorbed, thus proton-pump inhibitors can reduce absorption and an acidic drink such as fruit juice or soft drinks (especially cola) will ↑ absorption.

Most drugs are absorbed from the upper part of the small intestine. Thus changes in gut motility potentially affect absorption. Usually the total amount absorbed is unaffected, but the rate of absorption might be altered. This effect is used in some combination migraine products—eg including metoclopramide (an antiemetic) speeds up the rate of absorption of the analgesic.

Distribution

Some drugs are bound to proteins in the serum. Only free (unbound) drug is active. Protein binding is a competitive effect so one drug can displace the other from protein-binding sites. This interaction is only an issue with highly protein-bound drugs and is only significant if most of the drug remains in the plasma rather than being distributed into tissues (ie a low volume of distribution). Displacement of drug from protein-binding sites often only causes a small 'blip' in drug levels before equilibrium is restored (because the free drug is also now available for metabolism and excretion), but it could be significant for drugs with a narrow therapeutic index (eg warfarin).

Metabolism

Accounts for the majority of clinically significant pharmacokinetic interactions. Induction or inhibition of the cytochrome P450 (CYP450) system leads to changes in drug levels. CYP450 represents a large group of isoenzymes; drugs are rarely metabolized by a single enzyme, although one usually predominates. Equally, drugs can induce or inhibit several enzymes and some drugs can induce some enzymes and inhibit others (eg efavirenz). In addition, some (but not all) enzyme inhibitors or inducers can induce or inhibit their own metabolism.

When only two drugs are involved, the effect is fairly easy to predict, even if each drug is likely to affect the metabolism of the other. However, if three or more drugs, all of which are inducers or inhibitors, are involved, the effect is almost impossible to predict and this type of combination should be avoided if possible.

The full effects of enzyme induction and inhibition do not occur immediately.

• Enzyme induction takes about 2–3 wks to develop and wear off.
• Enzyme inhibition takes only a few days.

Thus, it might be necessary to delay dose adjustment or TDM until a few days (inhibition) or at least a week (induction) after starting or stopping the offending drug(s).

An emerging area of study is drug interactions involving induction or inhibition of p-glycoprotein. This probably includes interactions involving ↑ in bioavailability because it affects drug metabolism in the gut wall—eg grapefruit juice ↑ levels of ciclosporin by inhibiting gut-wall metabolism.

Excretion

Some drugs interfere with excretion (usually renal) of other drugs. If both drugs are excreted by the same active transport system in the kidney tubule, the excretion of each drug is ↓ by the other. This might be used as a beneficial effect—eg probenecid has been used to prolong the half-life of penicillin—or problematic—eg methotrexate and nonsteroidal anti-inflammatory drugs (NSAIDs).

Pharmacodynamic interactions

These occur if the pharmacological effects of two drugs are additive or opposing:

• Additive—the desired or adverse effects of the two drugs are the same. This can be beneficial or potentially harmful (eg ↑ sedation with alcohol plus hypnotics).
• Synergism—which is a form of additive effect. In this instance the combination of the two drugs has a greater effect than just an additive effect (eg ethambutol ↑ the effectiveness of other antitubercular drugs).
• Antagonism—at receptor level (eg a β-blocker should be prescribed with caution to an asthmatic patient who uses a β-agonist inhaler) or because of opposing effects (eg the desired effects of diuretics could be, at least partly, opposed by fluid retention caused by NSAIDs).

Predicting drug interactions
- Are the desired or adverse effects of the two drugs similar or opposing?
- If there is no information available for the drugs in question, are there reports of drug interactions for other drugs in the same class?
- Are both drugs metabolized by the liver, and if so, by which enzymes? Information on which drugs are metabolized by which CYP450 enzymes might be listed in the summary of product characteristics and can also be found on the following websites:
  - www.hiv-druginteractions.org
  - medicine.iupui.edu/flockhart/
- Drugs that are predominantly renally cleared are unlikely to interact with enzyme inducers and inhibitors.

Managing drug interactions

- Check whether or not the drug combination is new.
- If the patient has already been taking the drug combination, have they tolerated it? If yes, there is probably no need to change therapy, although monitoring might be required.
- Is the interaction potentially serious (eg significant risk of toxicity or ↓ drug effect)—in which case seek alternatives.
- Is the interaction potentially of low-to-moderate significance—in which case it might only be necessary to monitor for side effects, therapeutic effect, or arrange TDM.
- Remember that some drugs in the same class can have different potentials to cause interactions (eg ranitidine versus cimetidine).
- Remember that not only do interactions occur when a drug is started, but also unwanted effects can occur when a drug is stopped.
- The elderly are at greater risk of drug interactions, because of polypharmacy and impaired metabolism and excretion. Additive side effects can be a particular problem.
- Be aware of high-risk drugs and always check for potential interactions with these drugs:
  - Enzyme inhibitors and inducers (eg erythromycin, rifampicin, phenytoin, and protease inhibitors).
  - Drugs with a narrow therapeutic index (eg warfarin, digoxin, lithium, phenytoin, theophylline, and gentamicin).
- Remember that interactions can occur with nonprescription drugs, which the patient might not tell you about:
  - Herbal or traditional medicines.
  - Over-the-counter medicines.
  - Recreational drugs, including alcohol, tobacco and drugs obtained by other means, such as sildenafil purchased on the internet.

Anaphylaxis

Symptoms and signs

Anaphylaxis is defined as an immediate systems hypersensitivity event produced by IgE mediated release of chemicals from mast cells and basophils. Theoretically prior exposure to the agent is required and the reaction is not dose or route related, but in practice anaphylaxis to injected antigen is more frequent, severe, and rapid in onset.

Agents which commonly cause anaphylaxis include:

• Drugs eg penicillins, aspirin.
• Insect stings eg wasp and bee venoms.
• Food eg nuts.

Urticaria and angioedema are the most common and absence of these suggests the reaction may not be anaphylaxis.

Airways oedema, bronchospasm, and shock are life threatening and immediate emergency treatment is usually required.

The onset of symptoms following parenteral antigen (including stings) is usually within 5–30 minutes. With oral antigen, there is often a delay. Symptoms usually occur within 2 hours but may be immediate and life threatening. A late phase reaction may also occur with recrudescence of symptoms after apparent resolution. Recurrence is a fairly frequent phenomenon and health care workers should be aware of this. Patients should not be discharged too quickly as they may require further treatment.

End of needle reactions

Some patients may experience an anaphylactic-like reaction during rapid IV drug administration. This is known as an end of needle reaction. Initial symptoms may suggest anaphylaxis but in fact this is a vasopressor effect and can be distinguished from anaphylaxis as bradycardia occurs which is rare in anaphylaxis. Skin symptoms are also rare in end of needle reactions. Stopping or slowing down the infusion or injection usually leads to resolution of symptoms, and repeat administration at a slower rate usually avoids a repeat event.

Table 3.1 Signs and symptoms of anaphylaxis

F	Urticaria
R	Angioedema
E	Dyspnoea, wheeze
Q	Nausea, vomiting, diarrhoea, cramping abdominal pain
U	Flush
E	Upper airway oedema
N	
T	
R	Headache
A	Rhinitis
R	Substernal pain
E	Itch without no rash
	Seizure

Treatment of anaphylaxis

Anaphylaxis is a life-threatening condition; therefore, rapid recognition and treatment is essential. The first response is to secure the airway and lay the patient flat to reduce hypotension. If the patient cannot tolerate a supine position (because this can worsen breathing difficulties), a semirecumbent position is preferable.

In hospital and some community settings (eg home intravenous [IV] antibiotic therapy), it might be appropriate to keep an 'anaphylaxis box' for emergency use, which contains the following essential drugs:
- Adrenaline (epinephrine).
- An antihistamine (usually chlorphenamine injection).
- A steroid (usually hydrocortisone injection).

Adrenaline

In adults, 500mcg of adrenaline (1:1000 solution) should be administered intramuscularly if the patient is showing clinical signs of shock, airway swelling, or breathing difficulty (stridor, wheezing and cyanosis). The subcutaneous route is not used because absorption is too slow. IV adrenaline is hazardous and should only be administered in the hospital setting. The IV route is preferred if there are concerns about intramuscular absorption; however, time should not be wasted looking for IV access in the event of vascular compromise. For IV administration, use a dilution of at least 1:10 000 and administer the injection over several minutes. The 1:1000 solution is never used intravenously. In the community, patients and carers can be taught to administer adrenaline using a pre-loaded device, such as an EpiPen® (ALK-Abell) or AnaPen® (Celltech). Note that both types of pen contain a residual volume after use and patients should be warned about this (Table 3.2). Trainer pens can be purchased from the manufacturers. Adrenaline minijets are no longer recommended for self-administration. See Table 3.3 for doses of adrenaline for adults and children.

Emergency administration of adrenaline without a prescription

Adrenaline (1:1000 solution) is exempt from prescription-only control if it is used for the purpose of saving a life in an emergency. The code of ethics states that 'pharmacists must assist persons in need of emergency first aid or medical treatment'. The Royal Pharmaceutical Society of Great Britain (RPSGB) considers that a pharmacist is justified in supplying and administering adrenaline without a prescription in a life-threatening situation.

Chlorphenamine

In adults, a dose of 10–20mg chlorphenamine should be given after adrenaline and continued for 24–48h to prevent relapse. It should be administered intramuscularly or by slow IV injection to ↓ the risk of exacerbating hypotension.

Hydrocortisone sodium succinate

In adults, a dose of 100–300mg hydrocortisone is administered by intramuscular or slow IV injection after severe attacks to help prevent relapse. The onset of action is delayed for several hours. Asthmatics who have previously received a steroid are at special risk of delayed symptoms.

Additional treatment

Symptomatic and supportive care as needed: salbutamol or terbutaline nebules or IV aminophylline can be used to treat bronchospasm, with oxygen (O_2) or other respiratory support given as needed. Crystalloid infusion (eg sodium chloride 0.9%) might be needed to treat severe hypotension.

All patients treated initially in the community should be transferred to hospital for further treatment and observation.

Algorithms for the treatment of anaphylaxis in adults and children in hospital and community settings are available from the Resuscitation Council (UK) website[1].

Late sequelae

Patients should be warned of the possibility of symptom recurrence, and if necessary, kept under observation for up to 24h. This is especially applicable in the following circumstances:

- Past history of a recurrence (biphasic reaction).
- Severe reaction, with slow onset.
- Possibility that the allergen could still be absorbed (eg oral administration).
- Past history of asthma or a severe asthmatic component to the reaction.

Table 3.2 Adrenaline for self-administration (IM only)

EpiPen®/AnaPen®: for children and adults >30kg body weight, adrenaline 300mcg
Junior EpiPen®/Junior AnaPen®: children 15–30kg body weight adrenaline 150mcg
EpiPen®/Junior EpiPen®: 1.7mL remains in the pen after use (initial volume, 3mL)
AnaPen®/Junior AnaPen®: 0.75mL remains in the pen after use (initial volume, 1.05mL)

Table 3.3 Dose of IM of adrenaline for anaphylaxis (dose can be repeated at 5min levels, as needed)

Age	Dose	Volume of adrenaline in 1:1000 solution (1mg/mL)
<6months	50mcg	0.05mL
6months to 6yrs	120mcg	0.12mL
6–12yrs	250mcg	0.25mL
>12yrs/adults	500mcg	0.5mL
Doses of IV adrenaline injection for anaphylaxis		
Age	Dose	Volume of adrenaline in 1:10 000 solution (100mcg/mL)
Children	10mcg/kg body weight	0.1mL/kg body weight
Adults	500mcg	5mL (1mL/min; stop when response obtained)

1 The Resuscitation Council (UK). www.resus.org.uk/pages/reaction.htm

Prevention of anaphylaxis

The risk of an anaphylactic reaction can be reduced by good drug history taking and antigen avoidance:

- Check the patient's drug history for reports of allergy. If necessary, clarify the details of the reaction with the patient or a relative.
  A previous history of a mild penicillin-associated rash in infancy might not be a contraindication to future use, but bronchospasm would be.
- Be aware of cross-sensitivity between drug classes:
  - ≈10% of people allergic to penicillin are also allergic to cephalosporins.
  - Patients allergic to aspirin are frequently also allergic to other prostaglandin inhibitors.
- Advise patients with severe allergies to carry some form of warning information (eg MedicAlert® bracelet).
- Some drugs (eg NSAIDs, and ACE inhibitors) can exacerbate or ↑ the risk of a reaction. Avoid concomitant use of these drugs in situations where the patient could be exposed to the allergen (eg desensitization programmes).
- Remember that patients with peanut allergies should avoid pharmaceutical products containing arachis oil.

Clinical pharmacy skills

Guidelines for prescription endorsement of hospital or institutional drug charts by pharmacists

Administration/prescription chart review

- Pharmacists should initial and date all sections of drug charts where drugs have been prescribed when reviewing charts on the ward—this constitutes the 'clinical check' and assumes that all patient parameters are available to the pharmacist (ie drug history, medical notes, urea and electrolyte (U & E) levels-patient's own drugs, etc).
- If the pharmacist clinically checks the drug chart in the dispensary, the following applies:
  - All drug entries are clinically checked using the resources available in the dispensary (ie no access to patient's notes, limited access to U & E levels.
  - All entries are initialled and dated by the pharmacist, ideally in green ink, and any items supplied are endorsed with the quantity, strength and form supplied.
  - The ward pharmacist must then treat the drug chart as for a new patient (ie check drug history, patient's own drugs (pods), notes and U & E levels, as appropriate.
- Ideally, a drug history should be taken from the patient by the pharmacist. This should be indicated by DH, date and initial, and should be documented according to local policy.
- All endorsements by pharmacists are ideally made in green ink to distinguish pharmaceutical input from the prescribing process, although this is not a legal requirement.
- Pharmacists must check and write any identified drug allergies, sensitivities, intolerance or ADRs, in addition to the reaction, in the appropriate space section on the drug chart.
- If the patient's name, consultant, ward name or PAS number is missing, illegible or incorrect, this should be added or corrected by the pharmacist. If appropriate and if it is missing from the chart, the patient's weight and/or surface area should be added by the pharmacist.
- All sections of the drug chart should be checked, including 'once only' drugs, 'fluids' and 'patient-controlled analgesia' sections.

Drug name section

- All drugs should be endorsed by the pharmacist with their nonproprietary approved names, unless they are combination products with no approved names.
- Brand names must be added for ciclosporin, theophylline, mesalazine, interferon and lithium; brand names are also added for modified-release (M/R) nifedipine, diltiazem and verapamil. They are also desirable for carbamazepine, phenytoin, oral contraceptives, hormone-replacement therapy (HRT), multiple-ingredient skin products and inhalers.
- If M/R or enteric-coated E/C formulations are intended but not prescribed, drug names are endorsed M/R or E/C.
- When liquid formulations are intended but not prescribed, drug names are endorsed as liquid. The concentration should be specified. The dose in millilitres should be calculated and specified, if possible.
- When a dose is prescribed that requires a combination of strengths, the usual combination is clarified, eg, digoxin 187.5mcg, 3 x 62.5mcg or 62.5mcg+125mcg tablets.
- All changes agreed with the prescriber are endorsed 'confirmed with Dr [name]', dated and initialled. Do not use the abbreviation 'pc'.
- Nonformulary, clinical trial or 'named patient' items should be endorsed as such.

Advice for insulins

The source of insulin should be specified (ie human, bovine or porcine). The device used should also be endorsed (ie vial, 1.5mL or 3mL penfil, or disposable pen). Lastly, the mixture of insulin should be specified, if appropriate (eg 50/50).

Advice for inhalers

The strength of inhaler and the device (eg metered-dose inhaler [MDI], Easi-Breathe, Accuhaler, etc) should be specified.

Dose section

Doses are endorsed as whole units when not so prescribed (eg, 500mg not 0.5g).

Abbreviations are not used: doses prescribed as 'mcg' or 'µg' are endorsed as 'microgrammes'; doses prescribed as 'ng' are endorsed as 'nanogrammes'; and similarly, 'IU' or 'U' is endorsed as 'units'.

Dose times are amended, as appropriate:

- To suit meal times, Calcichew.
- Dose interval, antibiotics.
- At night, statins (not atorvastatin).
- Mane, fluoxetine/paroxetine.
- At 8am and 2pm to avoid nitrate tolerance, isosorbide mononitrate.

Note: changes to dose time do not need to be referred to the prescriber.

The dose and/or route is clarified where ambiguous—eg 'propranolol 1 tablet' or (sublingual) 'GTN po'. These details are confirmed with the patient or their notes, and do not have to be referred to the prescriber. Endorse that the details were confirmed with patient/GP/notes etc.

Endorsement of drugs administered weekly (eg methotreaxate and alendronate) must be clear, specifying the day of the week the drug is usually taken.

As required, drugs specifying multiple routes are not encouraged, but if prescribed, are endorsed with the appropriate dose for each route—eg prochlorperazine pr/po/im 25mg/5mg/12.5mg, respectively.

As required, drugs are endorsed with their maximum frequency or dose (eg analgesics) and/or instructions for use (eg antidiarrhoeals).

Prescriptions for IV drugs are endorsed with injection or infusion rates or special requirements for boluses (eg furosemide). High-dependency areas could be exceptions from this requirement.

The rates of currently running drug-containing infusions are checked, initialled and dated (as described below) in the pharmacy box.

Eye drops and ointments must have left/right/both eye(s) specified.

Pharmacy annotation section

All drugs are initialled and dated by a pharmacist, constituting the 'clinical check'. Supply endorsements are then made by the pharmacist:

- Stock(s) items.
- One-stop supply (28d).
- Controlled drugs (CD).
- Patient's own drugs (POD), including details of quantity and strength brought in and highlighting the date supplies were checked.

Symbols, such as triangle, circle and slash, are used to distinguish entries from people's initials.

- Although self-administration should be encouraged, such systems must be supported by specific protocols that have been agreed by your institution.
- 'Nonformulary', 'clinical trial' or 'named patient' is written in full in the drug name box.
- Prescriptions are endorsed with the date that a supply is made.
- Prescriptions are endorsed with the quantity supplied each time a supply is made and appropriate strength of the product supplied.
- When a chart is rewritten, the ward pharmacist must check each entry against the previous chart, initialling and dating each entry if it is correct. The pharmacist must add the appropriate endorsing information, as above, with the date of the last supply (for information).

Further information

- Drugs stored in the refrigerator are endorsed 'Fridge'.
- Endorse prescriptions with guidance on unusual or complex administration (eg disodium etidronate or alendronate).
- Clarify bioavailability differences if relevant (eg phenytoin capsules and suspension).
- Alert the prescriber to clinically significant drug interactions that are identified; communicate other potential interactions to the relevant doctor either by telephone or by documentation in the patient's notes.

Prescription screening and monitoring

In an ideal world, pharmacists would review prescriptions with all relevant patient information to hand and individualize drug therapy accordingly. In reality, time and circumstances do not allow this and pharmacists must be able to identify problems with only limited information. Time rarely allows for a full examination of all patient data, even if it is available, so pharmacists must learn to determine whether or not this is necessary.

The choice of information sources available could range from just the prescription, the patient or their representative or, possibly, prescription-medication records (PMR) in the community pharmacy to full laboratory data and medical and nursing notes in the hospital setting. The following discussion assumes all information is available but it can be adapted to situations in which there are more limited data.

First impressions

Look at the prescription and patient (if present). This might seem an obvious first step, but these simple observations can tell you a great deal.

- What does the prescription or chart tell you about the patient?
  - Age—think about special considerations in children (p.218) and the elderly (p.230)
  - Weight—is the patient significantly overweight/underweight? Will you need to check doses according to weight?
  - Ward name or consultant—may tell you the presenting illness (if this is not already obvious)
- Other charts can also provide important information—eg diet sheets, blood glucose monitoring, BP, and temperature.
- What does observation of the patient tell you?
  - Old, frail patients probably need dose adjustments because of low weight or poor renal function.
  - Take extra care checking children's doses; also check that the formulation is appropriate and consider licensing issues (p.222).
  - Unconscious patients cannot take drugs by mouth. Will you need to provide formulations that can be administered through a nasogastric or gastrostomy tube?
  - Do they have IV fluids running? Consider fluid balance if other IV fluids will be used to administer drugs (notably antimicrobials).
  - If the patient's weight is not recorded on the prescription, do they look significantly overweight/underweight. If you have concerns, ask the patient if they know their weight or weigh them.
  - Is the patient pregnant or breastfeeding?
  - Could the patient's racial origin affect drug handling—eg there is a higher incidence of glucose 6-phosphate dehydrogenase (G6PD) deficiency in people of African origin (p.214).

At this point, you might already have decided on points that need to be checked or monitored. Make a note of these as you think of them. In many hospitals a ward patient list is produced each day, which gives patient names, diagnosis and basic clinical details. This is a useful source of readily available patient information and you can make notes and pharmaceutical care points on your copy. Remember that the information on the list is confidential and you should be careful how you handle it. Do not leave it lying around for others to see and dispose of it by shredding or in a confidential waste bin.

Review prescribed drugs

Check each drug on the prescription carefully. Newly prescribed drugs are the highest priority, but it is important to periodically review old drugs.

- Are the dose, frequency and route appropriate for this patient, their weight and their renal function?
- What is the indication for the drug?
  - Is it appropriate for this patient?
  - Does it comply with local or national guidelines or formularies?
  - Could the drug be treating a side effect of another drug—if so, could the first drug be stopped or changed?
- Are there any potential drug interactions (p.24)?
  - Are they clinically significant?
  - Do you need to get the interacting drug stopped or changed or just monitor for side effects?
- Is TDM required?
  - Do you need to check levels or advise on dose adjustment?
  - Are levels being taken at the right time?
- Is the drug working?
  - Think about the signs and symptoms (including laboratory data and nursing observations) you should be monitoring to check that the drug is having the desired effect. Are any symptoms owing to lack of effect! Talk to the patient!
- Are any signs and symptoms owing to side effects?
  - Do you need to advise a dose adjustment, a change in therapy or symptomatic treatment of side effects? Remember that it is sometimes appropriate to prescribe symptomatic therapy in anticipation of side effects (eg antiemetics and laxatives for patients on opioids).
- Check that the patient is not allergic to or intolerant of any of the prescribed drugs. This is usually recorded on the front of hospital prescription charts or you might need to check the medical notes or talk to the patient. Community pharmacy PMR often record drug allergies or intolerance.

Ensure you have looked at all prescribed drugs. Hospital prescription charts usually have different sections for 'as required' and 'once only' ('stat') drugs and IV infusions. Many patients might have more than one prescription chart and some might have different charts for certain types of drug (eg chemotherapy).

By now, you will probably have added to your list of points to follow up and have some idea of which patients you should focus on.

Check the patient's drug history

When patients are admitted to hospital, it is important that the drugs they normally take at home are continued, unless there is a good reason to omit them.

- Check that the drugs the patient usually takes are prescribed in the right dose, frequency and form.
- Ideally, use a source of information that is different from the admission history (in case the admitting doctor has made any errors):
  - GP's referral letter or computer printout.
  - Copy of community prescription.
  - POD supplies.
  - Phone GP's surgery.
  - Talk to the patient/relative/carer.
- Talking to the patient often reveals drugs that might otherwise be overlooked (eg oral contraceptive pill, regular over-the-counter medicines or herbal medicines).
- If there are any discrepancies between what has been prescribed and what the patient normally takes that you cannot account for, ensure that the doctors are aware of this. Depending on your local practice, it might be appropriate to record discrepancies on the prescription chart or in the medical notes.

Talk to the patient

Patients are an important source of information about their drugs, disease and symptoms. Talk to them! You might find out important information that is not recorded in the medical notes or prescription chart. If you are reviewing charts at the bedside, always introduce yourself and explain your role and what you are doing. It is a good idea to ask the patient if they have any problems with or questions about their medicines. If the patient is on many drugs or complex therapy, check their adherence by asking if they are managing to take all their medicines at home.

Care plan

You will now have various notes of problems, questions and monitoring that you need to do. Resolve any problems and form a plan to continue monitoring the patient. Learn to prioritize. An elderly patient with renal impairment who is taking multiple drugs is at higher risk of drug-related problems than a young, fit patient who is only taking one or two drugs. If you are short of time, concentrate on the high risk patients. Check your notes, decide what jobs are essential and deal with these first.

In some hospitals, a formal pharmaceutical care plan is written for each patient. This can be quite time-consuming, but it is good practice if you can do it (for high risk patients if not for all).

Screening discharge prescriptions

- Are all regular drugs from all prescription charts prescribed? If not, can you account for any omitted?
- Are timings correct and complete (eg diuretics to be taken in the morning)?
- Are any 'as required' drugs used frequently and, ∴ needed on discharge?
- Are all the prescribed drugs actually needed on discharge (eg hypnotics)?
- Does the patient actually need a supply? They might have enough of their own supply on the ward or at home.
- Will the GP need to adjust any doses or drugs after discharge? If so, is this clear on the prescription or discharge letter?
- Is there any information that you need to pass on to the patient, carer, GP (eg changes to therapy or monitoring requirements)?
- Does the patient understand how to take the drugs, especially any new ones or those with special instructions (eg warfarin p.370)?
- Are adherence aids needed (p.6)?

Writing on medicine (drug) charts

All pharmacists should provide information to medical and nursing staff by writing on the drug chart. Information provided on the drug chart will vary according to local practice but should ideally include the following:

- Ensure patient details (eg name and ward) are complete and correct.
- Document drug history information on an appropriate page of the prescription chart. (If current drug chart doesn't have a dedicated area on chart, agree local practice).
- Drug history—a list of drugs, with specific details, must be recorded. Initial and date.
- ADRs/drug and food allergies.
- Additional instructions on administration:
  - IV administration.
  - Information about appropriate oral administration (e.g. with or after food).
  - Maximum daily dose.
  - 'Not with' (eg regular prescription).
- Brand name/form—if different version affects bioavailability (eg Sandimmun®/Neoral®, long-acting/M/R).
- Local formulary restrictions, as appropriate.
- Clarify dose if it is not clear or could cause confusion:
  - Change 0.5g to 500mg.
  - Liquid—annotate the concentration and volume required.
  - Ensure clarity for unusual frequencies (eg weekly or alternate days).
- Clinical information:
  - Drug interactions (eg drugs affecting warfarin levels).
- Monitoring requests or information:
  - Potassium (K^+) levels for drugs affecting.
  - Creatinine levels for drugs affecting/affected by creatinine.
  - Drug levels.
- Requests to doctors to review a prescription plan:
  - Length of course of antibiotics.

All information should be set out as following:

- Written in green ink or according to local practice.
  - Clear, legible and in indelible ink (if handwriting is poor, please print capitals).
  - Initialled and dated, including bleep number, as appropriate.
- Use only well-recognized abbreviations.

Understanding medical notes

'Are you taught to read doctors' handwriting?' is a question often asked when people first learn you are a pharmacist. However, it is not just poor handwriting that pharmacists must learn to decipher, but also the medical jargon and abbreviations that go with it.

When a patient is first admitted to hospital, a fairly standard series of questions, investigations and results relating to their physical examination is recorded in the notes. This is known as 'medical clerking' and is essentially the story (history) of the patient's illness to date. After interpretation of the initial clerking is mastered, it is usually fairly easy to understand subsequent entries in the notes because these are mostly brief updates. Notes written by GPs follow a similar format but are generally less detailed.

Medical clerking

Clerking usually uses the following format, although not every history includes every step:

- General information about the patient—name, age, gender, marital status and occupation.
- 'Complaining of' (C/O) or 'presenting complaint' (PC)—a statement of what symptoms or problems have lead to the patient's admission or attendance, ideally using the patient's own words.
- 'History of presenting complaint' (HPC)—more detail about the symptoms (eg timing, whether they have occurred previously, whether anything improves or worsens them, severity and character).
- 'Past medical history' (PMH)—does the patient have a past history of any medical complaint, including the following:
  - Previous hospital admission.
  - Surgery.
  - Chronic disease (eg diabetes mellitus or asthma).
- 'Drug history' (DHx)—the patient's current drugs and any drugs stopped recently are listed. Ideally, this should include any frequently used over-the-counter and herbal medicines. ADRs and allergies are also recorded here.
- 'Social history' (SH) and 'family history' (FH)—relevant details of the patients occupation, home circumstances and alcohol and tobacco consumption are recorded. Significant information about the medical history of close family members is noted:
  - Whether parents and siblings are alive and well (A&W).
  - Does anyone in the family have a medical problem related to the presenting complaint?
  - If close family members have died, at what age and what was the cause of death?

All the above information is found by asking the patient questions, before the doctor examines the patient. This is known as 'systems review' (S/R). Negative findings are recorded, in addition to positive findings.

- On examination (O/E)—this is a general comment about what the patient looks like (eg pale, sweaty or short of breath [SOB]).
- The doctor examines each body system in turn, recording what they have found by looking, listening and feeling. They concentrate on any systems that are most relevant to the symptoms described by the patient (eg if the patient has complained of chest pain, the cardiovascular system (CVS) and respiratory system [Resp] are most relevant). The following body systems are covered:
  - CVS
  - Resp
  - Gastrointestinal system (GI, GIT or abdo)
  - Central nervous system (CNS)
  - Peripheral nervous system (PNS)
  - Bones and joints (ortho).

Much of the information is recorded using abbreviations and medical 'shorthand'(Table 4.1 on p.48–53).
- 'Investigations' (Ix)—the results of any investigations, such as chest X-rays (CXRs), are recorded.
- 'Diagnosis' (Dx or Δ)—the doctor now draws a conclusion from the history and examination and records the diagnosis. If it is not clear what the diagnosis is, they might record several possibilities. These are known as 'differential diagnoses' (DDx or ΔΔ).
- The doctor now writes a plan for treatment, care and further Ix.
- Finally, the doctor signs the report and writes down their bleep number or other contact details.

Other clinical information

Remember that the complete clinical record is much more than the medical notes. To get a complete picture of the patient's history and progress you might need to use other information:
- Admission form (includes the patient's address, next of kin, and GP details).
- GP's referral letter.
- Nursing notes.
- Observation charts—eg temperature, BP, blood glucose levels and fluid balance.
- Laboratory data—might be paper copies in notes or on computer.
- Notes from previous admissions or out-patient attendances (including discharge summaries and clinic letters).
- Old drug charts.
- The current drug chart.

Table 4.1 Abbreviations commonly found in medical notes

+	increased, enlarged or present (more +s indicates increased severity)
↑	increase
↓	decrease
→	normal
⬡	represents the thoracic and abdominal areas
↔	normal
♀	female
♂	male
#	fracture
o	normal or none
†	dead or died
ABG	arterial blood gases
ACTH	adrenocorticotrophic hormone
ADH	antidiuretic hormone
AF	atrial fibrillation
AFB	acid fast bacilli
Ag	antigen
AIDS	acquired immunodeficiency syndrome
ALL	acute lymphoblastic leukaemia
AML	acute myeloid leukaemia
ANF	antinuclear factor
APTT	activated partial thromboplastin time
ARDS	acute respiratory distress syndrome
ASD	atrial septal defect
AST	aspartate transaminase
A&W	alive and well
AXR	abdominal X-ray
Ba	barium
BBB	bundle branch block
BMT	bone marrow transplant
BP	blood pressure
BS	breath sounds, bowel sounds
C/O	complaining of
Ca	carcinoma, cancer

Table 4.1 (*Contd.*)

CABG	coronary artery bypass graft
CAPD	continuous ambulatory peritoneal dialysis
CCF	congestive cardiac failure
CHD	congenital heart disease
CHF	chronic heart failure
CLL	chronic lymphoblastic leukaemia
CML	chronic myeloid leukaemia
CMV	cytomegalovirus
CNS	central nervous system
COPD	chronic obstructive pulmonary disease
CPAP	continuous positive airways pressure
creps	crepitations
CSF	cerebrospinal fluid
CSU	catheter specimen of urine
CT	computerized tomography
CVA	cerebrovascular accident
CVP	central venous pressure
CVS	cardiovascular system
CXR	chest X-ray
D&C	dilatation and curettage
D&V	diarrhoea and vomiting
DDx, ΔΔ	differential diagnoses (used if there is more than one possible diagnosis)
DHx	drug history
DIC	disseminated intravascular coagulation
DM	diabetes mellitus
DNA	did not attend or deoxyribose nucleic acid
DVT	deep vein thrombosis
D/W	discussed or discussion with
Dx, Δ	diagnosis
DXT	deep X-ray therapy, ie radiotherapy
EBV	Epstein–Barr virus
ECF	extracellular fluid
ECG	electrocardiogram

Table 4.1 (Contd.)

EEG	electroencephalogram
ELISA	enzyme-linked immunosorbent assay
EMU	early morning urine
ENT	ear, nose and throat
ERCP	endoscopic retrograde cholangiopancreatography
ESR	erythrocyte sedimentation rate
EUA	examination under anaesthesia
FBC	full blood count
FEV_1	forced expiratory volume in 1 second
FFP	fresh frozen plasma
FHx	family history
FSH	follicle-stimulating hormone
FSHx	family and social history
FVC	forced vital capacity
G6PD	glucose 6-phosphate dehydrogenase
GA	general anaesthesia
GABA	γ-aminobutyric acid
GFR	glomerular filtration rate
GGT	γ-glutamyl transpeptidase
GH	growth hormone
GI	gastrointestinal
GU	gastric ulcer, genito-urinary
GVHD	graft versus host disease
Hb	haemoglobin
HBV	hepatitis B virus
HCV	hepatitis C virus
HIV	human immunodeficiency virus
HLA	human leukocyte antigen
HPC	history of presenting complaint
HRT	hormone replacement therapy
HSV	herpes simplex virus
IBD	inflammatory bowel disease
ICP	intracranial pressure
IDDM	insulin dependent diabetes mellitus

Table 4.1 (*Contd.*)

Ig	immunoglobulin
IHD	ischaemic heart disease
IM	intramuscular
INR	international normalized ratio
ISQ	*idem status quo* (ie unchanged)
IT	intrathecal
ITP	idiopathic thrombocytopenic purpura
IUD	intra-uterine device
IV	intravenous
IVC	inferior vena cava
Ix	investigations
JVP	jugular venous pressure
KCCT	kaolin cephalin clotting time
LBBB	left bundle branch block
LFT	liver function tests
LH	luteinizing hormone
L°K°K°S°	liver, kidneys, spleen (° = normal)
LP	lumbar puncture
LVF	left ventricular failure
MC&S	microscopy, culture and sensitivities
MCHC	mean corpuscular haemoglobin concentration
MCV	mean corpuscular volume
MI	myocardial infarction
MND	motor neurone disease
MSU	midstream urine
N&V	nausea and vomiting
NAD	nothing abnormal detected
NG	nasogastric
NIDDM	non-insulin dependent diabetes mellitus
NKDA	no known drug allergies
O/E	on examination
OA	osteoarthritis or on admission
OC&P	ova, cysts and parasites
OGTT	oral glucose tolerance test

Table 4.1 (*Contd.*)

PC	presenting complaint
PCP	*Pneumocystis jirovecii* pneumonia
PCV	packed cell volume
PDA	patent ductus arteriosus
PE	pulmonary embolism
PEEP	positive end-expiratory pressure
PEFR	peak expiratory flow rate
PERLA	pupils equal reactive to light and accomodation
PID	pelvic inflammatory disease
PM	postmortem
PMH	past medical history
PR	per rectum or pulse rate
PT	prothombin time
PTH	parathyroid hormone
PTT	partial thromboplastin time
PUO	pyrexia of unknown origin
PV	per vaginum
RA	rheumatoid arthritis
RAST	radio-allergosorbent test
RBBB	right bundle branch block
RBC	red blood cell
RF	renal function
RIP	rest in peace (ie dead or died)
Rh	Rhesus
ROS	rest of systems
RS/RES	respiratory system
RTA	road traffic accident
RTI	respiratory tract infection
RVF	right ventricular failure
$S_1 S_2$	heart sounds (first and second)
SCD/SCA	sickle cell disease/anaemia
SIADH	syndrome of inappropriate diuretic hormone
SLE	systemic lupus erythematosus

Table 4.1 (*Contd.*)

SOA	swelling of ankles
SOB	shortness of breath
SOBOE	short of breath on exercise/exertion
ST	sinus tachcardia
SVC	superior vena cava
SVT	supraventricular tachycardia
TB	tuberculosis
TBG	thyroid binding globulin
TFT	thyroid function tests
THR	total hip replacement
TIA	transient ischaemic attack
TIBC	total iron binding capacity
TLC	tender loving care
TOE	transoesophageal echocardiogram
TOP	termination of pregnancy
TPN	total parenteral nutrition
TRH	thyrotrophin-releasing hormone
TSH	thyroid-stimulating hormone
TURP	transurethral resection of the prostate
U&E	urea and electrolytes
UC	ulcerative colitis
URTI	upper respiratory tract infection
UTI	urinary tract infection
VDRL	venereal diseases research lab (used to refer to the test for syphilis)
VF	ventricular fibrillation
VSD	ventricular septal defect
VT	ventricular tachycardia
W/R	ward round
WBC	white blood count
WCC	white cell count

Writing in medical notes

Pharmacists should write in the medical notes to communicate information relating to the pharmaceutical care of the patient to the medical staff if immediate action is not required, the information should significantly influence the care of the patient or to ensure that information is available to all members of the medical team. The notes are a legal document, and if the pharmacist has contributed to, or attempted to contribute to, the patient's care, this should be documented.

The following is appropriate information to write in the medical notes:
- Clinically significant interactions.
- Contraindications to medicine use.
- ADRs.
- Identification of a problem that could be related to medicine use.
- Amendments to DHxs.
- General medicines information about unusual medicines/conditions.
- Counselling details and outcome.

Pharmacists who are authorized (according to local practice) to make an entry in the patient's notes include the following:
- Registered pharmacists who have received suitable training.
- Junior pharmacists and locums should discuss potential entries with their seniors or clinical supervisor before making the entry.

The pharmacist should ensure that each entry into the notes is as follows:
- Directly relevant to that patient's care.
- At the appropriate point in the notes.
- Succinct and informative.
- Follows a logical sequence.
- Subjective—eg records relevant patient details.
- Objective—eg records clinical findings.
- An assessment of the situation.
- Recommendations are clearly expressed.

The entry should follow a standard format:
    27/3/05 Pharmacist

                    Amiodarone will ↑ plasma concentration of digoxin. As *BNF* states—halve dose of digoxin.

                    Tom Smith (sign) bleep 1178

Entries in the patient's notes should be as follows:
- Clear, legible and in indelible ink (many hospital pharmacists use green ink—providing the ink quality can be photocopied).
- Signed, with printed name, and dated.
- Include a contact number (bleep or extension).
- Use only well-recognized abbreviations.
- Include any discussion of the issue with medical or nursing staff.
- Not be informal.
- Not directly criticize medical/nursing care.

Medication review

Definition of medication review

A structured, critical examination of a patient's medicines by a healthcare professional, reaching an agreement with the patient about treatment, optimizing the use of medicines, minimizing the number of medication-related problems and avoiding wastage.

Regular medication review maximizes the therapeutic benefit and minimizes the potential harm of drugs. It ensures the safe and effective use of medicines by patients. Medication review provides an opportunity for patients to discuss their medicines with a healthcare professional. Medication review is the cornerstone of medicines management.

What does medication review involve?

- A structured, critical examination of a patient's medicines (prescription and other medicines, including alternatives) by a healthcare professional.
- Identification, management and prevention of ADRs or drug interactions.
- Minimizing the number of medication-related problems.
- Optimizing the use of medicines.
- Simplification of regimen.
- Ensuring all drugs are appropriate and needed.
- Avoiding wastage.
- Medication counseling.
- Adherence counseling—to ensure patients adhere to their drug regimens.
- Assessment of ability to self-medicate.
- Education of patient or carer—to help them understand their drugs better.
- Education of the patient on safe and effective medication use.
- Forum for suggesting effective treatment alternatives.
- Recommendation of compliance aids.

Principles of medication review

- Patients must be informed about their medication being reviewed.
- Patients should have the opportunity to ask questions and highlight any problems with their medicines.
- Medication review should improve the impact of treatment for an individual patient.
- A competent person (eg pharmacist) should undertake the review in a systematic way.
- Any changes resulting from the review are agreed with the patient.
- The review is documented in the patient's notes.
- The impact of any change is monitored.

Levels of medicine review

- Level 3 (clinical medication review)—face-to-face review of medication with the patient and their notes, specifically undertaken by a doctor, nurse or pharmacist. Provides an opportunity to discuss what medication the patient is actually taking and how medicine taking fits in with the patient's daily life.
- Level 2 (treatment review)—review of medicines, with reference to the patient's full notes, in the absence of the patient and under the direction of a doctor, nurse or pharmacist.
- Level 1 (prescription review)—technical review of a list of the patient's medicines in the absence of the patient and under the direction of a doctor, nurse or pharmacist.
- Level 0 (ad-hoc review)—unstructured, opportunistic review of medication.

Who to target

- Patients on multiple medications or complicated drug regimens.
- Patients experiencing ADRs.
- Patients with chronic conditions.
- Elderly patients.
- Nonadherent patients.

Benefits of medication review

- Identification, management and prevention of ADRs.
- Ensuring patients have maximum benefit from their medicines.
- ↓ risk of drug-related problems.
- ↑ the appropriate use of medicines.
- Improved clinical outcomes.
- Cost-effectiveness.
- ↑ quality of life.
- Optimizing therapy.
- ↓ waste of medicines.
- Enables patients to maintain their independence.
- ↓ admissions to hospital.
- ↓ in drug-related deaths.

Problems identified during a medication review

- Potential ADRs.
- Potential interactions (drug–drug or drug–food).
- Suboptimal monitoring.
- Adherence/lack of concordance issues.
- Impractical directions.
- Incorrect/inappropriate dosages.
- Drugs no longer needed (eg one medication used to treat the side effects of another).
- Difficulties with using certain dose forms (eg inhaler or eye drops).

Recording medication reviews
- There is no universally agreed way of documenting medication reviews.
- Local guidance for recording medication reviews needs to be followed.
- The minimum information that should be recorded is as follows:
  - Current medication history.
  - Problems identified.
  - Advice given.
  - Suggested timeframe for the next medication review.
  - Date, signature, name and, position

Futher reading

Room for review—A guide to medication review: the agenda for patients, practitioners and managers. (2002). www.medicines-partnership.org/medication-review/welcome

Intervention monitoring

Clinical pharmacists can audit their impact on patient care by intervention monitoring. Some hospitals undertake these audits at regular intervals and present the results internally or to the multidisciplinary team.

Data collection forms or electronic handheld systems are used to collect the relevant data on a pharmacist's interventions to improve patient care. Examples of data collected for this purpose include the following:

- Patient details and demographics.
- Area of work/specialization.
- Written details of the intervention.
- Date of intervention.
- Other healthcare professionals contacted.
- Evidence used to support the intervention.
- Who initiated the intervention—eg pharmacist, doctor, nurse or patient.
- Possible effect the intervention would have on patient care.
- Outcome of the intervention.
- Actual outcome on patient care that the intervention had.
- Significance of intervention.
- Category of intervention (see below for examples).

Examples of the categories of pharmacist interventions in drug therapy include the following (Table 4.2):

- ADRs.
- Additional drug therapy required.
- Patient adherence.
- Patient education.
- Communication with prescriber.
- Incorrect medication prescribed.
- Incorrect drug dose—either high or low.
- Optimization of drug therapy, including improving cost-effectiveness.
- Dose advice.
- Advice on drug choice.
- Drug interaction.
- Side effect/toxicity.
- TDM.
- Drug–disease interaction.
- Formulation.
- Compatibility.
- Formulary or protocol adherence.

Further reading

Becker C, Bjornson DC, Kuhle JW (2004). Pharmacist care plans and documentation of follow-up before the Iowa Pharmaceutical Case Management program. *Journal of the American Pharmacists Association* **44(3)**: 350–7.

McDonough RP, Doucette WR (2003). Drug therapy management: an empirical report of drug therapy problems, pharmacists' interventions, and results of pharmacists' actions. *Journal of the American Pharmacists Association* **43(4)**: 511–18.

Table 4.2 Example of an intervention monitoring form

Date	In-patient		TTO	Out-patient	
Hospital	Ward/area				

Contact source:

Doctor	Consultant	Specialist registrar	Senior house officer	House officer	GP
Nurse	Sister	Staff nurse	Auxiliary		
Other (specify)					

Category of intervention:

Incorrect dose

Dose advice

Drug choice

Drug interaction

Side effect/toxicity/ADR

TDM

Drug–disease interaction

Formulation

Compatibility

Patient adherence/education

Formulary/protocol adherence

Cost

Other (specify)

Solution	Outcome
Prescriber contacted	Advice ignored
Nurse contacted	Advice acted upon
Documentation in notes	Acknowledged no action
Other	Information only

Patient risk:

Low	1	2	3	4	5	High

Time taken:

<5mins	5–15 mins	15–30mins	30mins

Details of intervention:

Answer/outcome on patient care:

Drug-history (DHx) taking

Before taking a DHx from a patient ensure that relevant information is obtained from the medical and nursing notes that might aid the process. Consider whether it is beneficial to have the patient's carer present, particularly for very young or old patients, for those who have difficulty communicating, or if the carer administers the medication. It is preferable if the DHx taking is carried out in an area where interruptions from visitors or other healthcare professionals are minimized.

When taking the DHx, remember to obtain details of the following:
- Drug name.
- Dose.
- Frequency.
- Formulation.
- Duration of treatment.
- Indication.
- Any problems with medication, such as with administration (eg inhaler), ADRs or allergies

It is essential that details of all types of medication are obtained for a DHx, including the following:
- Medicines prescribed by the GP.
- Medicines prescribed by the hospital.
- Over-the-counter medicines.
- Alternative (eg herbal or homeopathic) medicines.
- All forms of medicines (eg tablets, liquids, suppositories, injections, eye drops/ointments, ear drops, inhalers, nasal sprays, creams and ointments).
- If a compliance aid (eg dosette box) is used, who fills it?

DHxs sometimes have to be verified if patients cannot remember the details of their medication and have not brought their medication with them. DHxs can be verified by the following means:
- Checking against the POD supply.
- Checking against GP letters.
- Checking records of prescriptions used in the community (FP10 prescriptions in UK).
- Telephoning the GP's practice.

During the DHx-taking process, it is also useful to establish whether the patient has any drug allergies, including symptoms.

The following information recorded from the DHx taking should be entered in the medical notes, or other record according to local procedure:
- Date and time.
- DHx, including the above details.
- Allergies.
- Pharmacist recommendations.
- Information provided to the patient as a result of this process.
- Signature.
- Name and profession in bold.

Drug-use evaluation (DUE)

DUE is a quality-assurance tool, which monitors and evaluates drug use against agreed criteria/standards, and if necessary, advises on a change of practice to improve the quality, safety and cost-effectiveness of prescribing. The process can be carried out retrospectively, prospectively or concurrently. DUE is usually used as a tool in areas where prescribing practice is not consistent with agreed standards.

Steps to undertake a DUE cycle include the following:
- Select a drug or therapeutic area for a DUE.
- Agree objective, measurable criteria and standards of use for the target area, if these are not set already.
- Design a sample data-collection sheet and pilot.
- Collect the prescribing data to evaluate current practice against the standards.
- Analyse the data.
- Evaluate the practice against the standards.
- Decide what intervention needs to be introduced to improve prescribers' compliance with the agreed criteria and action plan.
- Educate staff and introduce practice to correct any inappropriate prescribing.
- Evaluate the impact of the DUE.
- Communicate the results.

To ensure an effective DUE programme, a multidisciplinary approach should be taken. Doctors and pharmacists should agree the criteria, and accurate prescribing data should be collected. There should be critical evaluation of the data and an acceptable means of correcting any deficiencies in prescribing.

Suitable drugs or areas for a DUE study are as follows:
- Commonly used drugs to ensure cost-effective prescribing.
- Drugs for which there is a high cost or volume of usage.
- High potential for toxicity or ADRs.
- Narrow therapeutic index.
- Proposed formulary inclusion.
- Used in patient population probably at high risk of ADRs.
- Already included in a therapeutic policy (eg antibiotic policy).
- Drugs that could improve the quality of life or patient care.
- Areas where prescribing practice is not following the standards.
- To justify the use of resources.
- The drug is most effective when used in a specific manner.

Benefits of DUE

- Confirms appropriate quality of prescribing, with respect to safety, efficacy and cost to an organization.
- Financial benefits with the ↓ of inappropriate drug use.
- Improved quality of clinical pharmacy service, with respect to targeting clinical pharmacy activity and educational benefits.
- Essential component of clinical audit.
- Improves credibility of reports on drug expenditure.
- Support of the development, implementation and monitoring of drug formularies.

Dealing with mistakes

Medicines management policies and procedures should be in place to minimize the risk of medication errors occurring during the medication process (ie for prescribing, dispensing and administration).

Prescribing
- Adequate knowledge of the patient and their clinical condition.
- Clear, multiprofessional treatment plans.
- Complex calculations checked by two members of staff.
- Review drug treatments regularly.
- Implement electronic care records and prescribing systems.
- Legible prescriptions.
- Avoiding abbreviations.

Dispensing
- Training and competency assessment for checking prescriptions and dispensing.
- Checking medication with a patient when it is being issued and allowing patients the opportunity to ask questions about their medication.
- Formal dispensary procedures and checking systems.

Administration
- Risk management must be built into the previous steps to ensure medication is administered safely.
- Training of staff administering medication.
- Procedures for drug administration.
- High-risk areas of administration to have a double check by a second member of staff (eg for IV infusions or complex calculations).
- Involving patients or their carers in the administration process if appropriate.
- Storage of medication appropriately to minimize errors. Controlling the availability of high-risk drugs (eg potassium chloride ampoules).
- Using information technology to support prescribing, dispensing, and administration of medication.

Create a culture where staff can learn from their mistakes. Do not have a blame culture:
- Explore why a mistake has happened.
- Remain calm.
- Find out the facts.
- Focus on the processes that allowed the mistake.
- Provide support.
- Assume that the person wants to learn from their mistakes.
- See mistakes as part of a learning process.

Harness the power of mistakes:
- Create mechanisms to provide support when mistakes occur.
- Learn to question and challenge without antagonism.
- Create personal learning contracts to promote self-managed learning.
- Acquire a habit of active reflections.

Reporting mistakes:
- Use the appropriate reporting mechanism within your hospital.
- Inform a more senior member of staff of the mistake.
- Inform the multidisciplinary team of the mistake.
- Document the mistake and the steps leading up to the mistake.

Dealing with mistakes:
- Dealing with your own feelings, if you are the person who made the mistake—remember that we are all human and can make mistakes. You will probably feel remorse that you have made the mistake. Reflect on how the mistake was made, and plan how you will learn from the mistake to ensure that it isn't repeated.
- Dealing with people who don't acknowledge their own mistakes or who make repeated mistakes—the person's manager should be involved in dealing with the person who does not acknowledge their mistakes. Evidence must be used to discuss the mistakes, and performance-management strategies put in place to ensure that the mistakes are acknowledged and learnt from.
- Dealing with a more senior member of staff who has made a mistake—it is difficult for a junior member of staff to deal with mistakes made by a more senior member of staff. Whenever possible, it is best to speak directly to the member of staff who has made the mistake, informing them of the outcome and any action you have taken. If necessary, involve another senior member of staff or your manager in the discussion.

Remember

Mistakes can be fatal. Ensure you are aware of local policies and procedures to minimize the risk of mistakes occurring.

Further reading

Smith J (2004). *Building a Safer NHS for Patients: Improving Medication Safety*. London: Department of Health.

Financial reports and budget statements

On the basis of data provided from pharmacy computer systems, pharmacists often take responsibility for providing financial information to their clinical area. Reports are generally monthly or quarterly. At the end of the financial year, an annual finance report is usually produced. Reports are usually sent to the finance manager, clinical director and manager of a clinical area.

The objectives of a financial report are as follows:
- Relevant and timely information.
- Easy to understand and concise information.
- Verifiable and complete numbers.
- Format enables comparison.
- Reporting is consistent in form and content.
- Reports are adequate for the audience.
- Reports are periodic.
- Data is inclusive, analytical and comparative.
- Assumptions are attached.

Financial reports should include the following elements:
- Statistical data.
- Financial data.
- Current month.
- Actual versus budgeted.

The type of financial information that a pharmacist supplies is as follows:
- Overall drug expenditure for a financial year by month or quarter.
- Actual drug expenditure to date.
- Projected expenditure for that financial year and the next financial year.
- Comparison of expenditure with that of the previous financial year (eg by month, quarter or year).
- Analysis of expenditure by clinical areas, in-patient/out-patient/take-home medication.
- The top 20–50 high-expenditure drugs by month, quarter or year.
- High-expenditure therapeutic areas for a specified period of time (eg month, quarter or year).
- Explanation of any areas of unexpected high expenditure.
- Interpretation of financial information, detailing areas where cost-savings can be made.
- Detail where cost-savings have already been achieved.
- Interpretation of changes in expenditure or drug use.
- Exceptions to previous trends.

This information can be portrayed in a tabular or graphical form but should be presented in ways that are easy to interpret and include a commentary.

Before providing financial reports, check what the recipient actually wants in the report.

Hospital budget statements

- The finance department often produces budget statements, which are useful for pharmacists to understand.
- The financial year in the UK National Health Service (NHS) is April 1 to March 30.
- The budget statement reflects the budget that is available and the financial position at a point in a financial year.
- These budget statements include salary (pay), nonsalary (nonpay) and income budgets for a department or group of departments.
- Drug budgets usually sit in the nonsalary budget.
- The drug-budget expenditure is based on the cost of the pharmacy drugs issued.
- Budget statements usually include the following information for each of the budgets:
  - The total annual budget.
  - The budget available for the year to date.
  - The actual budget spent for the year to date.
  - The difference between the available budget and the actual budget spent (variance).
  - The percentage of budget spent to date.
  - The forecast spend for the financial year.
  - Total financial position.
- If a budget is overspent, it is usually represented as a positive number.
- If a budget is underspent, it is usually represented as a negative number.
- Finance department budget statements should be linked to financial reports prepared by pharmacy staff (see p.68).
- Pharmacists might be asked for a breakdown of drug-expenditure information.

Writing reports

Pharmacists can be required to write reports on a variety of subjects, such as the following:
- Drug expenditure analysis.
- Evaluation of a new drug.
- Proposal for a new project.

A well written and well presented report is more likely to be read and acted on than something that is messy and incoherent. Much of the guidance below also applies to writing business letters, e-mails and memos (Table 4.4).

Define the aim

- What is the purpose of the report and what are you trying to achieve? Is it simply to inform the reader or is some course of action expected as a result of the report?
- Use a title that describes the aim or the content. As appropriate, write aims and objectives:
  - Aims describe what you intend to do.
  - Objectives describe how you intend to achieve the aims.

Content

The content should all be relevant to the title/aims. Look through your notes and delete any unnecessary material.
- Ensure content is appropriate the readership:
  - Who are the readers?
  - What do they already know about the subject?
  - How much time will they have to read the report?
  - Might they have certain expectations of the report or preconceptions about the subject?
  - Why are you submitting this report to them?
- What type of information will you be including and how is this best presented:
  - Drug expenditure report—graphs and tables.
  - Review of papers—predominantly text.
- Review the information and classify it under headings or sections, following the suggested structure and the rules below:
  - Headings should follow a logical sequence:
    —problem/cause/solution.
    —chronological order.
    —priority— by urgency or need.
    —drug review—follow *BNF* headings, ie drug, indication, contraindications and cautions.
  - Headings should clearly tell the reader what that section is about.
  - Ideally, the maximum number of items in a section is seven otherwise there is too much information for the reader to take in at once. If necessary, subdivide sections.
  - Ensure content of each section is relevant to the heading.
  - Try not to repeat information in different sections.

Layout

Even a well-written report with good content can be overlooked if it is difficult to read. A large amount of type crowded on to a page is difficult to read and the eye soon becomes tired.

* Leave wide margins at both sides and ample space at the top and bottom of each page. This also gives the reader space to write notes and ensures that print on the left hand side doesn't disappear into the binding.
* Avoid left and right justification. Left justifying only creates spaces in the text, which is easier on the eye.
* Use 1½ or double spacing.

Bullet points and numbering

Putting information into lists using bullet points or numbering has the following benefits:

* Makes it easier to read.
* Has more impact.
* Cuts the number of words (and waffle).

Most word processing programmes offer a selection of bullet points. Keep things simple and only use one or two different types of bullet in your report.

Use a straightforward numbering system eg 1, 1.1, 1.2, 1.2.1 and avoid over numbering eg 1.2.1.1.1!.

Font

Use a font that is clear and easy to read. Use fonts without serifs ('sans serif'; eg Arial) and use a 12-point font size for the majority of the text eg ('**good writing**') (Gill Sans MT, 12 point) is easier to read than ('good writing') (Times New Roman, 12 point) or ('**good writing**') (Gill Sans MT, 10 point).

Avoid using capitals or underlining to highlight text: **bold** is easier to read than CAPITALS or <u>underlining</u>. People with poor literacy skills find uppercase text especially difficult to read.

For a lesson in how font style and layout affects ease of reading, compare *The Sun* newspaper to *The Times*!

Paragraphs

A paragraph should cover only one point or argument. As a rule, it should be about seven or eight lines long and certainly no longer than 10 lines. The most important information should be in the first or last sentence of the paragraph.

Charts and tables

These should be used to convey information—usually of numerical origin—that might be too complex to describe in words. However, overuse or inappropriate use can divert the reader from the main message, making your work confusing. When deciding whether to use a chart or table consider the following points:

* Will it save words?
* Will it clarify things for the reader?

- Is the information to be presented quantifiable in some way?
- Will it help the reader to make comparisons?
- Will it help to illustrate a specific point?

In general, bar charts are the simplest charts to produce and suit most data. They are easier to interpret and less prone to be misleading than pie charts, graphs or pictograms.

When using charts, consider, the following points:
- Give the chart a title.
- Make sure bars or axes start at zero.
- If comparing two charts, the axes should have the same scale.
- Label axes and bars.
- Show actual amounts on bars and pie chart slices.
- Use only two-dimensional versions—three-dimensional bars and slices can distort the relative proportions.
- Avoid overuse of colour or hatching , which might not reproduce clearly.
- Keep it simple!

Language

- Keep language simple and to the point.
- Avoid long sentences.
- Avoid foreign language phrases—eg *ad hoc* and *pro rata*.
- Use active rather than passive sentences—'*Use paracetamol regularly for pain*' is preferable to '*Paracetamol is to be used regularly for pain*'.
- Avoid double negatives as these can cause confusion—'*Paracetamol is not incompatible with breastfeeding*' could easily be misinterpreted as '*Paracetamol is not compatible with breastfeeding*'.
- Only use common abbreviations without explanation, such as 'eg'. Where you wish to use an abbreviation, write in full the first time, followed by the abbreviation—eg Royal Pharmaceutical Society of Great Britain (RPSGB). Thereafter, the abbreviation can be used.
- Avoid jargon and clichés.

Revision and editing

As much as 50% of the time spent writing a report should be devoted to revision and editing (Table 4.5 on p.76):
- Print the report and check for spelling mistakes and other obvious errors (do not just rely on computer spelling and grammar checks).
- Check punctuation.
- Work through the report using the editing checklist and revise, as necessary.
- Ask a colleague to read the report and make comments. Check that they interpret the information as you intended.

Table 4.4 Report structure

The following is a suggested structure. Depending on the type of
report, the structure can vary.

Title

Identification

Your name, department and contact details and the date

Distribution

It might be helpful to list the following:
- Those who need to take action.
- Those for whom the report is for information only.

Contents

Aims and objectives

Summary or abstract

Introduction
- Provides the background and context of the report.
- Explains why the report was written.
- Gives terms of reference.

Method/procedure

There should be sufficient information for the reader to understand what you
did, without giving every detail.

Results/findings

Discussion

The main body of the report; use section headings here.

Conclusions

A re-statement of the main findings.
Includes recommendations or proposals for future work.

References

Use a standard system, such as the Vancouver style,—ie author, date in brackets,
title of the article, journal title, volume and page numbers.

Appendices

These should include information that informs the reader but is not essential on
the first reading.

Glossary

Explain any unusual or scientific terms or unavoidable jargon.

Footnotes

Author name, date of preparation, review date and page numbers.

Table 4.5 Editing checklist

Aim

Is the aim clear?

Is the content at the right level for the reader?

If action is required as a result of the report, is this clear?

Content

Is the structure logical?

Do the conclusions follow the argument?

Is numerical data accurate and clearly presented?

Do graphs and tables achieve their aim?

Have you quoted references and sources appropriately?

Language

Are paragraphs the right length?

Have unnecessary words, double negatives, clichés and jargon been avoided?

Is spelling and punctuation correct?

Presentation

Are abbreviations and symbols explained and used consistently throughout?

Do page breaks fall at natural breaks in the text?

Are page numbers and footers etc included, as needed?

Does any of the text get lost on printing?

Does the whole report look tidy and professional?

Using medicines information services

The Medicines Information (UKMI) service is a countrywide network comprising 16 regional and 250 local MI centres. Local services range from one pharmacist, providing information part-time, to a large centre, with pharmacists, technicians and administrative staff. Most MI centres provide an information service to hospital based and community-based enquirers, including members of the public, but some only answer enquiries from within their NHS trust. For both community pharmacists and hospital pharmacists, it is a good idea to check who provides the MI service for your area.

Some regional centres provide a specialist information service (Table 4.6) but it is usually advisable to contact the local service first. Remember to also contact local specialists, because advice from a regional centre might not reflect local practice.

Before contacting your MI centre with an enquiry, do some basic research. Most MI centres expect pharmacist colleagues to have checked basic sources before contacting them—eg *BNF*, Summary of Product Characteristics and *Martindale*. Before contacting the MI centre, try to anticipate what background information they might require and have this ready. Depending on the type of enquiry, this might include the following:

- Drug details, including dose, route, formulation, brand and indication.
- Patient details, including underlying condition, relevant laboratory results, age, weight and past medical history.
- The identity of the original enquirer.
- Urgency.
- Contact details.
- Whether a written or verbal response is required.
- Any sources already checked for information and what was found.
- ADRs—nature of reaction, timing of the event, other drugs, any de-challenge/re-challenge and the outcome.
- Pregnancy—number of weeks gestation, whether or not the drug has already been taken by the mother and indication.
- Breast feeding—age, weight, medical status of infant and whether the treatment is short or long term.
- Drug interactions—which drugs/drug classes are involved and the nature of event, if a suspected interaction has already occurred.

After the enquiry is complete, it is really helpful if you feed back the outcome to your MI centre. It's rare that they hear what happened as a result of the answer given and it is useful information to add to their enquiry records. Remember to fill in a yellow card for any significant ADRs (p.13).

Further reading
www.ukmi.nhs.uk
www.druginfozone.uk

Table 4.6 UKMI specialist information centres

Specialist topic	Centre
Prescribing in pregnancy	Newcastle Regional MI
Drugs in breast milk	Sutton Coldfield and Leicester Regional MI
Complementary medicine	Cardiff Regional MI
Medicines in children	Alder Hey Childrens Hospital MI
Drugs in liver impairment	Leeds Regional MI
Drugs in renal impairment	Bristol Regional MI
Oncology	Royal Marsden Hospital MI
Ophthalmic drugs	Moorfields Hospital MI
HIV/AIDS	St Marys Hospital (London) MI Chelsea and Westminster Hospital MI

Phone numbers are in the *BNF* and on the UKMI website www.ukmi.nhs.uk

Ward etiquette

Starting work on a new ward

- If possible, speak to the pharmacist who previously covered that ward.
- Introduce yourself to the ward manager, key medical staff, nursing staff and other relevant staff (eg the ward clerk).
- Check how the ward functions.
- Find out the best time for your visit.
- Establish if there are any handover meetings or ward rounds that would be useful for you to attend.
- Check whether the ward has a pharmacy book in which nursing staff write down their supply requests or whether there is another system in place eg it is the responsibility of the pharmacist or medicines management technician to check supply needs.
- Find out the ward system that the multidisciplinary team use to know which patients are in which beds.
- Explain how much time you can spend on the ward and the degree of pharmaceutical care that you can provide.
- Establish what sort of pharmaceutical care service the ward is expecting from you.
- Be aware of local policies/guidelines that pertain to your ward work.
- Comply with any rules regarding hand washing and wearing an apron, gloves and mask.

Each ward visit

- Introduce yourself to the nursing co-ordinator.
- Check whether there are specific pharmaceutical care issues they would like you to follow up that day.
- Check which patients are new admissions and which ones aren't, to prioritize work if necessary.
- If the curtains are around a patient that you need to consult with, check why.
- If patients in side rooms have their doors shut, knock before entering.
- Make the nursing staff aware when you leave the ward.

Assertiveness

Assertiveness is an essential skill that can be learnt, developed and practised. Applying assertive strategies enables you to stand up for yourself and express yourself appropriately and constructively.

Definition of assertiveness

- Expressing thoughts, feelings and beliefs in a direct, honest and appropriate way.
- Having respect for yourself and others.
- Relating well to people.
- Expressing your needs freely.
- Taking responsibility for your feelings.
- Standing up for yourself if necessary.
- Working towards a 'win–win' solution to problems.
- Ensuring that both parties have their needs met as much as possible.

Assertive people effectively influence, listen and negotiate so that others choose to co-operate willingly. Assertiveness promotes self-confidence, self-control and feelings of positive self-worth, and it is the most effective means for solving interpersonal problems.

Assertive behaviour

- When you differ in opinion with someone you respect, you can speak up and share your own viewpoint.
- You stand up for your rights or those of others no matter what the circumstances.
- The ability to correct the situation when your rights or those of others are violated.
- You can refuse unreasonable requests made by friends or co-workers.
- You can accept positive criticism and suggestion.
- You ask for assistance when you need it.
- You have confidence in your own judgement.
- If someone else has a better solution, you accept it easily.
- You express your thoughts, feelings and beliefs in a direct and honest way.
- You try to work for a solution that, as much as possible, benefits all parties.
- Interacting in a mature manner with those who are offensive, defensive, aggressive, hostile, blaming, attacking, or otherwise unreceptive.

Nonassertive behaviour

- Aggressive behaviour—involves a person trying to impose their views inappropriately on others. It can be accompanied by threatening language and an angry, glaring expression, and communicates an impression of disrespect.
- Submissive behaviour—is the opposite of aggressive behaviour. The person plays down their own needs and is willing to fit in with the wishes of others to keep the peace. It shows a lack of respect for the person's own needs and communicates a message of inferiority. It can be accompanied by passivity, nervousness and lack of eye contact.
- Manipulative behaviour—occurs when a person seeks to ingratiate themselves with another through flattery and other forms of deceit. It can be accompanied by overattention and a simpering, smarmy voice.

Strategies for behaving more assertively

- Identify your personal rights, wants and needs.
- Use 'I' messages to let give people complete information to address a problem, to include three parts:
    - Behaviour—what it is that the other person has done or is doing?
    - Effect—what is happening because of their behaviour?
    - Feelings—what effect does their behaviour have on your feelings?
- Be direct and express your request succinctly.
- Choose assertive words.
- Use factual descriptions.
- Avoid exaggerations.
- Express thoughts, feelings, and opinions reflecting ownership.
- Convey a positive, assertive attitude using the following communication techniques:
    - Maintain good eye contact.
    - Maintain a firm, factual, but pleasant, voice.
    - Pay attention to your posture and gestures.
        —Stand or sit erect, possibly leaning forwards slightly, as a normal conversational distance.
        —Use relaxed, conversational gestures.
    - Listen, to let people know you have heard what they said.
    - Ask questions for clarification.
    - Look for a win–win approach to problem solving.
    - Ask for feedback.
- Evaluate your expectations and be willing to compromise

Examples of assertive language

- I am….
- I think we should….
- I feel bad when….
- That seems unfair to me.
- Can you help me with this?
- I appreciate your help.

Communication skills

Communication is a key skill for pharmacists. Every day pharmacists communicate with a variety of different groups:
- Patients/customers.
- Other healthcare professionals.
- Drug company representatives.
- Managerial staff.

Depending on the audience and circumstances, a different approach might be required, but the core skills are the same.

Planning and preparation

Before any encounter, a certain amount of planning and preparation is required, even if it is just a few words with a counter assistant to establish a customer's requirements:
- Establish the most appropriate means of communication—this might be written, in the form of a letter, memo or leaflet, or verbal, such as a conversation, seminar or oral presentation, or both.
- Know the subject—if necessary, do some background reading or research. Even if it means keeping a customer waiting, a quick look in the *BNF* could mean that ultimately your message is accepted more readily because it is well informed.
- Know the audience—understanding their background, knowledge base and requirements aids effective communication. Communicating with one person requires different strategies compared with communicating with a small or large group.
- Prepare the message—a simple, straightforward piece of information, such as dosage instructions, requires little, if any, preparation. However, a more complex message, such as the answer to a medicines information enquiry, might require some preparation:
  - Be clear in your own mind about what message or messages you want to get across.
  - Break the message down into a series of points.
  - Structure the message so that ideas are presented in order of importance.
  - Provide a one or two sentence summary/conclusion at the end.
- Think ahead—try to anticipate any questions that might arise and be prepared with the information needed to answer them.

Delivering the message

Whether communicating in writing or verbally, the same rules apply:
- Use language appropriate to the audience—avoid jargon and complex terms; use simple, direct words.
- Avoid vague terms—eg 'occasionally' or 'frequently' becauses these might mean different things to different people.
- Check understanding—by asking for feedback or questions.

Remember that verbal communication is made up of three aspects:
- 55% body language.
- 38% tone of voice.
- 7% words that make up the communication.

Listening skills

An essential part of communication is listening. Not only does this ensure your own understanding, it shows interest and concern and empowers the respondent by enabling them to fully participate in the communication process. The traditional active/passive roles of healthcare professional talking and patient listening respectively are not conducive to good communication. Good listening (by both parties) ensures that the encounter has the mutual participation of healthcare professional and patient. This should lead to the information elicited being of more value; any message is more likely to be remembered and acted upon.

- Reflecting back—clarify your understanding by repeating back ('mirroring') information, but in paraphrase.
- Summarizing—'What I think I hear you saying is….'
- Body language:
  - Use facial expressions and postures to show empathy;
  - Mirror facial expression.
  - Nod encouragingly.
  - Adopt a listening posture—as appropriate, lean towards the speaker while being careful to avoid invading their personal space.
  - Maintain eye contact.
  - Avoid signs of impatience or being in a hurry.
- Ask open-ended questions—e.g. how and why.
- Use closed questions, as appropriate–ie those with a 'yes' or 'no' response.
- Use silences appropriately:
  - Allow the speaker to finish what they want to say and avoid the temptation to jump in.
  - Do not interrupt or finish the speakers sentences.
  - If necessary, allow a short period of silence to elapse, especially if the speaker is slow or hesitant in their speech.
  - Silences can be helpful in giving thinking time.
- Use verbal or nonverbal signals to show you are listening and encourage the speaker—eg nodding and saying 'yes' or 'mm'.
- If necessary, note down key points while the other person is speaking but avoid scribbling throughout. Warn the speaker that you will be doing this so that they don't find it off-putting.
- In responding, avoid the following:
  - Exclamations of surprise, intolerance or disgust.
  - Expression of overconcern.
  - Moralistic judgements, criticism or impatience.
  - Being defensive and getting caught up in arguments.
  - Making false promises, flattery or undue praise.
  - Personal references to your own difficulties.
  - Changing the subject or interrupting unnecessarily.
  - Speaking too soon, too often or for too long.

Questioning

Questioning is also an important skill for communicating effectively. As pharmacists, this often involves direct questioning of a colleague regarding a course of action or prescribing decision. However, when dealing with patients, a broader approach might be required to get all the information required:

- Use open questions to enable the respondent to elaborate and give new information—eg 'how are you getting on with your medications'?
- Phrasing questions in different ways often elicits different information— eg asking 'do you have any problems with your medicines?' can elicit more information than asking 'do you have any side effects?'.
- Avoid leading questions—eg 'you're not getting any side effects are you' because usually the respondent will give the answer they think the questioner wants (in this case, 'no').
- Closed questions can be used to establish specific information— eg 'are you taking this medicine with food?'
- Be specific because the respondent might interpret certain terms differently to you—eg 'are you taking these medicines regularly' could mean the respondent is taking them once daily, once weekly or once monthly!
- Avoid questions that the respondent might interpret as being judgemental or critical.
- As appropriate, ensure you understand the answer by paraphrasing it back to the respondent— eg 'just to be clear, I think you are saying….'

Table 4.7 Barriers to good communication

Physical barriers:
- Speech problems
- Hearing impairment
- Communicating in a language that is not the audience's first language or through a translator
- Visual impairment
- Learning difficulties
- Noisy or distracting environment

Emotional barriers:
- Preconceptions and prejudice
- Fear
- Aggression

Table 4.8 Checklist of essential interpersonal skills to improve communication

- Body language:
  - Be aware of body language when interacting with people
  - Mirror body language
  - Ensure body language, tone and words are sending out the same messages
- Rapport with people
- Social poise, self-assurance and confidence
- Tact and diplomacy
- Consideration of others
- Assertiveness and self-control
- High standards
- Ability to analyse facts and solve problems
- Tolerance and patience
- Ability to make good decisions
- Honesty and objectivity
- Organizational skills
- Good listening habits
- Enthusiasm
- Persuasiveness
- Ability to communicate with different types of people

Table 4.9 10 ways to become a better listener

- Schedule a time and place to listen
- Create comfort
- Avoid distractions
- State the reasons for the conversation
- Use nonverbal signals
- Use reflection, paraphrasing and summarizing
- Listen for the message behind the emotions
- Be patient
- Write down any commitments
- Follow-up

Dealing with medical staff

Medical hierarchy

In the UK, doctors undertake a 5yr degree followed by a preregistration year as a **House Officer** before they become qualified. House officers undertake much of the day-to-day care of patients under the supervision of senior house officers.

The house officer year is followed by a rotation of at least 2yrs through different specialities as a **Senior House Officer**. During this time, doctors take their Part I and Part II clinical examinations. Senior house officers are responsible for prescribing and the day-to-day care of patients.

After a doctor has undertaken at least 2yrs of rotation and has passed the Part I and Part II examinations, they can specialize as a **Specialist Registrar**. They train for 4yrs in a speciality, some of which require successful examination before qualifying as a **Consultant.**

Medical staff work in teams, headed by one or more consultants. The specialist registrars often rotate between teams of the same speciality to ↑ their experience.

Dealing with medical staff

- Deal with the correct team of doctors; ideally, talk directly, to the prescriber if a change in the prescription is required.
- Be aware of the medical hierarchy, and deal with the appropriate grade of doctor.
- Be assertive.
- Be confident with your knowledge of the subject. If necessary, do some background reading.
- Try to anticipate questions and have answers ready.
- Explain succinctly.
- Repeat, if necessary.
- Understand and explore their viewpoint.
- Be prepared with alternative suggestions.
- Come to a mutual agreement.
- Do not be bullied.
- Be honest.
- Acknowledge if you 'don't know', and be prepared to follow up.
- If necessary, walk away from a difficult situation and seek the support of a more experienced colleague.
- Occasionally, you might need a discussion with a more senior grade of doctor if you are unhappy with the response from the junior doctor. This should be approached with tact and diplomacy.

Patient etiquette

Patient etiquette

When delivering pharmaceutical care to patients, it is essential that pharmacists follow an appropriate code of conduct, as described below:

- Introduce yourself to the patient, stating your name and job title or role.
- Ask if it is convenient for you to speak to the patient about their medication.
- Check the patient's identity against the drug chart/notes:
  - Ask them their name.
  - If necessary, check their date of birth.
- Ask the patient how they would like to be addressed—eg by first name or Mrs/Mr.
- Explain what you will be doing—eg checking the medicine chart, checking the POD, taking a medicines history, counselling patients on their new medicine. Use the term 'medicine' rather than 'drug' when talking to patients.
- Check whether the patient has any questions at the end of the consultation.
- If you are sorting out any problems with the medication, ensure the patient is kept fully informed.
- Avoid consultations while patients are having their meals. If it is essential to speak to the patient at that time, check that it is acceptable with the patient to interrupt their meal.
- If patients have visitors present, check with the patient if it is all right to interrupt. If so, check with the patient whether they are happy for the visitors to be present during the consultation. If the patient does not want the visitors present, ask the visitors to return after a set period of time.
- If the curtains are around the patient's bed, check with the ward staff as to the reason. If necessary, speak to the patient from outside the curtain to check whether it is all right for them to see you or whether you should return later.
- If the patient becomes distressed, or is too unwell, try to sort out the task with the help of the notes/ward staff/relative or return later when the patient can be involved with the consultation.
- Be polite at all times.
- Respect the patient's privacy.

Dealing with aggressive or violent patients

Most pharmacy staff experience some form of threatening behaviour from patients at some stage during their working lives. This can range from a patient becoming verbally abusive because of a long wait for medicines to be dispensed to an armed robbery of a community pharmacy. Even if there is no physical injury, the psychological effect of a violent or aggressive encounter can be significant and could affect the victim's attitude to work, co-workers and patients. The emotional distress can be ↑ in a healthcare setting because staff might feel unprepared for this type of behaviour from a patient or customer they are trying to help. There could be feelings of guilt, embarrassment, shame, fear of blame or denial. Incidents should not be accepted as 'part of the job' and should be reported, so that appropriate action can be taken to both protect and support the victim and other members of staff. If healthcare teams have strategies to review and discuss incidents of threatening behaviour, staff find this useful for coping and learning.

Facing an aggressive or violent patient can be a frightening and shocking experience and often the response is a 'fight or flight' reaction. Being prepared for this type of incident, and knowing strategies to deal with or defuse such a situation, is of great value.

The safety of staff and other patients/customers is of paramount importance:

- Be aware of and develop systems to avoid vulnerable times and situations —eg pharmacy opening and closing times, a lone pharmacist or dealing with patients with mental health problems.
- Don't attempt any heroics—your personal safety is far more important than the contents of the shop till. Hand over any money or goods demanded, because insurance cover can replace loss but not lives.
- Be aware of 'escape routes' and try not to let the patient get between you and the door.
- Ensure you are aware of any safety procedures—eg panic buttons and how to activate them.
- Aim to avoid situations where you are on your own with a potentially difficult patient. If you have to go into a room alone with them, leave the door open and make sure a colleague is close by to give you back up if necessary.

When dealing with an aggressive or verbally abusive patient, good handling of the incident can help defuse the situation or at least prevent it from escalating.

Don't

- Take the threatening behaviour personally.
- Be defensive or aggressive in return.
- Attempt to appease the patient by giving into their demands, although be prepared to compromise if appropriate.
- Ignore or tolerate the behaviour.
- Be overapologetic.
- Argue with the patient.
- Be overly sympathetic and take the patient's side.
- Use defensive or aggressive body language.

Do

- Remain calm and state your case clearly and concisely.
- Be assertive, without being aggressive.
- Maintain eye contact.
- Speak in a manner that is calm, clear, simple, slow and nonconfrontational.
- Listen to the patient and give them a chance to voice their complaints.
- Apologize if there clearly is some justification for the patient's complaint, without being overly apologetic or apportioning blame.
- Explain to the patient how to make a written complaint if they wish (frequently the patient will back down at this point).
- Call a more senior colleague if you feel out of your depth.

Limit setting

In some situations it might not be possible to avoid continued contact with a patient who has been aggressive or violent towards staff. This might be an in-patient who needs further medical care or someone attending for further out-patient appointments or repeat prescriptions,(eg injecting drug users on opioid replacement therapy). In these cases, it might be possible to avoid further threatening incidents by setting limits.

An effective system is to draw up a contract detailing what is expected of the patient and what behaviour is considered unacceptable, and, in return, what the patient can expect from the healthcare team. The contract should state what will happen if the patient breaks the limits—usually a single warning, followed by withdrawal of services if the limits are broken again. These contracts can be very helpful in controlling patient behaviour but it must be a two-way process—healthcare staff must also stick to their side of the contract both in terms of providing care and being prepared to carry out the threat of withdrawing care if the limits are broken.

Further reading

www.nhs.uk/zerotolerance

Dealing with distressed patients

Pharmacists might occasionally have to deal with patients who are distressed or agitated for the one of the following reasons:

- Their diagnosis.
- Difficulty in tolerating side effects.
- Witnessing an upsetting event with another patient.
- The behaviour of visitors, other staff or other patients.

If faced with this situation, even the busiest pharmacist should try to spend some time comforting or supporting the patient as best they can. Spending even a little time with the patient can bring considerable relief from distress:

- Do not ignore the patient, even if you are busy or unsure how to deal with the situation. If you feel you cannot deal with the situation yourself, acknowledge the patient's distress and ask if they would like you to call another member of staff.
- Ask the patient if they would like to talk to you about what it is that is upsetting them.
- Listen and don't interrupt.
- Never say 'I know how you feel'. Even if you have had to deal with the same situation yourself, it is presumptuous to state that you know how another person feels.
- If any misunderstandings or misconceptions are contributing to the patient's distress, try to correct these. If necessary, ask the medical team to talk to the patient.
- Answer any questions the patient has as honestly and openly as you can.
- Provide reassurance about symptoms that might be causing anxiety—eg pain can be controlled, morphine wont make them an 'addict', and side effects can be managed.
- If the patient's distress is caused by another colleague's behaviour, do not offer any comment or judgement. Listen and make a noncommittal comment, such as 'I'm sorry that's how you feel'. As appropriate, suggest that they might like to speak to a senior member of staff—eg ward sister or senior doctor.
- Remember that silence is often as helpful as conversation. Just sitting with a patient for a few minutes while they get their emotions under control can be very helpful.
- As appropriate, physical contact, such as holding the patient's hand or touching their arm, can be a source of comfort.
- Offer practical comfort—eg tissues, glass of water, a chair or privacy.
- Don't avoid the patient or the incident next time you see them, but be careful not to get too emotionally involved. A simple question like 'How are you today?' acknowledges the patient's previous distress and allows them to talk further if they wish.

Dealing with dying patients

Death is an almost daily occurrence on most wards. Although in general, patients spend most of the final year of life at home, 90% of patients spend some time in hospital and 55% die there.

As a pharmacist, you might not be as closely involved in the care of a dying patient as the nursing or medical staff, but it is still a situation that affects most pharmacists at some stage. Some pharmacists, such as those working in palliative care, oncology or intensive care units, might be quite involved in the care of both the dying patient and their family. Learning how to deal with your own feelings, in addition to those of the patient and their family, is important.

The patient

On being told that they are dying, a patient (or their relatives) usually go through the following stages (although not all people go through every stage):

- Shock/numbness
- Denial
- Anger
- Grief
- Acceptance.

It is important to let these processes happen, while supporting the patient and family sensitively.

Providing information about the illness enables the patient and family to make informed decisions about medical care and personal and social issues and this is where you can help. Patients and relatives might perceive doctors as being to busy to answer their questions or be embarrassed to ask. A pharmacist might be perceived as having more medical knowledge (and being less busy!) than the nursing staff but being more approachable than the medical staff.

When talking to dying patients and answering their questions, bear the following points in mind:

- Be honest—don't give the patient false hope. Answer questions as honestly and openly as possible. If the patient asks you directly whether they are dying, it is probably not appropriate for a pharmacist to confirm this. An appropriate response might be to ask why they are asking you this or to enquire what they have been already told and then formulate an appropriate response.
- Be sensitive—some patients might want lots of information about their diagnosis and care, but others might not be interested. Respect the patient's need for privacy at a difficult time but do not be afraid of talking to a dying patient—sometimes patients can feel lonely and isolated and even a discussion lasting a few minutes can be of real benefit. Remember that different cultures have different responses to death. Whatever your own views, respect patients' religious or secular beliefs.
- Be careful—patients might not wish family or friends to know the diagnosis or that they are dying, so be especially careful what you say if other people are present.

Patients often have questions about treatment:

- Will current treatment be continued or stopped?
- Can pain or other symptoms be controlled?
- Will they get 'addicted' to morphine?
- What happens if they can no longer take medication orally?

Answer these questions as fully as you can, without overloading the patient with information. Be practical with your information and remember that some cautions become irrelevant at this stage—eg do not insist on NSAIDs being taken with food if the patient is not eating. If you don't feel it is appropriate for you to answer a question, tactfully tell the patient that it would be better to ask someone more appropriate—eg the doctors. However, you could help the patient to formulate the question so that they feel better able to ask the doctors.

The information you provide will depend on the situation and your level of expertise. If you feel out of your depth, ask a senior colleague for advice.

Carers and relatives

Carers' and relatives' needs and questions will often be the same as the patient's and you might need to go over some issues more than once. If the patient is going to be cared for at home, there can be many practical questions and information needs that you can answer:

- A simpler (layman's) explanation of the diagnosis and symptom management (often carers, relatives and patients find it difficult to ask doctors for a simplified explanation).
- Coping with (potentially complex) medication regimens.
- Side effects and what to do about them.
- What to do if the patient vomits soon after taking a dose.
- Medicine storage.
- Obtaining further supplies.
- What to with unused medicines when the patient dies.
- What to do if symptoms are not controlled.
- What to do if the patient becomes too unwell to take oral medicines.

Yourself

It is important to recognize your own emotional needs, especially if your job means you are frequently involved in the care of dying patients or if a death is especially 'close to home'. The patient or the circumstances of their illness/death might remind you of the death of a close relative or friend. This can 'open up old wounds', which you must come to terms with. When a patient dies, you might experience various emotions:

- Sadness—a natural response to any death, but accept that it is a 'hazard' of working in healthcare.
- Relief—a prolonged or distressing illness is over.
- Grief or loss—you might have become quite attached to the patient and/or their family.
- Guilt/inadequacy—if symptoms weren't controlled or the patient's death was unexpected.

It is important to find ways to cope with this. Talking to a colleague, hospital chaplain or close friend might help, but bear in mind that you must maintain confidentiality.

If the patient is well known to the ward/community pharmacy staff the family might invite them to the funeral or memorial service. Attending the funeral can benefit healthcare workers, in addition to giving the family support. Consider whether your attendance could breach confidentiality. Avoid wearing a uniform, remove identification badges and bleeps and consider whether wearing a symbol, such as a red or pink ribbon, would be inappropriate. If you are unsure whether it would be appropriate to attend, discuss it with a senior member of staff—eg ward sister or your manager.

Euthanasia

It is extremely unlikely that a patient would directly ask a pharmacist to assist them to die. However, you might be aware that a patient has expressed this desire to other staff. Whatever your personal view on the morality of euthanasia, you should treat the patient the same as any other.

Euthanasia is still illegal in most countries. However, it is generally considered acceptable to give treatment that is adequate to control symptoms, even if this could shorten the duration of life, provided the primary intent is symptom control. If you have any concerns about the appropriateness of therapy/doses in this situation, you should discuss this with the prescriber and/or a senior colleague.

What if your patient is dead in the bed?

Although not a common occurrence, clinical pharmacists can be the first to realise that a patient has died, often quietly in their bed or a chair. Here are some things to bear in mind should this happen on your round:

- Do not panic, but remain calm.
- Withdraw yourself from that patient's area and close the bed curtains, if open.
- Speak to the member of the nursing team responsible for that patient, to check that they are aware of the situation.
- Consider what you feel about the incident.
- If necessary, speak to a member of the multidisciplinary team.
- Take a break to recover.
- Speak to a colleague for support.
- Continue with the day's work.

If a relative is with the patient, they might call the pharmacist to the bed if they are concerned that the patient has died. Inform the relative that you will get a nurse to attend. Find a nurse or a member of the medical team immediately to deal with the patient, as appropriate.

It might be useful, as part of the pharmacist induction, to visit the mortuary, because dealing with death requires professional support.

Managing meetings

To efficiently manage meetings, get the best results and use time effectively, follow the tips below:

- Ensure the agenda is understood in advance–circulate a written agenda, including the following points for each item to be discussed:
  - Topic
  - Duration
  - Responsibility.
- Circulate the agenda at least a week in advance, or more in advance if papers need to be read before the meeting.
- The meeting should have a chairman who must ensure that the meeting runs smoothly and to time, allowing all participants to be involved.
- Be clear with the participants why the meeting is being held and what it will achieve.
- Ensure that at least two-thirds of the participants have a role in every topic on the agenda. Consider rearranging the agenda so that people do not waste time listening to a topic they have no active interest in.
- Be clear what preparation is required in advance of the meeting.
- Always start and finish on time.
- Discourage AOB (any other business).
- Always use a flip chart and record actions on it for all to see.
- Try to ensure individuals record their actions in their diaries before leaving, and do not wait for the arrival of the 'minutes'.
- 'Minuting' depends on the culture of the organization—use common sense as to what is recorded, how it is recorded and by whom.
- Minutes should be circulated as soon as possible after the meeting, ideally delaying no longer than 2wks.

Oral presentation skills

Oral presentation skills

Pharmacists often make presentations to a variety of audiences. These can be both formal and informal. Below are some suggestions on how to prepare and effectively deliver an oral presentation:

- Find out the duration of the presentation.
- Find out format—eg workshop or formal presentation.
- Find out about facilities—eg availability of audiovisual aids.
- Prepare approximately one slide per 1–2mins of presentation.
- Find out whether you are expected to supply handouts to the audience, how many and what level they should be aimed at.
- Check whether you are expected to send the presentation slides in advance, and, if so, the timelines for this.
- Plan and prepare your presentation.
- A presentation usually consists of three parts:
  - Tell the audience what you are going to talk about.
  - Talk about it.
  - Tell the audience what you told them.
- Always take a back-up option for the presentation—have the presentation saved on disc or on a memory stick, and take overheads.
- Arrive at the presentation in plenty of time to ensure that the equipment can be tested or your presentation can be downloaded.
- Familiarize yourself with the venue and the equipment available—eg pointer or computer equipment.
- Ensure you are not blocking the audience's view of your slides from where you are standing.
- Check that your slides are in focus.
- Look at the audience and NOT the screen!
- Make sure you look at ALL of the audience, so that they all feel included.
- Minimize how much you move around.
- Ensure that the audience can hear you.
- Don't forget to introduce yourself, why you are presenting and your background experience to the subject.
- Involve the audience by asking questions or for input, as appropriate.
- Ask if the audience have any questions—depending on the time/ format, invite questions during the presentation and/or at the end.

Prioritizing

Pharmacists can be called upon to undertake a variety of tasks. Work often has to be prioritized, to use time effectively and complete tasks in a timely manner. The ability to understand the priorities of others and to prioritize your own work is a very important skill to learn. Below are some tips on prioritizing:

- When deciding the priority of a particular task, consider both its importance (is it worth doing?) and its urgency (does it need to be done right now?):
  - If a task is both urgent and important, drop everything else and do it. It is preferable to take care of important tasks before they become urgent.
  - If a task is important but not urgent, get it done before time becomes short to avoid unnecessary stress.
  - If a task is urgent but unimportant, get it done as quickly as possible and without elaboration.
  - If a task is neither important nor urgent, don't waste your time on it.
- When deciding whether to do a particular task, consider the number of people it affects and cost of undertaking the task.
- Numbered daily checklists are often helpful.
- To understand the priorities of others requires excellent communication skills, especially the ability to ask good-quality questions, listen to the answers and notice body language.
- Knowing where your plan fits into the plans of others is useful in predicting problems, solving problems and influencing.
- Knowing where your plan fits in your own organization's priorities ensures access to and release of resources.
- This is a useful tool for prioritizing your work—write tasks in the boxes according to whether they fit the labels (Fig. 4.1):
  - Urgent and important tasks take first priority.
  - Important tasks that are not urgent take second priority.
  - Unimportant tasks that are also not urgent take lowest priority.

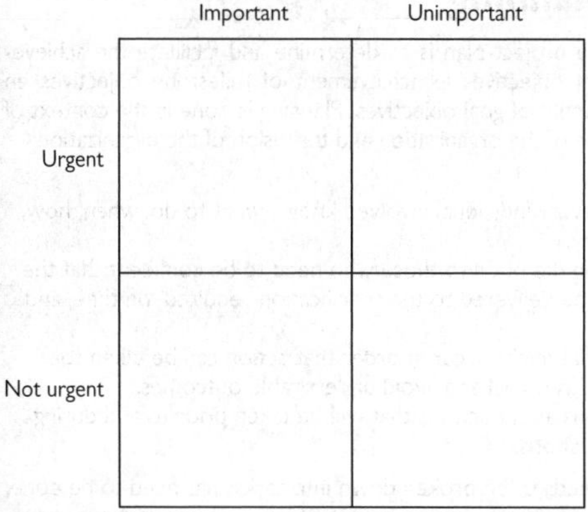

	Important	Unimportant
Urgent		
Not urgent		

Fig. 4.1 Tool for prioritizing work—write tasks in the boxes according to where they fit the labels.

Project planning

The purpose of a project plan is to determine and facilitate the achievement of a set of objectives ie achievement of milestone objectives en route to achievement of goal objectives. Planning is done in the context of the stated mission of the organization and the vision of the organization.

Planning is about:
- Ensuring that every individual involved knows what to do, when, how, where, and why.
- Communicating the plans to those who need to be confident that the ambitions will be delivered to the specification required, on time, and within budget.
- Forecasting what might occur in order that action can be taken to achieve the desired goal and avoid undersirable outcomes.
- Making decisions about actions that will be taken prior to and during anticipated situations.

A project plan needs to be broken down into tasks that need to be done, and then sequencing the tasks in a logical order. Tasks are actions. Accurate identification of the tasks is essential as they are the basis of:
- Developing schedules.
- Identifying milestones.
- Implementing change plans.
- Planning communication.
- Resource planning: manpower, materials, and machinery.
- Monitoring.
- Maintaining records.
- Managing risk.
- Measuring progress.
- Forecasting remaining work.

It can be useful to complete a one-page summary of each task that contains all the information needed to delegate the responsibility for completion of the task to one person, as each task is effectively a 'mini-project'.

The quickest and most effective way to produce outline plans is to do it in five phases:
1. Describe the scope of the project.
2. Identify the tasks.
3. Scheduling the tasks into a sensible order that will achieve the outcome of the plan.
4. Identifying milestones. Milestones are the significant objectives that are to be achieved on the way to completing the project, and serve as visible indications of progress. They enable people to know that the plan is being implemented without having to know the details.
5. Implement the plan.

When scoping the project, the questions to be considered are:
- Simple description.
- Why it is being considered at all?
- Where does it fit with other proejcts?
- What are the benefits to the organization?
- What are the downsides or penalities of not doing it?
- Major issues.
- Risks.
- Measures of success.
- Return on investment summary.
- Names of key stakeholders and stakeholder groups.
- An indication of whether to invest resource in a project plan.

Software is available to help with project planning and the production of time flow charts (Gant charts).

Time management

Quick techniques for managing time include the following:
- The four Rs of paperwork:
  - Recycle (bin)
  - Refer (out-tray and delegation)
  - Respond
  - Record (file).
- Invest time, don't spend it.
- De-clutter.
- Use a system for time management:
  - Use a list system to write down ideas, thoughts and tasks as you think of them.
  - Diary system.
  - Names and addresses system.
  - 'Bracket' tasks, appointments and travel time.
  - Set time limits, with interruptions.
  - Use 'scrap time' wisely.
  - Take frequent, quick breaks to ↑ productivity.
  - Do the most important tasks first.
  - Or, do the fastest and easiest tasks first.
  - Demand completed work from your staff.
  - Communicate upwards when you have problems:
    —Description of problem.
    —List of possible solutions.
    —Recommended solution.
    —List of necessary resources.
    —Implementation of the solution.

Ethical dilemmas

Medical ethics deals with situations where there are no clear course of action. This might be because of a lack of scientific evidence, but it is more frequently where moral, religious or other values have a significant influence on decision making. Thus, medical ethics differs from research ethics, the latter is concerned with evaluating whether clinical trials are appropriate, safe and in the best interests of the participants and/or the wider population. Many hospitals have medical ethics, in addition to research ethics, committees.

The issues debated by medical ethics committees are many and varied. They might produce guidelines to cover certain issues, but frequently a committee does not give a definite answer and simply provides a forum for debate. Issues debated by medical ethics committees include the following:

- Consent to or refusal of treatment, especially with respect to those unable to make decisions themselves—ie children or incapacitated adults.
- End of life issues, such as 'do not resuscitate' orders, living wills and withdrawal of treatment.
- Organ donation and transplantation.
- Contraception and abortion.

Like most other healthcare professionals, pharmacists are expected to conduct their professional (and to a certain extent their personal) lives according to ethical principles. In the UK, the RPSGB gives advice in a code of ethics, which covers many areas of pharmacy practice. However, there are occasions where pharmacists are faced with dilemmas for which there are no clear course of action:

- The pharmacist's religious beliefs or moral values are in conflict with what is expected of them—eg over-the-counter sale of emergency hormonal contraception.
- There is no clear scientific or evidence-based treatment available— eg use of unlicensed or experimental treatments.
- Business or economic issues clash with patient or public interests.

Ethical decision making attempts to deal with these dilemmas using the following considerations:

- The values or beliefs that lie behind them.
- The reasons people give for making a moral choice.
- Duty of care—to the patient, their family and to other healthcare professionals or yourself.
- Medical law.

In many instances, there is not a right or wrong answer and different people might make different—but equally justifiable—decisions based on the same set of circumstances.

It is best not to attempt to deal with ethical dilemmas alone. Depending on the situation, it is advisable to discuss the situation with the following people:
- A colleague.
- The multidisciplinary team.
- Other interested parties, such as management, patient advocates, clergy or legal advisers.

Consider the following points:
- What are the patients wishes? It is good to ask yourself 'do I know what the patient really wants?'.
- What do the patient's relatives or representatives think? Are they adequately informed to make a decision? Do they have the patient's best interests at heart? (Remember you need to have the patient's permission to discuss the situation with their family.)
- Would you be willing for a member of your own family to be subject to the same decision making process?
- Could the decision made in this situation adversely affect the treatment of other patients?
- Do issues of public health or interest outweigh the patient's rights?
- Is the decision or course of action legally defensible?
- Is the decision just and fair—eg are scarce resources being used appropriately?

It is also important to remember the following points:
- 'Do no harm' is a good basic principle, but sometimes some 'harm' must be done to achieve a greater individual or public good.
- Ensuring patient health should include mental and spiritual health, in addition to physical health.
- Acting with compassion is not necessarily the same as acting ethically.
- Slavishly following scientific or evidence-based decision making could lead to a morally inappropriate action (or lack of action).

Clinical trials

Definitions

The development of new drugs has four phases of clinical trials:

Phase I trials

These trials assess the maximum tolerated dose and toxicity of a drug used for the first time in humans. They are primarily concerned with the safety, pharmacokinetics and pharmacodynamics of the drug. The drug is usually administered as a single, low dose, and then the dose and duration are gradually ↑, depending on the side effects experienced by the volunteers. Phase I trials usually only involve small numbers of participants, and are usually undertaken in healthy volunteers, unless it is unethical eg cytotoxic drugs must be tested in cancer patients. Phase I studies provide information on the tolerability of a range of doses of the drug, early dose–response relationships and pharmacokinetics.

Phase II trials

Phase II trials are usually the first time that patients are exposed to the drug (with the exception of anti-cancer drugs). These trials assess the efficacy of a treatment and define the therapeutic dose range and dosing regimen for a specific indication, with minimum side effects. They also produce additional information on safety, pharmacokinetics and pharmacodynamics in the presence of the disease process. Relatively small numbers of patients are studied under close supervision, usually by specialized investigators. Phase II studies are usually just a trial of the drug and provide information on the small range of doses that should be used in phase III studies. Phase II studies do not assess the drug's efficacy versus another agent.

Phase III trials

Phase III studies assess real outcomes in a variety of patients approximating to the population of patients who will receive the drug once it is launched. Phase III trials are undertaken in large numbers of patients, often in multiple centres. Their aim is to compare new treatments with existing treatments and to demonstrate long-term safety and tolerance.

Phase IV trials

These studies are performed after a product licence is obtained. Their main aim is either to investigate the incidence of relatively rare ADRs or to compare drugs with comparative treatments, often to extend the range of approved indications.

Trial design, randomization and blinding (phase III and IV studies)

- The most robust trials include blinding and randomization. Randomized controlled trials form the cornerstone of phase III testing.

- Controlled clinical trials compare a test treatment with another treatment. Comparisons in controlled trials can be with either retrospective patients who have the same disease (historical controls) or a prospective control group. Prospective clinical trials can be designed as parallel or cross-over studies:
  - Parallel studies assign patients to receive one of the study treatments and two groups of patients continue in the study in 'parallel'.
  - Crossover studies assign both of the treatments to one group of patients. They receive one treatment for a period of time and, following a wash out period, the same patients receive the second treatment.
- Randomized trials assign treatments to successive patients in a predetermined, random way. Randomized trials aim to show that one treatment is superior to another, and they avoid investigator bias. There are several practices of randomization:
  - Simple randomization assigns equal numbers of patients to each group.
  - Unequal randomization can be used–eg if experience is required in a larger number of patients receiving a new treatment.
  - Stratification is used to avoid bias if a large difference in responses between groups is expected; separate randomization lists, containing different disease categories, are used. That is, if a patient factor could affect the patient response, stratification ensures equal allocation of patients with this factor to both treatment groups. Stratification occurs before randomization.
- In randomized controlled trials, patients are randomly allocated to either the new drug or an existing recognised treatment with which it is being compared. These trials are often blinded and there are two levels of blinding:
  - Single-blind study—the investigator or assessor does not know which treatment has been administered.
  - Double-blind study—neither the subject nor the investigator know which treatment has been given. This is the preferred type of study. Controlled, randomized, double-blind, parallel–group studies are the reference standard for comparing treatments.

There can be problems with blinding in a clinical trial:
- If the drugs have obvious differences–eg IV versus oral forms.
- When ADRs are associated with one arm of the trial.
- Ethical issues of withholding information from patients on the exact treatment they are receiving.

When trials are blinded, mechanisms are in place to ensure individuals can be unblinded in the case of emergencies.

Further reading

Clinical trials directive (2001/20/EC). www.mhra.gov.uk
Di Giovanna I, Hayes G (ed) (2001). *Principles of clinical research*. Guildford: Wrightson Biomedical Publishing Ltd.

Licensing

Before a clinical trial starts, the following authorizations/approvals must be obtained:
- Clinical trial authorization from a competent authority (in the UK this is the Medicines and Healthcare Products Regulatory Agency [MHRA]):
  - The competent authority must consider the application within 60 days (maximum). This application can run in parallel with the ethics opinion.
  - The competent authority must notify the sponsor within 35 days if there are grounds for refusal.
- A favourable opinion from one ethics committee.
- An opinion on the suitability of the local investigator and facilities from the local research ethics committee (LREC) for each site.
- Permission from the NHS trust for the trial to take place within that trust (R&D approval) for each site.
- A EudraCt number must be obtained from the EudraCt database for all trials commencing after May 1 2004. The EudraCt number is a unique number allocated to each trial by the competent authority (MHRA). The EudraCt database registers details of all trials approved in the European Union (EU).

The (MHRA) has the following role in clinical trial licensing:
- UK 'competent authority'.
- Grants licences to conduct trials.
- Monitors safety aspects of trials.
- Provides enforcement—mandatory inspections.

Further reading

Clinical trials directive (2001/20/EC). www.mhra.gov.uk

European directive

- Clinical trials are controlled by directive 2001/20/EC, which became part of UK law on May 1, 2004 as 'The Medicines for Human Use (Clinical Trials) Regulations, 2004'.
- The directive enforces controls on the preparation and testing of clinical trial materials (investigational medicinal products [IMPs]) on humans.
- The EU directive on good clinical practice (GCP) in clinical trials provides a legal framework and harmonizes standards for clinical trials.
- The MHRA enforces these standards in the UK by performing inspections of GCP and good manufacturing practice (GMP).
- There is no distinction between commercial and noncommercial trials, and there are no exemptions for any trials using a drug that is prescribed outside of its licence.
- To help the exchange of information between EU member states, there are secure networks linked to European databases of information on approved clinical trials and pharmacovigilance.
- All clinical trials must be covered by a clinical trial authorisation.
- Hospitals preparing clinical trial materials must hold an IMP manufacturer's licence (MA) issued by the MHRA. A Pharmacist is required to be named as the qualified person (QP), who is usually the quality-control pharmacist.
- The production pharmacist is named in the manufacturing licence as being responsible for the manufacture of the product.
- A representative from the hospital pharmacy department must have a place on the research ethics committee.
- An individual in the pharmacy department, who is separate from the above pharmacists, must be named as being responsible for clinical trials in hospitals managing clinical trials.
- The nominated co-ordinator of clinical trial materials in the pharmacy must liaise with the trust's research and development department to ensure that the trials are valid and acceptable. The co-ordinator is the contact person for any pharmaceutical company or investigator.
- Clinical trial protocols must be made available to the pharmacy department in advance of consideration by an ethics committee, so that the practical details, such as doses and method of administration, packaging, labelling and study documentation appropriate for each individual trial, can be checked. The protocol must specify the duration and responsibility for the storage of all pharmacy records relating to the trial.
- Trials have to be under the control of a named sponsor. The sponsor is the person legally responsible for the conduct of a clinical trial. This is usually the chief executive of the body registered as the sponsor. This person is responsible for ensuring that the required systems are in place and that all the regulations are complied with.
- All staff involved in clinical trials must have evidence of suitable training in their CPD log.

- The following requirements must be met before commencement of a clinical trial:
  - A favourable opinion from a Research Ethics Committee (REC).
  - Authorization from the competent authority to conduct the clinical trial.
  - The sponsor must receive authorization to conduct the trial with the IMP(s) specified.
- Failure to comply with the EU clinical trials directive is a criminal offence.
- The conduct of clinical trials must follow these requirements:
  - The sponsor must notify the competent authority within 90days of the conclusion of the trial.
  - If the trial terminates early, the sponsor must notify the competent authority within 15days.
  - The competent authority can suspend or terminate any trial if there are doubts about the safety or scientific validity.
- In summary, the regulations set standards for the following reasons:
  - Protecting clinical trial participants.
  - Establishing ethics committees on a statutory basis.
  - The manufacture, import and labelling of IMPs.
  - Manufacture and labelling of drugs compliant with GMP.
  - Provision for quality assurance of clinical trials and IMPs.
  - Safety monitoring of patients participating in trials.
  - Procedures for reporting and recording ADRs and events through the eudravigilance database in Europe.
  - Regulatory approval system for clinical trials in the EU.
  - Information exchange between member states by means of a database of trial information (EudraCT database).
- GCP documents for undertaking clinical trials include the following:

UK only:
  - Medicines for Human Use (Clinical Trials) Regulations, 2004.
  - Governance arrangements for research ethics committees (GAfREC).

European:
  - EU directive 2001/20/EC.
  - The guidance notes to support the directive (GCP and GMP).
  - ICH note for guidance on GCP.
  - Annex 13 of the GMP guidelines (labelling requirements).

Further reading

Clinical trials directive (2001/20/EC). www.mhra.gov.uk
Fenton-May V (2004). Clinical trials directive—it is nothing more than good practice. *Hospital pharmacist* **11**: 218.

Clinical trials and the European directive: hospital pharmacy guidance

Receipt of supplies

- Ensure all clinical trial supplies are received from an approved EU supplier.
- Clinical trial supplies must be verified by an EU-approved QP.
- Clinical trial supplies manufactured outside the EU must be imported into the EU with an import licence (available from the MHRA) and released by an EU-approved QP named on the importing licence.

Storage and handling

- The pharmacy department must manage all clinical trial medication.
- Clinical trial materials must be kept in a separate and secure storage area, with sufficient room to ensure that there is no confusion between trial materials.
- The designated pharmacist should ensure that the formulation, presentation and storage of clinical trial medications are appropriate.
- Clinical trial medication must be dispensed against appropriate prescription forms, which have been agreed by the trial investigators and pharmacy department. Each clinical trial drug prescription must contain the agreed title of the study and protocol number unique to the study.
- The pharmacy department should be involved in the reconciliation and disposal of unused medication. Guidance is available from the regional quality assurance pharmacists' document on waste disposal.

Labelling, packaging and stability issues

- All medication must be suitably labelled to comply with current labelling requirements for IMPs, as outlined in annex 13 of the GMP guide, and the European clinical trials directive 2001/20/EC.
- Pharmacists, and those working under their supervision, do not need to hold a manufacturing authorization to repackage or change the packaging of clinical trial materials, if this is done in a hospital or healthcentre for patients of that establishment.

Documentation and records

- The pharmacy department must keep appropriate records of the dispensing of clinical trial drugs and detailed drug accountability. Clinical trial documentation should be retained in the pharmacy for the life of the trial, and after that time, the sponsor is responsible for storage.
- All training must be documented and available for inspection.
- Records of storage conditions must be kept.
- Clinical trial randomization codes should be held in the pharmacy department. Arrangements for the codes to be broken outside of normal pharmacy working hours must be made. Criteria for code breaking should be available and records made in the relevant trial documentation.
- Departmental standard operating procedures must be in place, which are suitably version-controlled and reviewed at regular intervals.

Charging for clinical trials

- The pharmacy department should have a standard method of charging for clinical trials, which has been agreed with the R&D department.
- Arrangements should be made for the levy of prescription charges in accordance with current guidance:
  - Prescription charges do not apply to trials in which patients could receive an inert substance.
  - A prescription charge should be levied (subject to the usual prescription charge exemption criteria) for trials comparing active substances or different doses of an active substance.

Further reading

Clinical trials directive (2001/20/EC). www.mhra.gov.uk

Ethical committees

The EU directive (2001/20/EC) ensures there are national ethics committees operating within a legal framework, with firm deadlines for approval. The UK ethics review system is the GAfREC.

Definitions

- **Central office for research ethics committees (CORECs):**
  - Authorized by the UK Department of Health (DoH) to give operational advice and support to all RECs in England.
  - Issue standard operating procedures for RECs in the UK.
- **GAfREC:**
  - Defines REC and their composition.
  - Defines the research sites.
  - Defines investigators.
- **LREC:**
  - Reviews research proposals for studies that are not multicentre studies.
  - Provide site-specific assessments (SSAs) for multicentre trials.
  - Must work to SOPs and policy laid down by CORECs.
- **Multicentre research ethics committees (MRECs):**
  - Reviews trials taking place at more than one site—ie multicentre studies.
- **Office for research ethics committees (ORECs):**
  - 11 regions, each with an appointed OREC manager.
  - Lead the development process in the area.
  - Review and develop existing systems and structures to comply with the GAfREC and the EU directive.
  - Manage the REC system within the geographical area.
  - Manage internal and external communications relating to RECs in the area.
- **SSA:**
  - Suitability of the principal investigator and support staff.
  - Adequacy of the local facilities available for the research.
  - Arrangements for consent and provision of information in other languages.
- **United Kingdom ethics committee authority (UKECA):**
  - Establishes, recognises and monitors all ethics committees within the UK and accredits them.
  - Nondepartmental public body separate from government.
  - Oversees the regulations applicable to ethical review of clinical trials only.

Composition of an REC
- 12–18 members (lay and medical).
- Balanced age and gender distribution.
- Subcommittees encouraged.
- Lead reviewers suggested.
- Quorum of seven members stipulated and defined.
- Co-opted members allowed, as defined, to ensure the balance of the committee is maintained.

Rule of ethics committees
Ethics committees consider the following:
- The relevance of the clinical trial and trial design.
- Whether the evaluation of the anticipated benefits and risks is satisfactory and conclusions are justified.
- The protocol.
- The suitability of the investigator and supporting staff.
- The investigators brochure.
- The quality of the facilities.
- The consent form and patient information sheet.
- The procedure to be followed for obtaining informed consent.
- Justification for research on persons incapable of giving informed consent.
- The arrangements for the recruitment of subjects.
- Provision for indemnity or compensation in the event of injury or death.
- Insurance or indemnity to cover the liability of the investigator and sponsor.
- The arrangements for rewarding or compensating investigators and trial subjects, including the amount, and the relevant aspects of any agreement between the sponsor and the site.

Timelines for ethics committees
- Ethics committees meet monthly.
- The ethics committee has a maximum of 60 days from the date of receipt of the valid application to give 'its reasoned opinion'.
- Ethics committees must give favourable opinions within 35 days.
- There might be a single request for supplementary information.
- There is no extension to the 60 days period except for trials involving gene therapy, somatic cell therapy or xenogenic cell therapy.
- An LREC must notify a MREC of a decision on an SSA within 25 days of receipt of a valid application.

Further reading
Clinical trials directive (2001/20/EC). www.mhra.gov.uk
COREC www.corec.org.uk

Pharmacists advising ethics committees

Pharmacists advising ethics committees should be able to use their pharmaceutical expertise to advise on issues including:

- Quality assurance.
- GCP issues.
- GMP issues.
- Storage.
- Issues surrounding drug administration—eg blinding.
- Monitoring ADRs.
- Clinical trial design and randomization.
- Licensing arrangements for the trial.
- Indemnity arrangements for the trial.
- Safety and efficacy of any drugs involved.
- Appropriateness of the proposed dosage regimens.
- Appropriateness of the formulation.
- The method of monitoring compliance with drug regimens.
- Patient education.
- Continuing supply of medications for 2yrs following the trial.
- Availability of a QP.

Controlled drugs

Suspected loss of controlled drugs within hospitals

Ward or clinic level

Nursing staff suspecting loss of controlled drugs should report immediately to the nurse in charge of the shift on the ward/unit/department.

The nurse in charge should contact one of the following people:
- The ward sister/charge nurse of the ward, if the loss occurs during working hours.
- The senior nurse/operational manager if loss occurs during a night duty.
- A senior pharmacist, if the loss occurs during pharmacy opening hours.
- The on-call pharmacist, if loss occurs out of hours, who will report the loss to a senior pharmacist.
- Security, if necessary.

If the senior nurse/pharmacist believes police involvement is necessary in relation to the loss, your local policy for involving police must be followed. Advice can be sought from your security manager.

The pharmacy department should have a dedicated audit form to detail each report of possible loss of a controlled drug. The form must be completed immediately, in addition to a hospital incident form. The form should be handed to the relevant ward pharmacist (during normal working hours) or delivered by hand to the pharmacy within 24h (maximum) after the discovery of the loss.

A senior pharmacist manager should investigate the loss, make recommendations and copy the form to the lead nurse within the speciality, ideally within two working days. The lead nurse will then discuss this with the head nurse of the ward/unit/department and ward sister.

The head nurse for the ward/unit/department will add comments and return the completed form to the chief pharmacist. The chief pharmacist should organize a register of losses and monitor and analyse any trends.

The record of suspected losses should be reported to the clinical governance committee, or similar body, that has responsibility for one administration of medicines.

Notes for the investigating pharmacist

On investigating identified discrepancies, it is good practice to initially check the following:
- Arithmetic details in the register.
- Identify the time interval when the suspected drug balance was correct.
- Enquire about the probable number of staff that could have had access to the keys for controlled drug storage during the investigated period.
- Whether the senior nurse has organized that administrations for the drug to be checked against the patients drug chart.
- Ensure regular checks of controlled drug stocks to be performed.
- Check when nurse and pharmacist stock accountability was last undertaken.

Note that small discrepancies involving liquid preparations are not uncommon, but could need to be monitored in case a pattern emerges.

If an arithmetical error explains the loss, it is not usually considered necessary to complete an incident form or report the incident to senior managers.

Hospital pharmacy department

Suspicion of loss must be reported immediately to appropriate manager eg the dispensary manager or stores manager. The manager must undertake an inventory check and decide if staff are following the department's standing operating procedures for receipt and supply of controlled drugs.

It is GCP to check the following:

- Arithmetic details in the register.
- Identify the time interval when the suspected drug balance was correct.
- Department's standard operating procedures have been complied with — eg only designated staff have access to operate in controlled drug preparation area, including out-of-hours staff, and that all such staff have received appropriate training.
- Receipt and invoice procedures are in place.
- Access to the department by visitors is enforced and that visitors have no access to controlled drug preparation areas.
- All supply requisitions are checked.

If a discrepancy exists, the loss should be submitted in writing to the chief pharmacist, who should discuss review of standard operating procedures. The incident should be reported to the clinical governance committee, or similar body, that has responsibility for medicine management.

The decision to involve an external investigator must be undertaken with the involvement of the chief pharmacist.

Patient's own controlled drugs in a hospital setting

Patients admitted into hospital

If a patient is admitted with his/her own controlled drugs, two registered nurses should check these onto the ward.

The drug and its form, strength and quantity should be checked and the drug(s) then placed in a controlled drugs cupboard, with the details entered in a separate patient's own controlled drugs record book.

The patients name must be written on the label. If unlabelled strips of medicine are brought in, these should not be administered to the patient and the supplies should be highlighted to a pharmacist, who should organize their destruction or return to the patient, or their relative, on discharge.

Use of patient's own controlled drugs

Ideally, the use of the patients own supplies for in-patients should be restricted to the following:

- Nonformulary drugs.
- While awaiting supplies from the pharmacy.
- Administration records should be completed on the relevant page of the patient's own controlled drugs record book.

Nurses should be encouraged to order supplies from their pharmacy as soon as feasible.

Return of patient's own controlled drugs

When the patient goes home, their medicines must be signed out of the patient's own controlled drug record book by the patient's nurse and a witness and handed directly to the patient, assuming that the nurse has previously checked that the patient's drug and labelled dose schedule hasn't changed during the patient in-patient stay.

Returns belonging to deceased patients—disposal and destruction of controlled drugs

The PODs must be notified to the pharmacist responsible for the ward/unit/department; these controlled drugs can either be destroyed on the ward by the pharmacist or be returned to pharmacy, depending on local practice and policy.

Records of destruction

In both cases, an entry must be made in the patient's own controlled drugs record book on the appropriate page for the drug in question, specifying 'destruction' or 'return to the pharmacy', the quantity involved, the new stock balance and the signatures of the pharmacist and witness involved.

Evidence-based medicine

Evidence-based medicine (EBM) and clinical pharmacy

EBM has moved from esoteric to standard practice during recent years, although it is probably more widely practiced in primary care in the UK. The following definition of EBM can be adapted for clinical pharmacy.

Definition of EBM

> EBM is the conscientious, explicit and judicious use of current best evidence in making decisions about the care of individual patients.[1]

The authors of the definition go on to state that the practice of EBM requires the integration of individual clinical expertise with the best available external clinical evidence from systematic research.

The second definition comes from the McMaster University website:

> EBM is an approach to healthcare that promotes the collection, interpretation and integration of valid, important and applicable patient-reported, clinician-observed and research-derived evidence. The best available evidence, moderated by patient circumstances and preferences, is applied to improve the quality of clinical judgements.[2]

Evidence-based clinical pharmacy

Borrowing the Sackett definition above, a definition might be as follows: *Evidence-based clinical pharmacy is the conscientious, explicit and judicious use of current best evidence in making decisions about the care of individual patients.*

This entirely fits with the concept of pharmaceutical care (see p.257) and challenges clinical pharmacists not only to keep abreast of developments in their chosen speciality, but also to apply clinical developments to patient circumstances and preferences.

One of Bandolier's maxims is that EBM is essentially 'tools not rules'.[3] Pharmacists need to remember this when applying current best evidence to patient care.

Strengths of evidence

A hierarchy of evidence (Table 7.1) is helpful in avoiding types of studies that are inherently biased. There are a number of grading systems currently available which are useful in terms of identifying the level of evidence available and as a tool for categorizing recommendations made in clinical guidelines, for example. For updated information on this topic, see the GRADE website.[4]

---

1 Sackett DL *et al.* (1996) *BMJ* **312**: 71–2.
2 McMaster University. http://hiru.mcmaster.ca
3 www.ebandolier.com
4 www.gradeworkinggroup.org

Some evidence tables regard large randomized trials as Level I evidence. Evidence from levels IV and V should not be overlooked if it is all that is available. Conversely, recommendations should not be made on level V evidence if level I or II evidence is available.

Table 7.1 Type and strength of efficacy evidence

I.	Strong evidence from at least one systematic review of multiple well-designed randomized controlled trials
II.	Strong evidence from at least one properly designed randomized controlled trial of appropriate size
III.	Evidence from well designed trials without randomization, single group, cohort, time series or matched case-controlled studies
IV.	Evidence from well-designed non experimental studies from more than one centre or research group
V.	Opinions of respected authorities, based on clinical evidence, descriptive studies or reports of expert committees

Statistical versus clinical significance

Simply because a study finding was statistically significant, does not mean that the finding is important. Large trials or a large meta-analyses have the potential to find very small statistically significant differences between groups. An important consideration when interpreting significant findings is assessment of how clinically significant the finding is.

'*Clinical significance*' refers to a value judgement people must make when determining the meaningfulness of the magnitude of an intervention effect.

For example, if an expensive medication was found to significantly ↓ systolic BP by an average of 2mmHg, it would be important to consider the clinical merit of the intervention. Would there be any important health benefits to a patient of a ↓ in SBP of just 2mmHg? Would it be worth investing in an expensive intervention if it delivered such meagre ↓ in SBP? Are there any cheaper medications available that produce greater ↓ in BP?

Well-conducted, rigorous, randomized controlled trials should recruit enough participants to detect a difference between groups which is determined as clinically significant before the study.

Odds ratios and relative risk

What is an odds ratio?

The number needed to treat (NNT) is a very useful way of describing the benefits (or harms) of treatments, both in individual trials and in systematic reviews. Few papers report results using this easily interpretable measure. NNT calculations, however, come second to working out whether an effect of treatment in one group of patients is different from that found in the control groups. Many studies, particularly systematic reviews, report their results as odds ratios or as a ↓ in odds ratios, and some trials do the same. Odds ratios are also commonly used in epidemiological studies to describe the probable harm an exposure might cause.

Calculating the odds

The odds of an event occuring are calculated as the number of events divided by the number of nonevents. For example, 24 pharmacists are on call in a major city. Six pharmacists are called. The odds of being called are 6 divided by 18 (the number who were not called) or 0.33. An odds ratio is calculated by dividing the odds in the treated or exposed group by the odds in the control group. In general, epidemiological studies try to identify factors that cause harm—those with odds ratios > 1. For example, if we look at case-control studies investigating the potential harm of giving high doses of calcium-channel blockers to treat hypertension. Clinical trials typically look for treatments that ↓ event rates, and that have odds ratios of <1. In these cases, a percentage ↓ in the odds ratio is often quoted instead of the odds ratio. For example, the ISIS-4 trial reported a 7% ↓ in the odds of mortality with captopril treatment, rather than reporting an odds ratio of 0.93.

Relative risks

Few people have a natural ability to interpret event rates that are reported in terms of odds ratios. Understanding risks and relative risks seems to be easier to grasp.

The risk (or probability) of being called in the example above is 6 divided by 24 (the total number on call) or 0.25 (25%). The relative risk is also known as the 'risk ratio', and if reporting positive outcomes, such as improvement, it can be called 'relative benefit'.

Risks and odds

In many situations in medicine, we can get a long way in interpreting odds ratios by pretending that they are relative risks. When events are rare, risks and odds are very similar. For example, in the ISIS-4 study 2231 out of 29 ,022 patients in the control group died within 35days: a risk of 0.077 [2231/29 022] or an odds of 0.083 [2231/(29 022−2231)]. This is an absolute difference of 6 in 1000 or a relative error of ~7%.This close approximation holds true when we talk about odds ratios and relative risks, providing the events are rare.

Why use an odds ratio rather than relative risk?

If odds ratios are difficult to interpret, why don't we always use relative risks instead? There are several reasons for continuing with odds ratios, most of which relate to the superior mathematical properties of odds ratios. Odds ratios can always take values between zero and infinity, which is not the case for relative risks.

The range that relative risk can take, ∴, depends on the baseline event rate. This could obviously cause problems if we were performing a meta-analysis of relative risks in trials with greatly different event rates. Odds ratios also possess a symmetrical property: if you reverse the outcomes in the analysis and look at good outcomes rather than bad outcomes, the relationships have reciprocal odds ratios. This, again, is not true for relative risks.

Odds ratios are always used in case-control studies, where disease prevalence is not known: the apparent prevalence depends solely on the ratio of sampling cases to controls, which is totally artificial. To use an effect measure that is altered by prevalence in these circumstances would obviously be wrong, so odds ratios are the ideal choice. This, in fact, provides the historical link with their use in meta-analyses: the statistical methods that are routinely used are based on methods first published in the 1950s for the analysis of stratified case-control studies. Meta-analytical methods are now available that combine relative risks and absolute risk reductions, but more caution is required in their application, especially when there are large variations in baseline event rates.

A fourth point of convenience occurs if it is necessary to make adjustments for confounding factors using multiple regression. When measuring event rates, the correct approach is to use logistic regression models that work in terms of odds and report effects as odds ratios. All of which makes odds ratios likely to be in use for some time—so it is important to understand how to use them. Of course it is also important to consider the statistical significance of an effect, in addition to its size: as with relative risks, it is easy to spot statistically significant odds ratios by noting whether their 95% confidence intervals do not include 1, which is analogous to a<1 in 20 chance (or a probability of <0.05 or gambling odds of better than 19:1) that the reported effect is solely owing to chance.

Formula to calculate an odds ratio

$$\text{Odds ratio} = \frac{\text{odds on treatment}}{\text{odds on control}}$$

Where odds ratio = 1, this implies no difference in effect

Formula to calculate a relative risk

$$\text{Risk ratio} = \frac{\text{risk on treatment}}{\text{risk on control}}$$

Where risk ratio = 1, this implies no difference in effect

Binary and continuous data

Broadly, statistical tests can be grouped into those used to compare *binary* (also called 'dichotomous') outcome data and those used to compare *continuous* outcome data. Binary outcomes are those that can only take two possible values, such as dead or alive, pain or no pain, and smoker or nonsmoker. Statistical tests on binary data, such as relative risks compare the rate of an event in between the groups; it also makes the calculation of NNT possible. Continuous outcomes are derived from data that can take on any value on a scale. Some examples of continuous data include height, BP, time or the score in a test. Statistical tests on continuous data (eg 't' tests) compare the difference between means of each group (see p.142).

L'Abbé plots

L'Abbé plots are named after a paper by Kristen L'Abbé and colleagues and are an extremely valuable contribution to understanding systematic reviews. The authors suggest a simple graphical representation of the information from trials. Each point on a L'Abbé scatter plot represents one trial in the review. They are a simple and effective way to present a series of results, without complex statistics. The proportion of patients achieving the outcome with the experimental intervention is plotted against the event rate in the control group. Even if a review does not show the data in this way, it is relatively simple to determine this, if the information is available.

For treatment, trials in which the experimental intervention was better than the control are in the upper-left section of the plot, between the y-axis and the line of equality. If the experimental intervention was no better than the control, the point falls on the line of equality, and if the control was better than the experimental intervention, the point is in the lower-right section of the plot, between the x-axis and the line of equality (Fig. 7.1).

For prophylaxis, this pattern is reversed. Because prophylaxis ↓ the number of bad events–eg death after myocardial infarction following the use of aspirin–we expect a smaller proportion of patients harmed by treatment than in the control group. So if the experimental intervention is better than the control, the trial results should be between the x-axis and the line of equality.

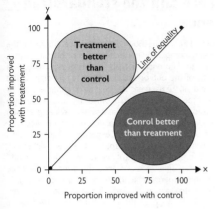

Fig. 7.1 L'Abbé plot for treatment.

Mean difference and the standardized mean difference

Analyses of continuous data often show the difference between the means of the groups being compared. In a meta-analysis, this can involve either comparing the mean difference of trials in two groups directly if the unit of measurement of the outcome is the same (eg if height is the outcome of interest and all trials measure height in centimetres) or standardizing the outcome measure and comparing the difference between the standardized means if different assessment scales are used to measure subjective conditions, such as mood, depression, or pain.

In a meta-analysis of continuous data, if an experimental intervention has an identical effect as a control (or comparison), the mean difference or standardized mean difference is = 0. ∴, if the lower limit of a confidence interval around a mean difference or standardized mean difference is > 0, the mean of the experimental intervention group is significantly greater than the control group. Similarly, if the upper limit of the confidence interval is < 0, the mean of the experimental intervention is significantly lower than the control. Whereas if the confidence interval incorporates the value 0, there is no significant difference between the means of the groups being compared.

Consider the output from a Cochrane review that compared the effect of very-low-calorie diets (VLCDS) with other interventions for weight loss in patients with type 2 diabetes mellitus (Fig. 7.2). In this case, weight loss is measured in kilogrammes so there is no need for standardization. As can be seen below, the meta-analysis of the two trials indicated that the mean difference in weight between the management with a VLCD and other interventions is −2.95 kg. This suggests that patients with type 2 diabetes mellitus on a VLCD are, on average, 2.95 kg lighter than patients with type 2 diabetes mellitus on the comparison interventions. However, the range of the 95% confidence intervals includes 0, which indicates that the difference in weight loss between the two groups is not statistically significant.

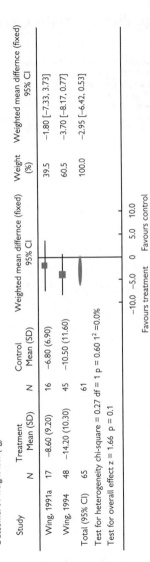

Review: Long-term non-pharmacological weight loss interventions for adults with type 2 diabetes mellitus
Comparison: 01 VLCD vs differnet intervention (1–10: fixed models. 11–20: random models, rho = 0.75)
Outcome: 01 weight loss (kg)

Study	Treatment		Control		Weighted mean differnce (fixed) 95% CI	Weight (%)	Weighted mean difference (fixed) 95% CI
	N	Mean (SD)	N	Mean (SD)			
Wing, 1991a	17	−8.60 (9.20)	16	−6.80 (6.90)		39.5	−1.80 [−7.33, 3.73]
Wing, 1994	48	−14.20 (10.30)	45	−10.50 (11.60)		60.5	−3.70 [−8.17, 0.77]
Total (95% CI)	65		61			100.0	−2.95 [−6.42, 0.53]

Test for heterogeneity chi-square = 0.27 df = 1 p = 0.60 I^2 =0.0%
Test for overall effect z = 1.66 p = 0.1

−10.0 −5.0   0   5.0 10.0

Favours treatment   Favours control

Fig. 7.2 Meta-analysis of a VLCD versus other interventions for weight loss in patients with type 2 diabetes mellitus.

Assessing the quality of randomized studies

Assessment tools for randomized studies are widely available and all have problems, because they do not cover all the issues that could be considered to be important. This simple method picks up on the main issues of randomization, blinding and patient withdrawal from studies (Table 7.2). The maximum quality score is 5 if all the criteria are fulfilled.

In addition a more general appraisal tool is presented (Table 7.3). It picks up details from the scoring system described above.

Table 7.2[1]

Is the study randomized?	Score
Yes	1
Is the randomization appropriate?	
Yes—eg random number tables	1
No—eg alternate patients, date of birth, or hospital number	−1
Was the study double blind?	
Yes	1
Was blinding correctly carried out?	
Yes—eg double dummy	1
No—eg treatments did not look identical	−1
Were withdrawals and drop outs described?	
Yes	1

Table 7.3 Assessment tool for a randomized trial

Was the method of randomization appropriate (eg computer-generated)?
Was the study described as 'double blind'? And was the method of blinding adequate (eg double dummy, or identical tablets)?
Was the trial sensitive, ie able to detect a difference between treatment groups eg use of a placebo, or additional active groups?
Were baseline values for each treatment group adequate for trialists to measure a change following treatment?
Were the groups similar at the start of the trial?
Similar patients?
Diagnostic criteria clearly stated?
Similar baseline measures?
Was the size of the trial adequate?
How many patients were there in each group?
Were outcomes clearly defined and measured appropriately?
Were they clinically meaningful?
Were they primary/surrogate outcomes?
Was the outcome data presented clearly?
If multiple tests were conducted, were single positive results inappropriately presented?

Quality score[1]			
Randomization	**Double-blinding**	**Withdrawals/ Drop outs**	**Total score**

1 Jadad A et al. (1996). Assessing the quality of reports of randomized clinical trials: is blinding necessary? Controlled Clinical Trials. **17**: 1–12.

Critical appraisal of systematic reviews

Systematic reviews are considered to be the best level of evidence if they are well conducted and evaluate a number of randomized trials. They can be particularly useful when seeking to answer clinical questions. However, they are only reliable if the process of the review has followed rigorous scientific principles. Authors should explicitly state the topic being reviewed and have made a reasonable attempt to identify all the relevant studies. The following 10 questions help in that assessment (Table 7.4). If the paper fails either of the first two questions, it is not worth proceeding further.

Table 7.4 10 questions to make sense of a review[1]

For each question answer : Yes, No or Don't Know

A. Are the results of the review valid ?

1. Did the review address a clearly focused issue (eg the population, intervention and/or outcomes)?

2. Did the authors look for the appropriate sort of papers?

   Check that the authors looked for randomized controlled trials or had clear reasons for including other types of studies.

Is it worth continuing?

3. Do you think the relevant important studies were included?

   Look for search methods, use reference list, unpublished studies and non-English language articles.

4. Did the authors do enough to assess the quality of the studies included?

   This would routinely be in the form of an assessment tool for randomized controlled trials.

5. If the results of studies were combined, was it reasonable to do so?

B. What are the results?

6. What is the overall result of the review?
   Is there a clear numerical expression?

7. How precise are the results?
   What were the confidence intervals?

C. Will the results help my local situation?

8. Can the results be applied locally?

9. Were all important outcomes considered?

10. Are the benefits worth the harms and costs?

---

1 Oxman AD et al. (1994). Users guide to the medical literature VI How to use an overview. *Journal of the American Medical Association* **272**(17): 1367–71.

Critical assessment of papers

When reading a clinical trial paper, it is too easy to quickly read the abstract and skim through the main text. Taking the time to critically evaluate the paper might seem daunting and too time-consuming. In many situations a quick read through is all that is needed. However, if the information gleaned from the paper is going to be used to decide on treatment options or might be used to support a formulary application, a more thoughtful approach is required. The information below specifically relates to critically evaluating a clinical trial paper, but the same process, adapted to the content, can be used for other types of clinical paper.

It is not necessary to be a statistician or an expert in trial design to critically evaluate a paper. Much of the evaluation is common sense. A full critical evaluation should take all the following points into account but even simply bearing them in mind will help you get more out of any paper you read.

- Title—does this accurately reflect the content of the paper? Ideally, the title should state the question under investigation, rather than potentially biasing readers by declaring the results. Cryptic titles are a popular way of attracting readers' attention, but if it is too obscure, could it be because that the authors don't really know what they are writing about? Before progressing, consider how useful this trial is in the clinical setting. If it is too esoteric, it might not be worth reading any further!
- Authors—should be from professions/institutions appropriate to the subject studied. Be cautious with papers authored by pharmaceutical industry employees, but don't dismiss these out of hand. Too many authors might mean that the work is scrappy. Multicentre studies should list the key authors and acknowledge other participants at the end of the paper. Is a statistician listed as an author or acknowledged? This should provide reassurance that the statistics are correct.
- Journal—don't assume that because a paper is published in a mainstream journal it is a good paper. However, be more cautious of papers from obscure journals.
- The introduction—should give relevant background information, building logically to the study topic. If the introduction is waffley or irrelevant, ask yourself if the authors really know what they are writing about.
- Method—a well-written method should give sufficient information for another person to reproduce the study. The information given should include the following:
  - Type of study (eg randomized controlled trial, cohort, or case study).
  - Numbers involved, ideally including details of powering.
  - Patient selection and randomization—details of patient demographics should be given and the baseline characteristics of each group should be roughly the same (and should be acknowledged if not).

- Inclusion/exclusion criteria—consider whether these are appropriate. If there are too many exclusion criteria, the study might not be relevant to the clinical setting.
- Outcome measurements—by now, the question the authors are trying to answer should be clear. The factors used to measure the outcome should be appropriate and if possible, directly related to the question. Be cautious of surrogate markers. In many clinical settings, it might be unethical, too invasive or take too long to use the target outcome. However, check that the surrogate marker closely reflects the target outcome as a whole and not just one aspect of it.
- An appropriate comparator drug should be used at its standard dose. Any new drug should be tested against standard therapy. If a drug is compared with placebo or an outdated or rarely used drug, ask yourself why. With the exception of the study treatment, all other interventions should be the same.
- A randomized controlled trial should ideally be double-blinded (ie neither the study participants nor the investigators know which subjects are receiving the study drug and which subjects are receiving the comparator). Sometimes, this is not feasible or ethical but there might be bias if the trial is open label (both subjects and investigator know who is receiving which treatment) or single-blind (the investigator but not the participants know who is receiving each treatment).
- Be cautious with cross-over trials—if the disease studied could improve with time without treatment (especially if self-limiting or seasonal), a cross-over trial is inappropriate. An adequate 'wash-out' period between treatments is essential.
- The details of statistical tests should be given—the tests should be appropriate to the type of data presented. Beware of trials that use numerous statistical tests. Why are so many tests needed? Is it that there is nothing to prove? Further discussion of statistical tests is beyond the scope of this topic. Consult relevant textbooks for further information.
- Results—should answer the question originally asked and be easy to comprehend:
  - Graphs and tables should be relevant and clear. Too many graphs and tables suggest that the authors are having difficulty proving their point! Watch labelling of axes on graphs. Sometimes labelling is skewed (eg not starting at zero) to give more impressive results.
  - If means are quoted, the variance and/or median should also be quoted. This helps determine whether the mean is a true 'average' or whether extreme values have skewed the results.
  - The results might be statistically significant, but are they clinically significant? Results presented as odds ratios, relative risks or NNT, are generally easier to apply to a clinical setting.

- The discussion—should logically build from the results to answer the original question, one way or another. If the authors make statements such as 'further study is required....' ask yourself why. Is this because the original study design was unsuitable? Any doubts or inconsistencies should be dealt with satisfactorily, not just explained away.
- The conclusion—should be appropriate to the data presented and give a definite final answer. If the conclusion is woolly, was there any point in the study in the first place or were the authors just 'paper chasing'?
- The bibliography—should be up to date and relevant. Beware of too many references from obscure journals. You should be able to satisfactorily follow up statements made in the rest of the paper by reference to the original papers quoted.
- Acknowledgements—Look for any specialists not in the author list, which might provide reassurance if you had any doubts about the authors expertise in any angle of the study. Watch out for funding or sponsorship from parties with a vested interest in the outcome of the study (notably the pharmaceutical industry!). However, don't dismiss pharmaceutical-industry-sponsored studies out of hand. Much good work is supported by the pharmaceutical industry.

Further reading
Sackett DL *et al.* (2005). *Evidence-based Medicine*. Churchill Livingstone.
Jones C (2002). Evidence-based medicine (1) Research methods. *Pharmaceutical Journal*, **268**: 875–7.
www.clinicalevidence.com

Bandolier's Knowledge Library for pharmacy

A good collection of evidence-based material, which is particularly relevant to the clinical pharmacist, has been collected together on the Bandolier website.[1]

This is a useful follow-up to material in this chapter and goes into some aspects in greater depth.

1 Bandolier's Knowledge Libraray for pharmacy. www.jr2.ox.ac.uk/bandolier/booth/booths/pharmacy.html

The number needed to treat (NNT)

The NNT is a measure of clinical significance and changes view from 'does a treatment work?' to 'how well does a treatment work?'. This concept is widely used and useful not only in its own right, but also to enable direct comparisons of treatments. The league table of treatments from the Oxford pain research unit illustrates the value of such an approach (Fig. 7.3). Ideally, we would want an NNT of 1. Although there are treatments that meet this criteria—eg anaesthetic agents,—in practice NNT are > 1 one for the reasons explained below.

The NNT is defined as follows: The number of people who must be treated for one patient to benefit. The NNT expressed in terms of a specific clinical outcome and should be shown with confidence intervals.

Calculating the NNT for active treatments

The NNT calculation is received from the understanding of risk ratios (Fig. 7.4). Although the NNT is the reciprocal of the absolute risk reduction, it is not necessary to understand this concept calculate the NNT', a worked example is included so that the process is transparent. The equation is quite simple and it is easy to calculate the NNT in published trials using a pocket calculator.

The NNT was initially used to describe prophylactic interventions. The NNT for prophylaxis is given by the following equation.

> 1/(proportion of patients benefiting from the control intervention minus the proportion of patients benefiting from the experimental intervention), and the NNT for active treatment is given by the following equation 1/(proportion by patients benefiting from the experimental intervention minus the proportion of patients benefiting from the control intervention).

From the equation in Fig. 7.4 it should be apparent that any response in the control arm leads to a NNT that is >1 one. People often ask what a good NNT is; it depends whether the NNT is for treatment—ideally in the range 2–4—or prophylaxis—the NNT is generally larger. Issues such as toxicity have an influence, including to cost. for example, a cheap and safe intervention that prevents a serious disease but has NNT of 100 might well be acceptable.

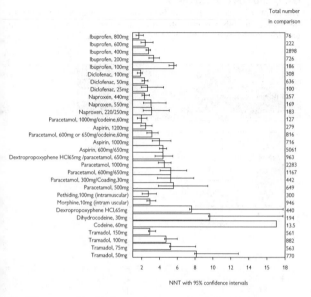

Total number
in comparison

Ibuprofen, 800mg	76
Ibuprofen, 600mg	222
Ibuprofen, 400mg	2898
Ibuprofen, 200mg	726
Ibuprofen, 100mg	186
Diclofenac, 100mg	308
Diclofenac, 50mg	636
Diclofenac, 25mg	100
Naproxen, 440mg	257
Naproxen, 550mg	169
Naproxen, 220/250mg	183
Paracetamol, 1000mg/codeine,60mg	127
Aspirin, 1200mg	279
Paracetamol, 600mg or 650mg/ocdeine,60mg	816
Aspirin, 1000mg	716
Aspirin, 600mg/650mg	5061
Dextropropoxyphene HCl65mg /paracetamol, 650mg	963
Paracetamol, 1000mg	2283
Paracetamol, 600mg/650mg	1167
Paracetamol, 300mg/Coading,30mg	442
Paracetamol, 500mg	649
Pethiding,100mg (intramuscular)	300
Morphine,10mg (intram uscular)	946
Dexpropoxyphene HCl,65mg	440
Dihydrocodeine, 30mg	194
Codeine, 60mg	13.5
Tramadol, 150mg	561
Tramadol, 100mg	882
Tramadol, 75mg	563
Tramadol, 50mg	770

NNT with 95% confidence intervals

Fig. 7.3 League table of NNT to produce ≥50% pain relief fo 4–6h compared with placebo in patients with pain of moderate or severe intensity.

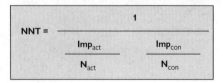

	Controls	Active treatment
Number of patients	N_{con}	N_{act}
Improved = clinical end point	Imp_{con}	Imp_{act}

$$NNT = \cfrac{1}{\cfrac{Imp_{act}}{N_{act}} - \cfrac{Imp_{con}}{N_{con}}}$$

Fig. 7.4 Number needed to treat (NNT)

Using the NNT to express harm

The number needed to harm (NNH) can also be helpful, in addition to the NNT. The NNH is calculated using a similar formula derived from data for adverse events rather than desired effect. (Fig. 7.5).

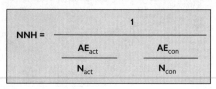

	Controls	Active treatment
Number of patients	N_{con}	N_{act}
AE-number with the adverse	AE_{con}	AE_{act}

$$NNH = \cfrac{1}{\cfrac{AE_{act}}{N_{act}} - \cfrac{AE_{con}}{N_{con}}}$$

Fig. 7.5 Number needed to harm (NNH)

Confidence intervals

Most pharmacists are aware of p values in terms of an answer being significant (in a statistical sense) or not. However, the use of 'p' is increasingly redundant and new methods of reporting significance have emerged.

The most method common is the confidence interval, which enables us to estimate the margin of error.

If, for example, we measured BP in 100 adults, we could derive a mean result. If we then took a further 100 adults and repeated the experiment, we would arrive at a similar but not equal, figure. The confidence interval, expressed as a percentage, enables calculation of the margin of error and tells us how good our mean is. Generally, the figure is set at 95% so we can be confident that the true mean lies somewhere between the upper and lower estimates (Fig. 7.6). Expressed a different way, there is only a 5% chance of the result being outside the calculated limits.

The statistics involved are derived from a range of 1.96 standard deviations above and below the point estimated. For a 99% confidence interval, the figure of 2.58 standard deviations is used.

Calculating confidence intervals

Although the formulae are available in standard statistic works, there are a number of confidence interval calculators on the web that require the use of the calculated point estimate and the number of samples to derive the confidence interval at a given percentage.

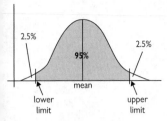

Fig. 7.6 Illustration of the data incorporated within a 95% confidence interval

Herbal medicines

Herbal medicinal products of current interest

Echinacea purpurea

Echinacea is widely used throughout Europe for the prevention and treatment of colds and other upper respiratory tract infections and is thought to have immunostimulant properties. A recent Cochrane review reported that some products might have an effect greater than placebo, but overall the results were inconclusive.

Garlic (Allium sativum)

Systematic reviews and studies using garlic extract (600mg) have investigated the effects of garlic preparations in lowering raised serum cholesterol concentrations. Generally, the studies report beneficial results for garlic. However, the evidence at present is insufficient to recommend garlic as routine treatment for hypercholesterolaemia. One of the major problems in assessing the evidence available for garlic is the wide variation in the chemical composition of the products available, compared with fresh garlic. Further controlled studies using standardized preparations are needed to investigate efficacy in reducing serum lipids, BP, platelet aggregation and antimicrobial activity.

Ginger (Zingiber officinale)

Some clinical studies reported ginger to be an effective prophylactic treatment for motion sickness, although subsequent studies found ginger to be ineffective.

Ginkgo biloba

Ginkgo leaf extract is widely used in France and Germany in authorized herbal medicinal products for the treatment of (peripheral and cerebral) circulatory insufficiencies. Currently, no licensed herbal medicinal products containing ginkgo are available in the UK.

Several systematic reviews have analysed the available evidence for the effects of ginkgo in cerebral insufficiency, dementia, tinnitus and intermittent claudication. Overall, the results suggest some beneficial effects, but further studies are needed.

Panax ginseng

Ginseng is widely renowned for its adaptogenic properties in Eastern countries, where it is used to help the body cope with stress and fatigue and promote recovery from illness or imbalance, such as hypertension or hypoglycaemia. Generally, it is only recommended for use in certain individuals with specific illnesses. By contrast, in the UK, ginseng is mainly self-administered and taken in the form of tablets or capsules containing dried extracts of the root. Ginseng products available in the UK are sold as food supplements, often in combination with vitamins and minerals. A wealth of research, describing a wide range of pharmacological activities, particularly in the hypothalamic and pituitary regions of the brain, has been documented for ginseng.

Saw palmetto (*Serenoa serrulata*)

Saw palmetto is widely used in Europe, particularly in Germany, for symptoms associated with benign prostatic hypertrophy (BPH). In the UK, saw palmetto is licensed in a number of products for the symptomatic relief of short-term, male urinary discomfort. Results of clinical trials indicate that saw palmetto is a potential agent for the symptomatic treatment of BPH.

Valerian (*Valeriana officinalis*)

Valerian is widely used in Europe for nervous tension and for promoting sleep. The therapeutic indications include relief of temporary, mild nervous tension and temporary difficulty in falling asleep. A systematic review of randomized, double-blind, placebo-controlled trials of valerian reported inconsistencies in methodologies between studies, and the evidence for efficacy was deemed inconclusive.

Herbal drugs

The efficacy and safety of herbal drugs present a number of issues to pharmacists. Herbal drugs are more often complex mixtures of active constituents that vary in quality as a consequence of a number of reasons, such as environmental and genetic factors. Furthermore, the constituents responsible for the claimed therapeutic effects are frequently unknown or only partly explained.

The position is further complicated by the traditional practice of using combinations of herbal drugs, and it is not uncommon to have as many as five or more herbal drugs in one product. There is potential risk from impurities/adulterations of herbal medicine mixed with toxic plant extracts from misidentification or intentional addition of allopathic drugs.

The European pharmacopoeia includes 120 monographs on herbal drugs. Control of the starting materials is essential to ensure the reproducible quality of herbal medicinal products. Herbal drugs must be accurately identified by macroscopical and microscopical comparison with authentic material. Herbal drugs are referred to by their binomial Latin names of genus and species; only permitted synonyms should be used. Different batches of the same herbal ingredient can differ in quality because of a number of factors:

- Inter species or intraspecies variation.
- Environmental factors.
- Time of harvesting.
- Plant part used—active constituents usually vary between plant parts, and it is not uncommon for an herbal drug to be adulterated with parts of the plant not normally used.
- Storage conditions and processing treatments can greatly affect the quality of an herbal ingredient.
- Instances of herbal remedies adulterated with other plant material and conventional medicines.
- Extraction/drying methods.
- Identity tests establish the botanical identity of a herbal drug.
- Chemical (eg colour or precipitation) and chromatographic tests are used for identification of the ingredients.
- Assay—a herbal drug with known active principles should have an assay established to set the criterion for the minimum-accepted percentage of active substance(s).

Legislation of herbal drugs

Although herbal drugs have been used as traditional remedies for centuries and are perceived by many to be without major safety problems, the UK has a series of controls to limit general availability.

Hazardous plants, such as digitalis, rauwolfia and nux vomica, are specifically controlled under the Medicines Act as prescription-only medicines (POMs).

Certain herbal ingredients are controlled under The Medicines (Retail Sale and Supply of Herbal Remedies) Order, 1977, SI 2130. This Order (part I) specifies 25 plants that cannot be supplied except by a pharmacy, and includes well-known toxic species, such as Areca, Crotalaria, Dryopteris and Strophanthus.

Herbal remedies exempt from licensing fall under two main categories:

- Subject to the provisions of section 12 of the Medicines Act, 1968, products can be compounded and supplied by a herbalist on their own recommendation.
- If no medical claims are made that are attributable to the herbal product, it can be sold as a food supplement.

Efficacy

Herbs used medicinally normally have a traditional reputation for their uses, but, generally, there is little scientific documentation of their active constituents, pharmacological actions or clinical efficacy.

The current emphasis on EBM requires evidence of efficacy from rigorous randomized controlled trials. Several systematic reviews have been prepared by the Cochrane Collaboration. These reviews highlight that, in some cases, the evidence base is weak and studies are often flawed. Evidence from randomized controlled trials has confirmed the efficacy of St John's wort products versus placebo in the treatment of mild-to-moderate depression.

If the active constituents of a herbal drug are known, it is possible and, in most cases, desirable to standardize the extract. The aim of standardization is to obtain an optimum and consistent quality of a herbal drug preparation by adjusting it to give a defined content of a constituent or group of constituents with known therapeutic activity. Examples include senna, frangula, digitalis, belladonna and horse chestnut.

In the case of St John's wort, early studies concentrated on the hypericin constituents but more recent work suggests that hyperforin and, possibly, flavonoids also contribute to the antidepressant properties.

Safety and adverse effects

Information on herbal medicines is lacking in many areas that include active constituents, metabolites, pharmacokinetics, pharmacology, toxicology, adverse effects, long-term effects, use by specific patient groups and contraindications:

- Herbal drugs could present a potential risk to health from exposure to contaminants present in the herbal product and result in ADRs (Table 8.1).
- Reliance on self-administration of herbal drugs or products could delay a patient seeking qualified advice or cause a patient to abandon conventional treatment without appropriate advice.
- Herbal medicines could, in some cases, compromise the efficacy of conventional medicines through herb–drug interactions.

Table 8.1 Examples of ADRs that can occur with herbal drugs

Potential adverse effect	Constituent/herbal ingredient
Allergic/hypersensitivity reactions	Sesquiterpene lactones: arnica, chamomile feverfew and yarrow
Phototoxic reactions	Furanocoumarins: angelica, celery and wild carrot
Immune	Canavanine: alfalfa
Cardiac	Cardiac glycosides: pleurisy root, squill and digitalis.
Endocrine	
Hypoglycaemic	Alfalfa and fenugreek
Hyperthyroid	Iodine: focus
Hormonal	
Mineralocorticoid	Triterpenoids: liquorice
Oestrogenic antiandrogen	Isoflavonoids: alfalfa, red clover
	Saponins: ginseng, saw palmetto
Irritant	
Gastrointestinal	Numerous compounds, including anthraquinones (purgative), capsaici-noids, diterpenes, saponins and terpene-rich volatile oils
Hepatotoxic/carcinogenic	Pyrolizidine alkaloids: comfrey and liferoot
	β-Asarone: calamus
	Lignans: chaparral, safrole, sassafras and kava kava
Mitogenic	Proteins: mistletoe and pokeroot
Cyanide poisoning	Cyanogenetic glycosides: apricot
Convulsant	Camphor/thujone-rich volatile oils

Chinese herbal medicine

Most of the substances used in Chinese herbal medicine originate from China. The Chinese pharmacopeia lists over 6000 different medicinal substances; there are currently over 600 different herbs in common use today. Herbs are used for their abilities to treat specific Chinese diagnoses and alleviate specific complaints. For example, there are assortments of herbs that can alleviate coughing, but each one is appropriate for a cough because of a different Chinese diagnosis. The variety and degree of different combination of the herbal medicines makes Chinese herbal medicine very complex.

Combination of herbal products

The one characteristic of Chinese herbal medicine that most sets it aside from other types of herbal medicine is the degree of combination undertaken. Chinese herbalists very rarely prescribe a single herb to treat a condition; instead, a mixture could contain > 20 herbs. Pre-made formulas are available; however, these products are usually not as potent as the traditional preparation of 'decoction'.

Decoction is the traditional method of preparing herbal medicine. A decoction is a concentrated form of tea. The practitioner weighs out a day's dosage of each herb and combines them in a bag. A patient is given a bag for each day the herbal formula must be taken. The herbs are then boiled in water by the patient at home; the boiling process takes 30–60min and the resulting decoction is consumed several times during the day.

Quality issues

The quality and safety of Chinese herbs has repeatedly come into question after media coverage of concerns over heavy-metal contamination, adulteration and use of endangered animal species. Heavy-metal contamination has been detected in several Chinese herbal products, usually as a result of poor manufacturing. Adulteration of herbal medicines with prescription drugs has been found in a few herbal products. The use of endangered animals in Chinese herbal medicine is very rare.

Herbal interactions

Information on herb–drug interactions (Table 8.2) are generally limited to case reports, although recognition is improving, with the result that clinically important interactions are being increasingly identified and prevented by healthcare professionals.

Variability of constituent ingredients and pharmaceutical quality of unlicensed herbal products can often be the main reason for the low incidence of reported interactions.

Types of interaction

Pharmacokinetic interactions with drugs
- Absorption
- Distribution
- Metabolism
- Excretion.

Pharmacodynamic interactions with drugs
- One substance affecting the response of another at its site of action.

Herb–disease interaction
Certain underlying diseases could be exacerbated by ingestion of herbal ingredients with the following properties:
- Hypertensive properties.
- Hyperglycaemic/hypoglycaemic activity.

Table 8.2 Some important herb–drug interactions

Herb	Drug interaction	Considerations
Black cohosh (*Actaea racemosa*)	Antihypertensives	May ↓ BP
Chamomile (*Chamaemelum nobile*)	Anticoagulants	Consider discontinuing 2wks before surgery
Echinacea purpurea	Immunosuppressant (eg corticosteroids)	Immune suppression can result from prolonged use >14 days
Ephedra (Ma Huang)– active constituent is ephedrine	Will have the same interactions as ephedrine	Misuse has resulted in death
Evening primrose oil	Could interact with anticoagulants or antiplatelet drugs Can ↓ seizure threshold	
Feverfew (*Tanacetum parthenium*)	Could interact with anticoagulants or antiplatelet drugs	Consider discontinuing 2wks before surgery
Fish oil supplements (omega-3 fatty acids)	Reports of ↓ platelet aggregation	Unlikely to have clinical significance
Garlic (*Allium sativum*)	Could interact with anticoagulants or antiplatelet drugs	Consider discontinuing 2wks before surgery
Ginger (*Zingiber officinale*)	Could interact with anticoagulants or antiplatelet drugs	Consider discontinuing 2wks before surgery
Ginseng (*Panax ginseng*)	Could interact with anticoagulants or antiplatelet drugs Interacts with hypoglycaemic drugs Avoid concurrent mono-amaine oxidase inhibitors	Varying effects on BP Hypoglycaemia Could potentiate action of monoamine oxidase inhibitors. Limit use to 3months
Hops (*Humulus lupulus*)	Could have additive effect with CNS depressants	Avoid in depressive states
Horse chestnut (*Aesculus hippocastanum*)	Could interact with anticoagulants or antiplatelet drugs	↑ risk of bleeding
Kava kava (*Piper methysticum*) (this is in the process of being withdrawn from UK market)	Kavalactones potentiate effects of other CNS depressants, including opioids, barbiturates and benzodiazepines ↓ effectiveness of levodopa Additive effect with anticoagulant and antiplatelet drugs Use with caution with mono-amine oxidase inhibitors	Limit use to 3months Avoid in depression Consider discontinuing 2wks before surgery

Table 8.2 (Contd.)

Herb	Drug interaction	Considerations
Passion flower (*Passiflora incarnate*)	Additive effects with CNS depressants Avoid concurrent monoamine oxidase inhibitors	Reports of hepatic and pancreatic toxicity
Saw palmetto (*Serenoa serrulata*)	Caution with finasteride	Potential of additive effect
St John's wort (*Hypericum perforatum*)	Anticonvulsants Ciclosporin Digoxin Protease inhibitors and non-nucleoside reverse transcriptase inhibitors Oral contraceptives Theophylline Warfarin Irinotecan	Loss or ↓ in therapeutic effect of the drug therapies. probably induction of CYP enzymes by St John's wort constituents)
Valerian (*Valeriana officinalis*)	Additive effects with CNS depressants	
Milk thistle (*Silybum marianus*)	CYP3A4 enzyme inducer Protease inhibitors and NNRTI's Phenytoin	↓ blood levels and, hence, chance of treatment failure

Please note that this is not an exhaustive list but a point of general reference. New information about herbal interactions can be obtained from www.mca.gov.uk.

Perioperative considerations for herbal drugs

- Herbal medicines have the potential to pose problems in the perioperative setting because patients often fail to communicate concurrent herbal remedies during DHx taking by healthcare professionals.
- Few data exist in the medical literature regarding the use of herbal products and the development of ADRs or interactions associated with anaesthesia.
- The most important risks associated with herbal products during the perioperative and immediate postoperative periods are cardiovascular, coagulation and sedative effects:
  - Cardiovascular effects–ephedra, ginseng and garlic:
    —Ephedra can cause a dose-dependent ↑ in heart rate and BP.
    —Ginseng ↑ in BP and its use is not recommended during surgical period in patients with cardiovascular disease.
    —Garlic could reduce BP, but its effects are normally brief and usually require high dosages.
  - Bleeding effects–garlic, ginseng, gingko, evening primrose oil, feverfew, fish oils, ginger, horse chestnut and kava kava.
  - Sedative effects–chamomile, kava kava, valerian, hops, passion flower and St John's wort.

Although there continues to be debate on the incidence of reactions to herbal products during perioperative period, it might be prudent to recommend discontinuation of these agents for at least 2wks before surgery.

Table 8.3 Perioperative considerations for herbal drugs

Herbal drug	Use(s)	Proposed mechanism of action/effects	Drug interactions	Other considerations
Black cohosh	• Treatment of PMS and dysmenorrhoea • Alleviate menopausal symptoms	• Active components are triterpene glycosides and formononetin (an isoflavanoid), which can have oestrogen-like hormonal activity • Suppresses leutenizing hormone secretion in menopausal women	• Caution when administered with other drugs than can ↓ BP	• Can lower BP • Side effects are generally mild (GI, headache, weight gain and dizziness) • Limit use to 3 months
Chamomile	• Anxiolytic/sedative • Treatment of gastrointestinal spasm or irritation • Treatment of menstrual disorders	• Also contains bioflavinoids, which are considered to be active • Apigenin competitively inhibits binding of several benzodiazepines	• No reports of coagulation disorders, but effects on coagulation system have not been studied; avoid concurrent administration of (or closely monitor) warfarin • Can make other drugs less effective when administered concurrently	• Sedative effects noted from a 6oz cup of strong tea • Can cause skin irritation, allergic conjunctivitis and/or severe allergic reactions • Long-term consumption could have cumulative effects • Consider discontinuing 2wks before surgery

Table 8.3 (Contd.)

Herbal drug	Use(s)	Proposed mechanism of action/effects	Drug interactions	Other considerations
Echinacea	• Anti-infective	• Enhances 'non-specific' cell immunity by enhancing release of cytokines and phagocytic activity • Stimulates autoimmune processes	• Could counteract immunosuppressant drugs (eg corticosteroids); do not administer together	• Hepatotoxic effects might be associated with prolonged use or if administered with other hepatotoxic agents • Immune suppression can result from prolonged use (>10–14 days)
Ephedra (Ma Huang)	• Treatment of asthma • Nasal decongestant • Appetite suppressant	• Active constituent is ephedrine • CNS, weight loss or athletic enhancement stimulant effects are potentiated by the addition of caffeine-containing botanicals (cola nut, mate and guarana) • High doses produce euphoria	• Probably have the same drug interactions as ephedrine • ↑ BP and blood glucose, especially when combined with caffeine-containing botanicals	• Can see palpitations, ↑ BP; misuse has resulted in death • Combined with caffeine-containing botanicals to promote weight loss or enhance athletic performance Ma Huang and St John's wort

Evening primrose oil	• Treatment of PMS • ↓ serum cholesterol • Allergic/inflammatory conditions (eczema, psoriasis) • Autoimmune disease (multiple sclerosis and lupus)	• Extract contains 60–80% linoleic acid and 8–14% linolenic acid (an omega-6 fatty acid formed by desaturation of linoleic acid) • ↓ platelet aggregation	• Can interact with anticoagulant or antiplatelet drugs to ↑ risk of bleeding • Use caution when administered with drugs that lower seizure threshold (eg phenothiazines, and tricyclic antidepressants)	• Side effects are generally infrequent (GI and headache) • Can ↓ seizure threshold
Feverfew	• Prevention and treatment of migraines • Anti-inflammatory agent (used to treat fever, menstrual problems and arthritis)	• Possible serotonin release during aggregation of platelets; inhibits platelet aggregation • Antagonizes actions of autocoids and vascular agonists potentially involved in migraines and chronic inflammation • Antipyretic and antiplatelet effects might result from phospholipase inhibitor that prevents the release of arachidonic acid, a precursor to prostaglandins and leukotrienes	• Can interact with anticoagulant or antiplatelet drugs to ↑ risk of bleeding • Use caution when administering with drugs that raise serotonin (eg fluoxetine and sumatriptan)	• Abrupt discontinuation can cause rebound headache or pain with stiff joints and muscles • Can cause mouth sores and loss of taste • Do not take for >4 months • Consider discontinuing 2wks before surgery

Table 8.3 (Contd.)

Herbal drug	Use(s)	Proposed mechanism of action/effects	Drug interactions	Other considerations
Fish oil supplements (omega-3 fatty acids)	• Management of severe dyslipidemia, ↓ risk of coronary heart disease and ↓ BP	• Possibly through effects on prostaglandins, thromboxanes and leukotrienes • ↓ platelet aggregation, ↓ thromboxane A₂ and ↑ bleeding times • Incorporated in RBCs, leading to ↓ blood viscosity	• Although no drug interactions have been reported, it would be prudent to avoid anticoagulant and anti-platelet drugs	
Garlic	• ↓ serum cholesterol • ↓ BP	• Active constituents are sulphur compounds and the alliin-splitting enzyme allinase • Inhibits cholesterol synthesis • Has vasodilator and antioxidant properties • Effects on coagulation include inhibition of platelet aggregation, antithrombotic activity, mean plasma viscosity and haematocrit	• Can interact with anti-coagulant and antiplatelet drugs to ↑ risk of bleeding • Can potentiate antihypertensive drugs	• Report of spontaneous epidural haematoma and post-operative bleeding • Can ↑ INR • Chronic or excessive doses can ↓ production of haemoglobin • Side effects include GI discomfort, dizziness, allergic reactions, headache, sweating and garlic odour of breath/skin • Hypoglycaemic effects • Consider discontinuing 2wks before surgery

| Ginger | • Prevention of nausea and vomiting
• Digestive problems
• Muscle pain and swelling | • Potent agonist at the serotonin receptor
• Exerts effect in GI tract, not in CNS
• Multiple effects on platelet aggregation (potent inhibition of thromboxane synthetase and prostacyclin agonist) | • Can interact with anti-coagulant and anti-platelet drugs to ↑ risk of bleeding
• ↑ calcium uptake by heart and can alter calcium-channel blocker effects | • Can ↑ bleeding time
• Can affect blood glucose
• Can affect BP
• Consider discontinuing 2wks before surgery |
| Ginkgo biloba | • Treatment of dementia symptoms or other conditions associated with cerebral or peripheral vascular insufficiency
• Treatment of vertigo or tinnitus of vascular or involutional origin | • Medicinal extracts contain 22–27% flavanoid glycosides, 5–7% terpene lactones (ginkgofides A, B and C and bilobalide) and <5ppm ginkgolic acids
• Several active constituents are potent antioxidants and free radicals scavengers
• Inhibits age-related decline of muscarinic cholinergic receptors and a_2-adrenergic receptors
• Ginkgolides, especially ginkgolide B, inhibit platelet activating factor and antagonize thrombus formation | • Can interact with anti-coagulant and antiplatelet drugs to ↑ risk of bleeding
• Ginkgo toxin in ginkgo leaf and seed can ↓ effectiveness of carbamazepine, phenytoin and phenobarbital in epileptic patients
• Do not use with drugs that lower seizure threshold | • Several cases of spontaneous bleeding reported (subdural and subarachnoid haematomas and bleeding from iris into anterior chamber of the eye)
• Consider discontinuing 2wks before surgery |

Table 8.3 (Contd.)

Herbal drug	Use(s)	Proposed mechanism of action/effects	Drug interactions	Other considerations
Ginseng	• Heighten resistance to stress • Enhance physical and mental performance	• Active ingredients thought to be ginsenosides • ↑ activity of CNS • Active ingredients thought to be ginsenosides by lowering their removal from neuronal synapse; ↑ in serotonin useful when treating anxiety and depressing disorders • Can potentiate activity of GABA • Steroidal mechanism of action has been suggested; possi-bility of hormone-like or hormone-inducing effects cannot be ruled out • Ginsenosides inhibit platelet aggregation and enhance fibrinolysis	• Can interact with anti-coagulant and anti-platelet drugs to ↑ risk of bleeding • Avoid concurrent administration of hypoglycemic drugs • Avoid concurrent administration of monoamine oxidase inhibitors	• Varying effects on BP • Hypoglycaemic effect; caution in diabetes mellitus • Avoid in patients with manic–depressive disorders or psychosis (resulting from steroid effects) • Can potentiate action of monoamine oxidase inhibitors • Limit use to 3 months
Hops	• Sedative–hypnotic, digestive aid	• Acts as a mild depressant on higher nerve centres • Contains substances with oestrogenic activity	• Can have additive effects with other CNS depressants • Drugs metabolized by the cytochrome P450 liver enzyme system	• Avoid in depressive states

Horse chestnut	• ↓ leg oedema • Improve symptoms of chronic venous insufficiency	• Main active constituent is aescin • Contains coumarin constituents	• Can interact with anti-coagulant and antiplatelet drugs to ↑ risk of bleeding	• Side effects include nausea, stomach discomfort, allergic skin reactions, itching and muscle spasms • Can turn urine red • Can cause kidney or liver damage • Can cause severe bleeding or bruising • Consider discontinuing 2wks before surgery
Kava kava (in the process of being withdrawn from the UK market)	• Sedative • Anxiolysis	• Active constituents are the kavalactones (kawain, dihydro-kawain, methysticin and dihydromethysticin) • Kavalactones might act on central gaba and bzd binding sites; can ↓ excitability of the limbic system • Can antagonize dopamine and inhibit monoamine oxidase uptake • Kawain (a kavalactone) has been shown to have antiplatelet effects resulting from lowering platelet aggregation 2° to inhibition of cyclo-oxygenase	• Kavalactones potentiate effects of other CNS depressants, including opioids, barbiturates and benzodiazepines • ↓ effectiveness of levodopa (by dopamine antagonism) • Theoretical additive effects with other anticoagulant and antiplatelet drug to ↑ risk of bleeding • Use caution with monoamine oxidase inhibitor and other psychopharmacological agents	• Avoid in depression; can ↑ suicide risk because of its CNS depressant effects • Can impair motor function • Continuous heavy use can cause changes in blood chemistry, pulmonary hypertension, exaggerated kneecap reflex, reddened eyes, shortness of breath, weight loss and dry, flaking, discoloured skin • Limit use to 3 months • No evidence of potential for dependency • Consider discontinuing 1–2wks before surgery

Table 8.3 (Contd.)

Herbal drug	Use(s)	Proposed mechanism of action/effects	Drug interactions	Other considerations
Passion flower	• Relaxation • Sleep	• Active constituents might be glycosides (harmala compounds), maltone and ethyl-maltone and flavanoids • Chrysin (primary component; a flavanoid) has bzd receptor activity	• Possible additive effects with other CNS depressants • Avoid monoamine oxidase inhibitors	• Reports of hepato-toxicity and pancre-atic toxicity • No evidence of potential for dependency
Saw palmetto	• Treatment of benign prostatic enlargement	• Thought to act similarly to finasteride (antiandrogenic activity); can have antioestrogenic activity • Anti-inflammatory and antioxidant actions in experimental models of additive inflammation	• Can be prudent to avoid concomitant use of other hormonal therapies because of potential of additive effects	• Can cause HTN and GI disturbances
St John's wort	• Treatment of mild–moderate depression and anxiety	• Hypericin (presumed active ingredient) shows affinity for serotonin, GABA and BZD receptors • Inhibits monoamine oxidase A and B (monoamine oxidase inhibitor effects are thought to be minor) • 1° mechanism of action of hypericin is thought to be inhibition of serotonin reuptake, in addition to down-regulation of serotonin receptors and neurohormonal mechanisms	• Although no drug–drug or drug–food interactions have been reported, it might be prudent to avoid concomitant use with mono-amine oxidase inhibitor, meperidine and sympathomimetics, in addition to traditional antidepressants	• Considered an atypi-cal antidepressant • Can cause (dose-related) photo-sensitivity in fair-skinned people • Can potentially cause serotonin syndrome • Can prolong effects of anaesthesia

		• Hypericin and pseudohypericin can induce hepatic enzymes (there are case reports of ↑ theophylline clearance resulting in a subtherapeutic theophylline level)	• Does not seen to affect driving ability, potentiate effects of alcohol or result in morning hangover • Side effects include headache and morning grogginess • Can cause cardiac disturbances • Can cause liver damage • Effects are not immediate (2–4wks) • Does not seem to cause dependence
Valerian	• Sedative • Anxiolysis	• Interacts and binds with GABA; a valerenic acid component can inhibit breakdown of GABA, thereby enhancing activity • Japanese valerian contains kessyl gycol diacetat, which has BZD-like anxiolytic effects and antidepressant effects (possibly resulting from blockage of monoamine oxidase uptake) • High concentration of glutamine in valerian extracts could explain sedative properties; glutamine is metabolized to GABA after it crosses the blood–brain barrier • Possible direct relaxing effect on smooth muscle (thought to result from GABA present in valerian) • Can also weakly antagonize BZD receptors • Too high initial dose can cause excitability	• Can have additive effects with other CNS depressants, including barbiturates, benzodiazepines and opioids • Will probably potentiate effects from barbiturates • Antabuse; there is alcohol in many of the extract products

a) Herbs are classified as dietary supplements and not approved by the MHRA to be used as drugs. The uses, proposed mechanism of action, effects, drug interactions and other considerations are desired from reports in the literature. The body of literature does not always agree on each herb's specific properties, effects and uses.

b) This is a very conservative recommendation for discontinuing these herbs before surgery, thereby allowing normal metaotologic function to return. Gingko biloba is believed to be the herbal product with the most serious side effects, with several case reports in the literature of spontaneous bleeding. In two cases, the patient was also taking chronic aspirin or warfarin.

c) Anticoagulant drugs include warfarin, heparin and low-molecular-weight heparin.

d) Antiplatelet drugs include aspirin, NSAIDs, dipyridamole, ticlopidine, clopidogrel and sulfinpyrazone.

Medical gases

Clinical uses

Air
Clinical indications
- In ventilators and incubators—to provide uncontaminated and controlled airflows.
- Replacement for contaminated atmospheric air.
- Carrier for volatile anaesthetic agents.
- Power source for pneumatic equipment.

Carbon dioxide
Clinical indications
- To rapidly ↑ depth of anaesthesia when volatile anaesthetic agents are administered.
- To facilitate blind intubation in anaesthetic practice.
- To facilitate vasodilatation, lessening the degree of metabolic acidosis during the induction of hypothermia.
- To ↑ cerebral blood flow in arteriosclerotic patients undergoing surgery.
- To stimulate respiration after a period of apnoea.
- To prevent hypocapnia during hyperventilation.
- For clinical and physiological investigations—eg insufflation into fallopian tubes.
- For tissue-freezing techniques.

Entonox (50:50 mixture of nitrous oxide:oxygen[O_2])
Clinical indications
Used exclusively for the relief of pain:
- Trauma
- Dental work
- Wound and burn analgesia
- Childbirth analgesia.

Administration of entonox
The gas is administered using a face mask or mouthpiece; gas flow is controlled by a sensitive demand-valve which is activated by the patient's inspired breath. This enables pressurized gas from the cylinder to flow through a pressure regulator into the lungs at a steady rate. Longer and deeper breaths enable greater volumes of gas to be taken into the lungs, if necessary.

The gas is rapidly absorbed on inhalation, providing analgesia within minutes. The patient safely controls the dosage and, under normal conditions, there is no risk of overdose because the patient's level of consciousness governs his/her ability to maintain the flow of gas.

Helium

Clinical indications

Helium is used with at least 21% O_2:

- To assist O_2 flow into the alveoli of patients with severe respiratory obstruction.
- To prevent atelectasis.
- For gas-transfer lung function tests.

Oxygen

Clinical indications

- To provide life support by restoring tissue O_2—levels eg asthma, (Myocardial infarction MI) and sickle cell crisis.
- Management of sudden cardiac or respiratory arrest.
- Resuscitation of the critically ill.
- Anaesthesia.

Typical dosing for O_2 in acute conditions

- Cardiac or respiratory conditions—100%.
- Hypoxaemia with $PaCO_2$ <5.3kPa—40–60%.
- Hypoxaemia with $PaCO_2$ >5.3kPa—24% initially.

Long-term O_2

Used to improve mortality and morbidity in patients with chronic hypoxia caused by chronic obstructive pulmonary disease (COPD), pulmonary malignancy, heart failure and other lung diseases, such as cystic fibrosis and interstitial lung disease. Should be considered if arterial PaO_2 <7.3kPa or 7.3–8kPa, if the patient has polycythaemia or evidence of pulmonary hypertension.

Nitrous oxide

Clinical indications

- Nitrous oxide is used as an inhalation anaesthetic in combination with either a volatile or an IV anaesthetic agent.
- In combination with 50% O_2 as an analgesic agent.

Table 9.1 O_2 delivery systems

Type	Flow rate	Inspired O_2 concentration
Low flow (Ventimask-controlled)		24%/28%/31%
Nasal prongs	1–2L	24–28%
High-flow mask	1–15L	24–60%
Nonrebreathing mask		≤ 90%
Anaesthetic mask or endotracheal tube		100%

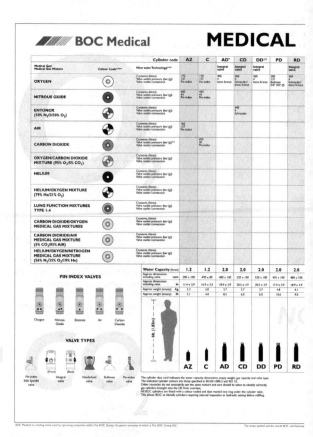

Fig. 9.1 Medical cylinder data. Information current August 2006 and is UK specific. Reproduced with permission from BOC Medical, part of the BOC Group PLC. www.bocmedical.co.uk

CYLINDER DATA

ZD	D	E	AF(1)	DF(1)	F	LF	VF	AV	HX	ZX	G	AK	J	L
Integral valve				Integral valve					Integral valve	Integral valve				
	145 127 Pin-index	680 137 Pin-index	1360 137 Bullnose 5/8" BSP (f)	1360 4 Schraeder/ 6mm firtree	1360 137 Bullnose 5/8" BSP (f)				1300 4 Schraeder/ 6mm firtree	3040 4 Schraeder/ 6mm firtree	3400 137 Bullnose 5/8" BSP (f)		6000 137 Pin-index (side spindle)	
	900 44 Pin-index	1800 44 Pin-index			3600 44 Handwheel 11/16" x 20tpi (m)						9000 44 Handwheel 11/16" x 20tpi (m)			
794 4 Schraeder	500 137 Pin-index				2000 137 Pin-index (side spindle)				2300 4 Schraeder	3970 4 Schraeder	5000 137 Pin-index			
		640 137 Pin-index			1280 137 Bullnose 5/8" BSP (f)						3200 137 Bullnose 5/8" BSP (f)		4400 137 Pin-index (side spindle)	
		1800 50 Pin-index				3600 50 Handwheel 0.860" x 14tpi (m)	3600 50 Handwheel 0.860" x 14tpi (m)							
					1360 137 Bullnose 5/8" BSP (f)						3400 137 Bullnose 5/8" BSP (f)		4800 137 Bullnose 5/8" BSP (f)	
	300 137 Pin-index				1200 137 Bullnose 5/8" BSP (f)									
								1760 4 Schraeder/ 6mm firtree						
								1300 200 Side outlet Handwheel 5/8"BSP(f)+H(f)			6000 200 Side outlet Handwheel 5/8"BSP(f)+H(f)			
								1460 200 Side outlet Handwheel 5/8" BSP (f)						6780 200 Side outlet Handwheel 5/8" BSP (f)
								1350 200 Side outlet Handwheel 5/8" BSP (f)						6780 200 Side outlet Handwheel 5/8" BSP (f)
								1310 200 Side outlet Handwheel 5/8" BSP (f)						6580 200 Side outlet Handwheel 5/8" BSP (f)
2.0	2.32	4.68	9.43	9.43	9.43	9.43	9.43	10.0	10.0	10.0	23.6	40.0	47.2	50.0
485 x 100	535 x 102	865 x 102	670 x 175	690 x 175	930 x 140	930 x 140	930 x 140	680 x 180	940 x 140	940 x 143	1320 x 230	1540 x 230	1520 x 229	1540 x 230
19.1 x 3.9	21.1 x 4	34.1 x 4	26.4 x 6.9	27.3 x 5.3	36.6 x 5.5	36.6 x 5.5	36.6 x 5.5	26.8 x 7.1	37.0 x 5.5	37.0 x 5.6	52 x 7	60.6 x 9.1	59.8 x 9	60.6 x 9.1
3.1	3.4	5.4	9.9	10.0	14.5	14.5	14.5	15.5	15.5	10.0	34.5	51.0	68.9	51.0
6.6	7.5	11.9	21.8	22.0	32.0	33.0	32.0	34.2	34.2	22.0	76.1	112.4	151.9	112.4

ZD	D	E	AF	DF	F	LF	VF	AV	HX	ZX	G	AK	J	L

□ Suitable for use in MRI environment.
□ Most common cylinders used within the hospital.
□ Specialist use cylinders used within the hospital.
□ Other medical cylinders used within the hospital.

(1) Domiciliary use only.

NOTES: * The indicated cylinder is for specialist applications and availability is restricted.
** Vapour pressure of liquified gas at 15 degrees celsius.
*** Integral valve feature a low content gauge, on/off handwheel, built-in flowmeter and regulator. Schraeder outlets are product specific, to accept perform to BS 5682.
**** Always identify the cylinder content by the information on the label.

BOC Medical
Customer Service Centre
Priestley Road
Worsley
Manchester
M28 3UT
Tel 0800 111 333
Fax 0800 111 555
www.bocmedical.co.uk
bocmedical-uk@boc.com

Fig. 9.1 (Contd.)

Cylinder identification coding

Cylinders are made either from steel or, more recently, from aluminium wrapped with kevlar. Each cylinder is marked with a specific colour for each gas type, according to standards BS1319C and ISO 32, and fitted with outlet valves of various types. The top of the cylinder has a tapered thread into which is permanently fitted a valve. The valve can be opened by a handwheel, thumbwheel or special key. The gas outlet from this valve is connected to a pressure-reducing regulator, pressure gauge and other devices, depending on the application.

Four main types of cylinder outlet valves are in use: bull-nosed, pin index, handwheel, and valve and side spindle pin-index valves. More recently, cylinders have been introduced that carry an integrated valve/regulator. These are also known as 'Star valves' or 'Combi-valves'.

The most important valve in use is the pin-index valve, which has a system of noninterchangeable valves designed to ensure that the correct gas is filled into the cylinder and that the cylinder can only be connected to the correct equipment.

Medical gas flowmeters

Medical O_2 and air flowmeters normally have differently calibrated flow tubes, but the fitting the cylinder onto the regulator is the same. The entonox® cylinder is fitted with a demand valve, because administration is dependent on patient demand.

The cylinder labelling includes details of the following (Fig. 9.1):
- Product name, chemical symbol and pharmaceutical form.
- Safety phrases.
- Cylinder size code.
- Nominal cylinder contents in litres.
- Maximum cylinder pressure in bars.
- Product shelf-life and expiry date.
- Reference to the medical gas data sheet (which details clinical indications dosage schedules and contraindications – ensure you are aware of location of this information in the pharmacy).
- Storage and handling precautions.

At the pressures used, some gases liquefy within the cylinder, and, ∴, behave differently during storage and delivery.

O_2 and Entonox® remain gases, whereas nitrous oxide and carbondioxide (CO_2) liquefy. The liquids will cool considerably during expansion and this can cause problems, although this drawback is put to good use in cryosurgery where nitrous oxide evaporation and expansion are used as the energy source. In the case of Entonox®, it should not be stored below freezing point ($0°C$) because the mixture (50% nitrous oxide and 50% O_2) can separate.

Patient management issues

Drug use in liver disease

The liver is the main site of drug metabolism and the principal location for CYP450 metabolism (see p.25). In most cases, metabolism leads to inactivation of the drug, although some drugs have active metabolites (eg morphine) or require metabolism to be activated (eg cyclophosphamide). Despite this, it is frequently not necessary to modify the dose (or choice) of drug in liver disease because the liver has a large reserve of function, even if disease seems severe. However, special consideration of drugs and doses are required in the following situations:

- **Hepatotoxic drugs**—whether the hepatotoxicity is dose-related or idiosyncratic, these drugs are more likely to cause toxicity in patients with liver disease and so should be avoided if possible.
- **Protein binding**—the liver is the main source of synthesis of plasma proteins (eg albumin). As liver disease progresses, plasma protein levels fall. Thus, with less protein available for binding, there is more free drug available, which can lead to ↑ effects and toxicity, especially if the therapeutic index is narrow or the drug is normally highly protein-bound (eg phenytoin). If albumin levels are significantly ↓, serum levels measured for TDM might have to be adjusted to give a corrected level.
- **Anticoagulants/drugs that cause bleeding**—the liver is the main source of synthesis of clotting factors and there is an ↑ risk of bleeding as liver function deteriorates. Anticoagulants should be avoided (and are rarely indicated because of the ↓ in clotting factors) and drugs that ↑ the risk of bleeding (eg NSAIDs, selective serotonin reuptake inhibitors [SSRIs]) should be used with caution. Avoid intramuscular injections because there is a risk of haematoma.
- **Liver failure**—patients with clinical signs of liver failure (eg significantly deranged liver enzymes, ascites or profound jaundice) usually have altered drug handling (Table 10.2). In addition, drugs that could worsen the condition should be avoided:
  - Hepatic encephalopathy could be precipitated by certain drugs. Avoid all sedative drugs (including opioid analgesics), drugs causing hypokalaemia (including loop and thiazide diuretics) and drugs causing constipation.
  - Oedema and ascites could be exacerbated by drugs that cause fluid retention (eg NSAIDs and corticosteroids). Drugs with high sodium content (eg soluble/effervescent formulations, some antacids and IV antibacterials) should also be avoided.

Table 10.1 Terminology in liver disease

Hepatocellular injury	Damage to the main cells of the liver (hepatocytes)
Hepatitis	Inflammation of the liver, a type of hepatocellular injury. Could be caused by viruses, drugs or other agents, or could be idiosyncratic
Cirrhosis	Chronic, irreversible damage to liver cells, usually caused by alcohol or hepatitis C. If the remaining cells cannot maintain normal liver function (compensated disease), ascites, jaundice and encephalopathy can develop (decompensated disease)
Cholestasis	Reduction in bile production or bile flow through the bile ducts
Liver failure	Severe hepatic dysfunction where compensatory mechanisms are no longer sufficient to maintain homeostasis. Could be acute and reversible or irreversible, eg end-stage cirrhosis

Drug dosing in liver disease

The effects of liver disease, and consequent impairment of drug handling, are diverse and often unpredictable. Unlike renal disease, drug clearance does not ↓ in a linear fashion as liver function worsens. In addition, whereas in renal disease measuring creatinine clearance gives a good predictor of drug clearance, in liver disease there is no good clinical factor that predicts drug clearance and thus dose adjustment.

Impaired elimination is usually only seen in advanced liver disease. The following markers indicate significant impairment:

- ↓ Albumin (↑ or ↓ in acute liver disease).
- ↑ Prothrombin time.
- ↑↑ Liver function tests (LFTs).

Four main factors discussed below affect drug clearance.

Hepatic blood flow

Hepatic blood flow might be altered in liver disease because of cirrhosis (fibrosis inhibits blood flow), hepatic venous outflow obstruction (Budd–Chiari syndrome) and portal vein thrombosis. Even in the absence of liver disease, hepatic blood flow might be ↓ in cardiac failure or if BP is massively ↓ (eg in shock).

The clearance of drugs that are highly metabolized by the liver (high extraction/high clearance drugs) is directly related to blood flow. When these drugs are administered orally, their first-pass metabolism is significantly ↓ (if hepatic blood flow is ↓) and so bioavailability ↑. Administration by nonenteral routes, especially IV administration, avoids the effect of first-pass metabolism and ∴ bioavailability is unaffected. The effect of liver impairment on the clearance of these drugs is thus fairly predictable, being directly related to hepatic blood flow.

Drugs that are poorly metabolized (low extraction/low clearance drugs) are unaffected by changes in hepatic blood flow. Clearance of these drugs is affected by a variety of other factors.

In both situations doses should be titrated according to clinical response and side effects (Table 10.2).

↓ hepatic cell mass

Extensive liver cell damage can occur in both acute and chronic liver disease. High-extraction drugs are metabolized less efficiently and ∴ doses should be ↓ because peak plasma levels are ↑. Low-extraction drugs will have ↓ systemic clearance, leading to delayed elimination. Thus the dose should remain the same but the dose interval should be ↑ (Table 10.2).

Table 10.2 High/low-extraction drugs

High-extraction drugs
Dose at 10–50% normal for oral administration
Dose at 50% normal for IV administration
↑ dose interval in portal systemic shunting

- Chlormetiazole
- Glyceryl trinitrate
- Lignocaine
- Metoprolol
- Morphine
- Pethidine
- Propranolol
- Verapamil

Low-extraction drugs
Dose at 50% normal (all routes)
↑ dose interval

- Ampicillin
- Atenolol
- Chloramphenicol
- Chlordiazepoxide
- Cimetidine
- Diazepam
- Digoxin
- Furosemide
- Lorazepam
- Naproxen
- Prednisolone
- Spironolactone
- Tolbutamide
- Warfarin

Portal systemic shunting

If cirrhosis or portal hypertension are present, a collateral venous circulation could develop, which bypasses the liver. This means that drugs absorbed by the GI tract might directly enter the systemic circulation. Thus, there is minimal first-pass metabolism of high-extraction drugs and peak concentrations are ↑. For both high-extraction and low-extraction drugs, the half-life is prolonged and so the dose interval should be ↑.

Cholestasis

In cholestasis, substances that are normally eliminated by the biliary system accumulate. This includes some drugs that are eliminated by bile salts (eg rifampicin and sodium fusidate). Because lipid absorption is dependent on bile salt production, it is theoretically possible that there is a ↓ in absorption of lipid-soluble drugs.

In cholestasis, bile salts accumulate in the blood. This could ↑ bioavailability of protein-bound drugs because of competition for binding sites.

Analgesia in liver failure

The choice of analgesic drug in liver failure is problematic because both NSAIDs and opioids are contraindicated. The analgesic of choice is paracetamol because hepatotoxicity only occurs in overdose, when glutathione is saturated. In liver failure, glutathione production is maintained. It is advisable to avoid maximum daily doses of paracetamol because this can ↑ prothrombin time.

Further reading/information

Remington H et al. (1992). Drug choice in patients with liver disease. *Pharmaceutical Journal*, **248**: 845–8.
Cavell G (1993). Drug handling in liver disease. *Pharmaceutical Journal*, **250**: 352–5.
British National Formulary Appendix 2. www.bnf.org
Summaries of product characteristics
Leeds medicines information centre

Table 10.3 General guidelines for prescribing in liver disease

- Avoid hepatotoxic drugs (note many herbal medicines/adulterants are potentially hepatotoxic)
- Use renally cleared drugs in preference
- Monitor closely for side effects of hepatically cleared drugs
- Avoid drugs that ↑ the risk of bleeding
- Avoid sedating drugs if there is a risk of encephalopathy
- Avoid constipating drugs if there is a risk of encephalopathy
- In moderate or severe liver impairment consider the following options:
  - ↓ the dose of highly metabolized drugs
  - ↑ the dose interval for all hepatically cleared drugs
- If albumin levels are low, consider ↓ the dose of highly protein-bound drugs
- Drugs that affect electrolyte balance should be used cautiously and monitored carefully
- In preference, use older, well-established drugs if there is experience of use in liver impairment
- Start with the lowest possible dose and ↑ cautiously, according to response or side effects

Hepatorenal syndrome (HRS)

HRS is defined as the development of unexplained renal impairment in patients with severe liver disease. The kidneys are morphologically normal and recover if liver function recovers (eg following liver transplantation). However, the condition has a poor prognosis, with a mortality of 95% and mean survival of <2wks.

HRS seems to be caused by ↓ renal blood flow and perfusion consequent to the circulatory changes associated with severe liver impairment. It is characterized by oliguria, hyponatraemia and uraemia.

Management

- Maintain renal perfusion:
  - Correct hypovolaemia—human albumin solution 4.5% is preferred (avoid glucose 5% solution because it exacerbates hyponatraemia).
  - Maintain BP—if necessary, using pressor agents. Terlipressin has been used to ↑ BP, but this is an unlicensed indication.
- Investigate and correct other causes of renal failure:
  - Stop diuretics and all potentially nephrotoxic drugs.
  - Start empiric broad-spectrum antibacterials, investigate possible septic focus and perform blood cultures.
  - Avoid paracentesis without colloid cover.
- Institute renal-replacement therapy:
  - Because of the poor prognosis, the decision to institute dialysis should not be taken lightly and only instituted if other organs are functioning well.
  - Continuous haemodialysis/filtration is required because intermittent therapy can lead to significant disturbance of haemodynamics and intracranial pressure.
  - Renal-replacement therapy is usually necessary until liver function improves.
  - Molecular adsorbent recirculating system (MARS) is a form of dialysis that removes albumin-bound toxins. Early studies have shown improved survival versus haemofiltration.
- Liver transplantation is the only treatment shown to significantly improve survival but is usually inappropriate by the time HRS is established.

Table 10.4 Suggested treatment regimen for HRS

Day 1	Terlipressin, 0.5mg IV twice daily
	Albumin, 1g/kg body weight
Days 2–5	Albumin, 20g/daily
	If no fall in serum creatinine after 48h, ↑ terlipressin dose to 1mg four times daily

Drugs in renal impairment

Patients with renal impairment (which frequently includes elderly patients) can experience various problems with drug use and dosing. In addition to the obvious problem of ↓ excretion and thus ↑ toxicity, considerations are as follows:

- Pharmacokinetics of some drugs can be altered, including altered distribution and protein binding.
- Sensitivity to some drugs is ↑, although excretion is not impaired.
- Side effects can be tolerated less well by renally impaired patients.
- Some drugs (notably those that rely on urinary excretion for effect) can be ineffective if renal function is impaired.

This section mainly concentrates on the problem of ↓ excretion because this is what most pharmacists come across in their daily work. For additional information, consult the texts listed below.

Distribution

Oedema/ascites could ↑ the volume of distribution of highly water-soluble drugs, so an ↑ dose might be required. Conversely, dehydration or muscle wasting can lead to a ↓ volume of distribution, thereby requiring a ↓ dose.

In uraemic patients, plasma protein binding might be ↓, leading to ↑ levels of free drug but a shorter half-life. This might be significant for drugs with a narrow therapeutic index. In some instances, it is necessary to make compensatory adjustments when assessing plasma levels of certain drugs (eg phenytoin).

Metabolism

There are only two clinically significant examples of drug metabolism being affected by renal impairment:

- Insulin is metabolized in the kidney and thus ↓ doses might be required.
- Conversion of 25-hydroxycholecalciferol to 1,25-dihydroxycholecalciferol (ie active vitamin D; calcitriol) takes place in the kidney. This process might be inhibited in renal impairment; ∴, patients with renal failure might require supplementation with α-calcidol or calcitriol.

Excretion

This is the most significant effect because ↑ renal impairment leads to ↓ clearance and the potential for drug toxicity. This includes not only the original drug, but also toxic or active metabolites (eg morphine).

Assessing renal function

Renal function is assessed by measuring the glomerular filtration rate (GFR). An estimate of the GFR can be gained by measuring or calculating the creatinine clearance rate. Creatinine is a by product of muscle metabolism and is excreted by glomerular filtration. Provided muscle mass is stable, any change in plasma creatinine levels is directly related to GFR. Thus, measuring the rate of creatinine clearance gives an estimate of GFR.

Measuring creatinine clearance requires 24h urine collection (ie all of the patient's urine during a 24h period must be collected). The concentration of creatinine in the urine and total volume of urine is measured to establish the creatinine clearance. This process is inconvenient, involving a $\geq$ 24h delay in obtaining results. A reasonable estimate of the rate of creatinine clearance can be achieved by using the Cockroft and Gault equation (Table 10.5). This equation takes into account the fact that muscle mass (and, $\therefore$, serum creatinine levels) vary according to gender and weight.

Calculating the rate of creatinine clearance in this way gives a better estimate than simply using serum creatinine, but it is not exact and tends to under or overestimate the rate by up to 20%. Ideal body weight should be used in obese or fluid overloaded patients. The equation is especially inaccurate in pregnant women, children and patients with marked catabolism or rapidly changing renal function. For children a more accurate estimated CrCl can be calculated (Table 10.5).

Remember that elderly patients nearly always have some degree of renal impairment because of the normal ageing process. Despite its limitations, the Cockroft and Gault equation is extremely useful for assessing renal impairment in this setting and is preferable to using serum creatinine alone. For example, a serum creatinine of 120 micromol/L might be normal in a fit young man but could represent significant renal impairment in a frail elderly woman.

The rate of creatinine clearance normal in adults is ~80–120mL/min (for infants and children Table 10.6). In the UK, the following ranges of GFR are considered to represent various degrees of renal impairment:

- Mild–50—20mL/min.
- Moderate—20-10mL/min.
- Severe—<10mL/min.

Table 10.5 Calculating creatinine clearance

Adults[1]

$$\text{Creatinine clearance (mL/min)} = \frac{F\,(140-\text{age}) \times \text{weight (kg)}}{\text{serum creatinine (micromol/L)}}$$

Where, F = 1.04 in females and 1.23 in males.

Children[2]

$$\text{Estimated creatinine clearance (mL/min/1.73m}^2) = \frac{40 \times \text{height (cm)}}{\text{serum creatinine (micromol/L)}}$$

Neonates[3]

$$\text{Estimated creatinine clearance (mL/min/1.73m}^2) = \frac{30 \times \text{length (cm)}}{\text{Serum creatinine (micromol/L)}}$$

---

1 Cockroft DW, Gault MH (1976). The estimation of creatinine clearance from serum creatinine concentration. *Nephron*, **16**: 31–8.
2 Morris MC, Allanby CW, Toseland P, *et al.* (1982). Evaluation of a height/plasma creatinine formula in the measurement of glomerular filtration rate. *Archives of Diseases in Children*, **57**: 611–15.
3 Schwartz GJ, Feld LG, Langford DJ. (1984). A simple estimate of glomerular filtration rate in full terms infants during the first year of life. *Journal of Paediatrics*. **104**: 849–54.

Dose adjustment in renal failure

The kidney is involved in the elimination of most drugs, either in their active/unchanged form or their metabolites, although for some drugs this might be only a very small proportion of the dose. Drugs for which the kidney is a major site of elimination usually require dosage adjustment to avoid accumulation and thus toxicity. Remember that some of these drugs might also be nephrotoxic and drug accumulation can make renal impairment worse.

In patients with mild renal impairment it might only be necessary to monitor closely for side effects, with or without further deterioration in kidney function. However, in moderate or severe renal impairment an alternative drug should be used if possible. The ideal drug in renal failure would have the following attributes:

• <25% excreted unchanged in the urine.
• No active/toxic metabolites.
• Levels/activity minimally affected by fluid balance or protein-binding changes.
• Wide therapeutic margin.
• Not nephrotoxic.

Unfortunately, it is frequently not possible to find a suitable drug that fits these criteria, in which case dose adjustment is usually necessary. Two methods of dose reduction are used, either alone or in combination:

• Give a smaller dose at the same dose interval
• Give the same dose at a longer dose interval

It is possible to calculate a corrected dose/dose interval, but a more practical option is to use drug-dosing guidelines. The reader is referred to the sources on p.205.

Renal impairment prolongs the half-life of any drug excreted by the kidney. The time to steady-state concentration is ~five times the half-life. Thus, just as in patients with normal renal function, a loading dose might be needed if an immediate effect is required. This is especially true if the dose interval has been ↑. The loading dose in patients with renal impairment is the same as in patients with normal renal function.

Certain drugs should always be checked if there is any suspicion of renal impairment (Table 10.7). In many instances, not only are these drugs primarily excreted by the kidneys, but some are also potentially nephrotoxic, such that accumulation could lead to further renal impairment. In addition, side effects caused by accumulation might be mistaken for disease deterioration, and the pharmacist should be alert to this and advise medical staff accordingly. Wherever possible, avoid using potentially nephrotoxic drugs in patients with renal impairment.

Remember that renal function might improve or further deteriorate according to the patient's condition and, consequently, doses could need to be re-adjusted accordingly.

Table 10.6 Normal creatinine clearances in infants and children

Age	Creatinine clearance (mL/min/1.73m^2)
<37wks gestation	<25
Neonate	15–35
1–2wks	35–60
2–4 months	60–80
6–12 months	80–110
12 months to adult	85–150

Table 10.7 Checklist of drugs requiring dose adjustment in renal impairment

Commonly used drugs for which dose reduction is always necessary in moderate or severe renal impairment*

- Aciclovir
- Aminoglycosides
- Capecitabine
- Cisplatin
- Imipenem
- Meropenem
- Methotrexate
- Penicillin
- Thiazide diuretics
- Vancomycin

Commonly used drugs for which dose reduction should be considered in moderate or severe renal impairment*

- Allopurinol
- Amoxicillin
- Cephalosporins
- Cyclophosphamide
- Flucloxacillin
- Digoxin
- Ethambutol
- Frusemide
- Lomustine
- Melphalan
- Opioids
- Quinolones
- Sulphonamides (including co-trimoxazole)

* These lists are not comprehensive—check specialist references (p.205) for further information.

Drug dosing in renal replacement therapies

Renal replacement therapies are used in patients with chronic renal failure whose renal function is so poor that the kidneys are barely functioning. It can also be used temporarily in patients with acute renal failure. There are four types of renal replacement therapy in common use:
- Intermittent haemodialysis (HD).
- Continuous ambulatory peritoneal dialysis (CAPD).
- Continuous arteriovenous haemodialysis (CAVD).
- Continuous arteriovenous haemofiltration (CAVH).

Each method works on the principle of removing toxins from the blood by diffusion or osmosis across a semipermeable membrane into a dialysis solution. The factors that affect drug removal are, ∴, much the same for HD, CAPD and CAVD. CAVH is a slightly different technique and influenced by slightly different factors.

Dialysis-related factors

The following factors influence drug removal by dialysis or filtration:
- Duration of dialysis.
- Blood flow rate in dialyser.
- Type of dialyser membrane.
- Flow rate and composition of dialysate.

However, these characteristics are difficult to quantify and ∴ it is hard to predict exactly what effect they will have on drug removal.

In CAPD, frequent exchanges (eg every 1–4h) ↑ drug clearance.

Drug-related factors

It is possible to judge whether or not a drug will be significantly cleared by dialysis according to the pharmacokinetic parameters. Factors that favour drug removal are as follows:
- Low molecular weight–removal ↑ as molecular weight falls below 500 Da.
- Low protein binding (<20%).
- Low volume of distribution (<1L/kg).
- High water solubility.
- High degree of renal clearance in normal renal function.

The exception is CAVH, where molecules with a higher molecular weight (up to that of insulin) are preferentially removed, but there is less removal of smaller molecules (eg K^+ and urea).

Drug dosing in renal replacement therapies

Accurately quantifying drug clearance during renal replacement therapies is of limited value. The equations tend to assume constant conditions, but in practice both patient and dialysis conditions can vary. For example, the patient's clinical status, (eg BP or renal function) could change, which has an affect on drug clearance. In CAPD, peritonitis affects peritoneal permeability and thus clearance.

Table 10.8 Theoretical GFR in renal replacement therapy

Renal replacement therapy		Typical theoretical GFR achieved (mL/min)
HD	During dialysis	150–160
	Between dialysis periods	0–10
CAVD		15–20
CAVH		10
CAPD (4 exchanges daily)		5–10

The most practical approach is to use empirical dosing according to theoretical GFR achieved by the dialysis technique used (Table 10.8). This should be backed up by close monitoring for drug response and toxicity, including TDM.

In patients receiving HD, drugs should be given after the dialysis session to avoid the possibility that the drug might be removed before it has time to act. Because CAVH and CAVD are continuous processes, doses do not need to be scheduled around dialysis sessions. The same is true for CAPD, but the dose might need to be titrated up or down if the frequency of exchanges is ↑or ↓.

Further reading/information

Ashley C, Currie A (eds) (2004). *The Renal Drug Handbook*. Radcliffe Medical Press, 2nd ed..

Bennet MW *et. al.* (1999). *Drug Prescribing in Renal Failure*. American College of Physicians.

Summaries of Product Characteristics

British National Formulary, Appendix 3. www.bnf.org

Bristol Regional Medicines Information Centre.

Drugs in pregnancy

A drug is defined as teratogenic if it crosses the placenta, causing congenital malformations. Teratogenic effects usually only occur when the fetus is exposed during a critical period of development. Even then, not all fetuses exposed will be affected—eg <50% of fetuses exposed to thalidomide developed congenital abnormalities.

Various textbooks and reference sources (see p.209) give information on using drugs in pregnancy, but these sources do not always take into account all the relevant factors when assessing risk. To fully evaluate the risk/benefit of a drug in pregnancy, the following factors should be taken into account:

Other possible causes

- ≤10% of pregnancies result in an 'abnormal' outcome (including miscarriage and stillbirth) of which only 2–3% are caused by drugs or environmental factors.
- Maternal morbidity or an acute exacerbation/relapse of the disease could present a higher risk to the fetus than the drug.
- The underlying maternal disease might be associated with congenital abnormalities (eg epilepsy).
- Smoking and alcohol use during pregnancy can lead to congenital abnormalities, growth retardation and spontaneous abortion.

Drug characteristics

- Most drugs cross the placenta.
- High molecular weight drugs do not cross the placenta—eg heparin and insulin.
- Nonionized, lipophilic drugs (eg labetolol) cross the placenta to a greater extent than ionized, hydrophilic drugs (eg atenolol).
- A drug can cause fetal toxicity without crossing the placenta—eg any drug that causes vasoconstriction of the placental vasculature.

Timing

- If the drug is taken during the first 12 days (pre-embryonic phase), there is an 'all or nothing' effect—ie if most cells are affected, this leads to spontaneous miscarriage, and if a few cells are affected, this leads to cell repair/replacement and a normal fetus.
- Exposure during the first trimester (especially weeks 3–11) carries the greatest risk of congenital abnormalities.
- During the second or third trimester the main risks are growth defects or functional loss, rather than gross structural abnormalities. However, cerebral cortex and renal glomeruli continue to develop and are still susceptible to damage.
- Shortly before or during labour there is a risk of maternal complications (eg NSAIDs and maternal bleeding), or neonate complications (eg opioids and sedation).

Table 10.9 Some drugs that should be avoided* in pregnancy[1]

Drugs known to cause congenital malformations

- Anticonvulsants
- Cytotoxics
- Danazol
- Lithium
- Retinoids (systemic)
- Warfarin

Drugs that can affect fetal growth and development

- ACE inhibitors (after 12wks)—fetal or neonatal renal failure
- Barbiturates, benzodiazepines and opioids (near term)—drug dependence in fetus
- NSAIDs (after 12wks)—premature closure of ductus arteriosus
- Tetracyclines (after 12wks)—abnormalities of teeth and bone
- Warfarin—fetal or neonatal haemorrhage

* Note that if the benefit clearly outweighs the risk (eg life threatening or pregnancy threatening disease), these drugs can be used in pregnancy.

Some drugs that have a good safety record in pregnancy

- Analgesics: codeine (caution near term), and paracetamol
- Antacids containing aluminium, calcium or magnesium
- Antibacterials: penicillins, cephalosporins, erythromycin, clindamycin, and nitrofurantoin (avoid near term)
- Anti emetics: cyclizine and promethazine
- Antifungal agents (topical and vaginal): clotrimazole and nystatin
- Antihistamines: chlorphenamine and hydroxyzine
- Asthma: bronchodilator and steroid inhalers (avoid high doses in the long term), and short-course oral steroids
- Corticosteroids (topical, including nasal and eye drops)
- Insulin
- Laxatives: bulk forming and lactulose
- Levothyroxine
- Methyldopa
- Ranitidine

1 Welsh Medicines Resources Bulletin (2000) **7**(3): 1–5.

Other considerations

- Presence or absence of teratogenic effects in animals does not necessarily translate to the same effects in humans. Think logically, if the agent causes tail shortening in rats, is this relevant in humans? Some studies use higher doses in animals than would be used in humans.
- Drugs associated with abnormalities at high doses/during the first trimester might be lower risk at low doses/during the second or third trimester (eg fluconazole).
- If treatment cannot be avoided during pregnancy, in preference use established drugs that have good evidence of safety. (NB: sometimes a lack of reports of teratogenicity for a well-established/frequently used drug can have to be taken as evidence of safety.)
- Some teratogenic effects are dose-related (eg neural tube defects with anticonvulsants). Higher doses or combining more than one drug with the same effect will ↑ the risk.
- Consider non drug treatments (eg acupressure wrist bands for morning sickness) or whether treatment can be delayed until after pregnancy.

Maternal considerations

- Maternal drug handling changes during pregnancy; take special care with drugs that have a narrow therapeutic index.
- Remind the mother that some over-the-counter, herbal and vitamin products should be avoided in pregnancy.
- Many women do not comply with drug treatment during pregnancy because of safety concerns, so discuss this with the mother and reassure her.

Handling potentially teratogenic drugs

There is little published evidence on whether occupational exposure to potentially teratogenic drugs can ↑ the risk of congenital abnormalities. In the absence of evidence or specific guidelines, sensible precautions should be taken to reduce the risk of exposure, especially by pregnant ♀ and ♀ planning a pregnancy. A risk assessment should be performed (using, COSHH (Control of Substances Hazardous to Health) data, as appropriate) and pregnant ♀ should be excluded from any task that poses even a low risk.

Handling blister-packed versions of a teratogenic tablet present (virtually) no risk and film-coated or sugar-coated versions present a low risk. A high-risk procedure might involve preparation of cytotoxic infusions or handling crushed tablets of a known teratogenic drug. This type of procedure should not be carried out by pregnant ♀. ♀ (and ♂) of child-bearing potential (especially if planning a pregnancy) should take appropriate precautions (eg apron, mask and gloves). Ideally, potentially teratogenic infusions should be prepared by centralized pharmacy reconstitution service, where the use of cytotoxic cabinets further ↓ the risk of exposure.

Further reading

Briggs GG, Freeman RK, Yaffe SJ (eds) 7th edition (2005). Drugs in Pregnancy and Lactation. Lippincott Williams and Wilkins

Folb PL and Dukes MNG (eds) (1990). *Drug Safety in Pregnancy*. Elsevier.

Lee A, Inch S, Finnigen D (ed) (2000). *Therapeutics in Pregnancy and Lactation*. Radcliffe Medical Press.

National Teratology Information Service, tel 0191 2321525 for advice after exhausting other sources.

Toxbase drug monographs, including pregnancy risk (password required).

www.spib.axl.co.uk

www.motherisk.org

Drugs in breastfeeding

Breastfeeding has many advantages over bottle feeding. Even if the mother is taking a drug that is excreted in breast milk it can be preferable to continue breastfeeding.

The main questions to consider are as follows:
- Is the drug excreted into breast milk in quantities that are clinically significant?
- Do these drug levels pose any threat to the infant's health?

To answer these questions, the following factors must be considered.

Factors that affect drug transfer into breast milk

- **Maternal drug plasma level**—usually the most important determinant of breast milk drug levels. Drugs enter the breast milk primarily by diffusion. For most drugs, the level in the maternal drug compartment is directly proportional to the maternal plasma level. Thus, the higher the maternal dose, the higher the drug level in the breast milk. Diffusion of drug between plasma and milk is a two-way process and is concentration dependent: at peak maternal plasma levels (T_{max}) drug levels in breast milk are also at their highest. As the level of the drug in the plasma falls, the level of the drug in breast milk also falls as drug diffuses from the milk back into the plasma. Drugs that only have a short half-life thereby only appear in breast milk for a correspondingly short time.
  - During the first 4 days after delivery, drugs diffuse more readily into the breast milk because there are gaps between the alveolar cell walls in mammary capillaries. These gaps permit enhanced access for most drugs, in addition to immunoglobulins and maternal proteins. This results in ↑ drug levels in breast milk during the neonatal stage. After the first 4–7 days, these gaps close.
  - Some drugs pass into breast milk by an active process, such that the drug is concentrated in the milk. This occurs with iodides, especially radioactive iodides, making it necessary to interrupt breastfeeding.
- **Lipid solubility, of the drug**—Fat-soluble drugs (eg benzodiazepines, chlorpromazine and many other CNS-active drugs) preferentially dissolve in the lipid globules of breast milk. As a general rule, ↑ lipid solubility leads to ↑ penetration into milk. However, lipid solubility is not a good predictor of milk levels overall because fat represents a relatively small proportion of total milk volume.
- **Milk pH levels**—Breast milk has a lower pH than blood. Thus, drugs that are weak bases (eg isoniazid and atropine-like drugs), are ionized in milk, which makes them more water soluble and thus less likely to diffuse back into the plasma. This can lead to accumulation in the breast milk of these drugs. Conversely, weakly acidic drugs (eg penicillins, aspirin and diuretics) tend not to accumulate in breast milk.

Table 10.10 General principles to ↓ risk to breastfed babies

- Consider whether nondrug therapy is possible
- Can treatment be delayed until the mother is no longer breastfeeding or the infant is older and can tolerate the drug better?
- Use drugs where safety in breastfeeding has been established
- Keep the maternal dose as low as possible
- In preference, use drugs with a local effect (eg inhalers, creams or drugs not absorbed orally, such as nystatin)
- Use drugs with a short half-life and avoid sustained-release preparations
- Avoid polypharmacy—additive side effects and drug interactions potentially ↑ the risk
- Advise the mother to breastfeed when the level of the drug in breast milk will be lowest. This is usually just before the next dose is due

- **Molecular size/molecular weight of the drug**—As a general rule, 'bulky' drugs do not diffuse across capillary walls because the molecules are simply too big to pass through the gaps.
- **Drug protein binding**—highly protein-bound drugs (eg phenytoin and warfarin), do not normally pass into breast milk in significant quantities becuase only free, unbound drug diffuses across the capillary walls. Bear in mind that if a new drug is added that displaces the first drug from protein-binding sites, this could (at least temporarily) ↑ milk levels of the first drug.

Infant factors

- **Bioavailabilty**—drugs that are broken down in the gut or are not absorbed orally (eg insulin and aminoglycosides), should not cause any adverse effect because the infant's absorption of the drug is negligible, if any. Similarly, infant serum levels of any drug that has high first-pass metabolism are likely to be low. However, these drugs can sometimes have a local effect on the infants gut causing GI symptoms, such as diarrhoea.
- **Infant status**—must be taken into account. If the baby is premature or sick, they might be less able to tolerate even small quantities of the drug. Consider whether drug side effects could exacerbate the infant's underlying disease. For example, opioids in breast milk may be a higher risk for a baby with respiratory problems than a healthy baby.
- **Metabolism and excretion** of some drugs is altered in infancy, especially in premature infants who might have impaired renal and hepatic function. Thus, the drug effects can be greater than expected because the clearance of the drug is ↓. This can be especially marked for drug with a long half-life.
- **Drugs that are often administered to infants**—eg paracetamol, are generally safe if absorbed breast milk. As a general rule, < 1% of the maternal dose reaches the infant. Thus, if the normal infant dose is >1% of the maternal dose, it is usually safe, but side effects can still occur (eg antibiotic-induced diarrhoea).

Other factors to consider

- Some mothers and healthcare workers assume that because the infant was exposed to the drug during pregnancy, it will be safe in breast feeding. However, in pregnancy it is the maternal organs that clear the drug from the infant's circulation, but during breastfeeding the infant is clearing the drug. In addition, some adverse effects, such as respiratory depression, are not relevant during pregnancy but become relevant after delivery.
- Some mothers are resistant to using conventional medicines during breastfeeding because of perceived risks and decide to use alternative therapies. Mothers should be reminded that herbal or homeopathic medicines might be excreted in breast milk and cause adverse effects on the infant.
- Remember also to advise mothers that over-the-counter medicines, alcohol and other recreational drugs may be excreted in breast milk.
- Some drugs can inhibit or even stop breast milk production. This includes bromocriptine and other dopamine agonists, diuretics and moderate-to-heavy alcohol intake. Drugs that ↑ breast milk production, eg chlorpromazine, haloperidol and other dopamine antagonists, can lead to concern from the mother that the baby is not taking the full amount.
- Sometimes breastfeeding might have to be interrupted or stopped completely if there is no alternative to administering a potentially risky drug. For short courses, it might be possible to stop breastfeeding temporarily. Using a breast pump and discarding the pumped milk until such time as it is safe to resume breastfeeding should encourage continued breast milk production. Some mothers might find bottle feeding difficult because of more complex processes involved, cost or cultural issues and might need extra support.

Further reading/information

Briggs GG, Freeman RK and Yaffe SJ (eds) 6th edition (2005). *Drugs in Pregnancy and Lactation*. Lippincott, Williams & Wilkins.

Hale TW (ed) (2004). *Medications and Mother's Milk*. Pharmasoft Publishing.

Lee A, Incha S, and Finnigan D (eds) (2005). *Therapeutics in Pregnancy and Lactation*. Radcliffe Medical Press.

Sutton Coldfield and Leicester Regional Medicines Information Centre

Glucose 6-phosphate dehydrogenase (G6PD) deficiency

G6PD is an enzyme that produces reduced glutathione, which protects red blood cells against oxidant stress. G6PD deficiency is an X-linked genetic disorder. Thus, ♂ are either normal or deficient, whereas ♀ are normal, deficient or intermediate.

G6PD deficiency is distributed worldwide, with the highest prevalence in Africa, Southern Europe, the Middle East, South East Asia and Oceania. Thus, patients originating from any of these areas should be tested for G6PD deficiency before being administered an at-risk drug.

There are varying degrees of G6PD deficiency, with people of African origin generally having a lower level of deficiency (and, ∴, more able to tolerate oxidizing drugs) and those of Oriental and Mediterranean origin generally having a high level of deficiency. Mild deficiency is defined as 10–15% of normal activity. Note that young red cells are not deficient in G6PD. Thus, false-normal levels can occur during or immediately after an acute haemolytic attack, when new red cells are being produced.

Although many people remain clinically asymptomatic throughout their lives, they are all at risk of acute haemolytic anaemia in response to one of the following trigger events:
- infection
- acute illness
- fava (broad) beans
- oxidizing drugs

A haemolytic attack usually starts with malaise, sometimes associated with weakness, lumbar and abdominal pain. This is followed several hours or days later by jaundice and dark urine. In most cases, the attack is self-limiting, although adults (but rarely children) can develop renal failure.

Drug treatment in G6PD deficiency

- Patients in at risk groups should be tested for G6PD deficiency. The normal range is 1.2–1.72 units/10^{10}RBC (3.2–6.4 units/gHb)
- Patients with severe deficiency should not be prescribed highly oxidizing drugs (Table 10.11) and drugs with a lower risk should be prescribed with caution.
- Patients with a lesser degree of deficiency may be able to tolerate even the drugs listed in the Table 10.11 but exercise caution.
- The risk and severity of haemolytic anaemia is almost always dose-related. Thus, even severely deficient patients can tolerate low doses of these drugs, if there is no alternative. For example, for treatment of *Plasmodium vivax* or *ovale*, a dose of primaquine 30mg once weekly for 8wks, can be used instead of the usual dose of primaquine, 15mg once daily for 14–21 days.
- Drug manufacturers do not routinely carry out testing to identify the potential risk of their drug to G6PD-deficient patients. Do not assume with new drugs that if there is no warning in the data sheet, the drug is safe.

Treatment of a haemolytic attack

- Withdraw drug.
- Maintain high urine output.
- Blood transfusion, if indicated.

Table 10.11 Drugs to be used with caution in G6PD deficiency

Drugs with *definite* risk of haemolytic anaemia in most G6PD deficient patients (avoid)

- Dapsone and other sulphones
- Methylthioninium chloride (methylene blue)
- Nalidixic acid
- Nitrofurantoin
- Primaquine
- Quinolones
- Sulphonamides

Drugs with *possible* risk of haemolytic anaemia in some G6PD-deficient patients (caution)*

- Aminosalicylic acid
- Amodiaquine
- Ascorbic acid
- Aspirin (doses >1g/day)
- Chloramphenicol
- Chloroquine**
- Dimercaprol
- Hydroxychloroquine
- Isoniazid
- Levodopa
- Menadione (water-soluble vitamin K derivatives)
- Penicillins
- Probenecid
- Pyrimethamine
- Quinidine
- Quinine**
- Streptomycin

* Use with caution, low doses probably safe
** Acceptable to treat acute malaria at usual doses

Patient specific issues

Medicines for children: introduction

Children represent a significant proportion of patients in both primary and secondary care. In the UK, the National Service Framework (NSF) for Children[1] lists a number of areas in which pharmacists can have an important role. These include the following areas:

- Developing and providing high-quality medicines information, especially with respect to unlicensed use or formulations.
- Promoting concordance.
- Ensuring good communication between primary and secondary care, especially with respect to unusual or unlicensed preparations.
- Advising on clinically appropriate, safe and cost-effective use of medicines in children.

It is important to remember that children are not small adults, neither are they a homogenous group. Drug handling in children can be quite different to that in adults and can also be different at different ages. For medical and pharmaceutical purposes, children are usually grouped according to the following ages:

- Premature—born before 40wks gestation.
- Neonate— ≤ 4wks old (if premature, add the number of weeks premature—eg if born 2wks premature, the baby would be considered a neonate until 6wks old).
- Infant—4wks to 2yrs.
- Child—2yrs to (usually) 12yrs.
- Adolescent—(usually) 12yrs to 18yrs.

From 12yrs old onwards, drug handling and dosing is usually the same as adults, but adolescents require special consideration in terms of social and emotional needs.

1 www.dh.gov.uk/PolicyAndGuidance/HealthAndSocialCareTopics/ChildrenServices/ChildrenServicesInformation/fs/en

Medicines for children: pharmacodynamics and pharmacokinetics

Virtually all pharmacokinetic parameters change with age. An understanding of how drug handling changes with age is essential to avoid toxicity or underdosing.

Absorption

GI absorption may be slower in newborns and infants than adults. Newborns have a prolonged gastric-emptying time. Lower levels of gastric acid in newborns might ↓ absorption of some drugs (eg itraconazole). Drugs, that bind to calcium or magnesium should not be given at the same time as milk feeds.

Intramuscular absorption requires muscle movement to stimulate blood flow and so could be erratic in newborns who are relatively immobile. In addition, blood supply to the muscles is very variable.

Topical absorption of agents is enhanced in neonates and infants because the skin is thinner and better hydrated. This, age group also has a proportionally larger body surface area for weight than older children. Thus, topical agents applied over a large area can provide a significant systemic dose.

Distribution

Total body water changes with age:
- Premature—80% of body weight.
- Newborn—70% of body weight.
- Children—60–65% of body weight.
- Adults—60% of body weight.

This affects the volume of distribution of water-soluble drugs and higher doses per kilogramme might be required for premature or newborn infants.

Protein binding

In neonates, protein binding of drugs is less than in adults, but within a few months after birth it is similar to adult levels. ↓ protein binding might account for the ↑ sensitivity of neonates to some drugs (eg theophylline).

Metabolizm

Premature and newborn infants metabolize drugs more slowly than adults. However, young children have a faster rate, which ↓ to adult levels with ↑ age. Thus, doses of highly metabolized drugs are proportionally lower per kilogramme for neonates and infants and higher for young children.

As the child grows, doses should be frequently recalculated not only to allow for differing rates of drug metabolizm, but also to allow for ↑ in height and weight.

Premature infants and neonates have immature renal function, with the neonatal GFR usually ~30% of the adult rate. Thus, doses should be ↓ accordingly. After infancy, plasma clearance of some drugs is significantly ↑ because of both ↑ hepatic elimination (as above) and ↑ renal excretion.

Table 11.1 Tips on making medicines more palatable

- Chill the medicine (but do not freeze it)*.
- Take the medicine through a straw.
- Use an oral syringe to direct the medicine towards the back of the mouth and away from the tongue (and, ∴, away from the highest concentration of taste buds).
- Chocolate disguises many flavours—try mixing the medicine with a small amount of chocolate milk, spread or syrup.*
- Coat the tongue and roof of the mouth with a spoonful of peanut butter or chocolate spread before taking the medicine.
- Suck an ice cube or ice lolly immediately before taking the medicine.
- Brush teeth after taking the dose.
- Eat strongly flavoured food after the dose—eg crisps, Marmite® or citrus fruit (small amounts of these foods should not adversely affect drug absorption).

---

* Check drug compatibility and storage temperature requirements.

Medicines for children: licensing

Up to 40% of prescribing in children is unlicensed or 'off licence'—ie the drug is not licensed for use in that age range, route, dose or indication. Extemporaneous preparations and imported and specials products are effectively 'named patient' and thus unlicensed. Until such time as a wider range of formulations is available or drug manufacturers do the relevant trials to obtain licences for paediatric use or indications, this is an un-avoidable practice. The Royal College of Paediatrics and Child Health and the Neonatal and Paediatric Pharmacists Group (NPPG) have issued a joint declaration stating the following:

> 'The informed use of unlicensed medicines, or of licensed medicines for unlicensed applications, is necessary in paediatric practice.'

Pharmacists should ensure that licensed preparations are used wher-ever possible. If there is no alternative, they should ensure that both prescribers and parents (and the child, as appropriate) are informed of unlicensed or off-label use. It is especially important to ensure that par-ents or carers do not feel that the medicine is 'sub-standard' or 'second best' because it is unlicensed. In general, it is not considered necessary to obtain formal consent for the use of unlicensed medicines in this context. The NPPG has produced leaflets suitable for parents and older children to explain the need to use unlicensed and off-label medicines. These are available on the NPPG website (p.226). Local guidelines on documenta-tion and consent for use of unlicensed medicines should be complied with.

It is important that pharmacists ensure a continued supply of unlicensed, extemporaneous and special medicines by liaising with and providing product information to GPs and community pharmacists.

Medicines for children: calculating children's doses

A reputable reference source should be used for children's doses. Different sources quote doses in different ways and it is important to be clear how the dose is calculated to avoid the risk of overdose. Doses are usually quoted as follows:

• The total dose in mg/kg body weight per day, and the number of doses it should be divided into.
• The individual dose in mg/kg body weight per dose, and the number of doses that should be given each day.

Most doses are based on weight, although doses based on body surface area are more accurate because this takes into account the child's overall size (Table 11.2). Body surface area dosing is more frequent for drugs if accurate dosing is critical (eg cytotoxic drugs). Nomograms for calculating body surface area can be found in paediatric drugs handbooks or the following equation can be used:

$$\text{Body surface area (m)}^2 = \sqrt{\frac{\text{body weight (kg)} \times \text{height (m)}}{3600}}$$

Very rarely it is impossible to find a published and validated children's dose for a drug, in which case it can be estimated from the adult dose (Table 11.3). This should only be used as a last resort. This method tends to give an underdose. Calculated doses should usually be rounded up, rather than down, and the dose titrated according to clinical response, as necessary.

Table 11.2 Approximate surface area and weight*

	Weight (kg)	Surface area (m^2)
Newborn	3	0.2
1yr	10	0.5
3yrs	15	0.6
5yrs	20	0.7
9yrs	30	1.0
14yrs	50	1.5
Adult	70	1.7

* Note many children in developing countries might only weigh 60–80% of the average weight

Table 11.3 Estimating children's doses as a proportion of the adult doses*

Weight	Age	Proportion of adult dose
3–5kg	0–5 months	1/8
6–10kg	6 months–1yr	1/4
11–20kg	1–6yrs	1/3
21–30kg	7–10yrs	1/2
>30kg	11–15yrs	3/4

* Note this method tends to result in an underdose

Medicines for children: adherence

Counselling on medicine use and adherence issues is important for children. Parents might be familiar with taking medicines themselves. However, this doesn't necessarily mean they will cope with giving medicines to their child, especially if they are distressed by the child's diagnosis or the child is uncooperative. The toddler age-group is often the most difficult because at this age they can be uncooperative but lack the language ability and insight needed for parents to reason with the child.

- Wherever possible and within the child's level of understanding, pharmacists should aim to involve the child in discussions about their medicines.
- Ideally, counselling about medicine use and adherence should involve both parents (or two carers), especially if the therapy is complex and/or long term. As appropriate, also involve school nurses, for example, though it is best to avoid giving doses during school time if at all possible.
- The most appropriate delivery form should be selected. Most parents find an oral syringe easy to use but some children can object to this and once measured the medicine might have to be transferred to a spoon.
- Parents and carers might find it easier to give the medicine mixed with a small amount of food or drink. They should be taught how to do this correctly so that the child takes the full dose. Medicines should not be added to baby's bottle feeds because the full quantity might not be taken.
- Be aware that some patient information leaflets might be for indications other than the one for which the medicine is being used.
- Explain to the child why they need to take their medicine in simple terms, allowing for any limitations on disclosure of the diagnosis—eg a child may not have been told they have HIV but might have been told that they need medicine to help them fight infection.
- Encourage parents to involve the child in the administration process. From quite a young age (and with appropriate supervision and support), children can be taught to measure doses of liquid medicines, make up a dosette box or even self-administer insulin.
- Help parents to think ahead to how medicines will be administered during the school day or on a school or youth organization residential event. Tailoring the regimen to once-daily or twice-daily dosing means that drug administration during school hours can usually be avoided.
- Adolescents might wish to discuss their medicines without their parents present. Nonadherence in adolescents is not uncommon as a way of expressing independence and requires sensitive handling.

Further reading

Costello I (ed) British National Formulary for Children. (2005). London: Pharmaceutical Press. www.bnfc.org

Royal College of Paediatrics and Child Health and the Neonatal Paediatric Pharmacists Group (2003). Medicines for Children London: RCPCH Publications Ltd.

Advice on administering medicines to children, formulae for extemporaneous preparation. www.pharminfotech.co.nz

Website of the Neonatal and Paediatric Pharmacists Group. www.nppg.demon.co.uk

National paediatric drug information advisory line (DIAL). www.dial.org.uk

UK NHS Stability Database and UK Formulary of Extemporaneous Preparations. www.stmarys.demon.co.uk

'Pill school': teaching children how to take tablets and capsules

Preparation

- Discuss the child's ability to swallow food, especially hard or chewy food with the parents. Ask whether they think the child would be able to swallow tablets or capsules.
- Ask whether the child has had any previous experience of taking tablets and capsules and whether this was successful.
- Check any dietary issues, with respect to the placebo capsules to be used, eg allergies to food colouring or consumption of gelatin products.
- Ask parents to ensure that the child has not eaten or drunk anything immediately before the session so that they are not too full to swallow the capsules or water.
- Arrange the appointment for a time when the child will be alert and co-operative, eg not straight after school or nursery when they may be tired.
- Advise parents and other health care workers not to tell the child in advance what the session is about because this might create anxiety and resistance.
- To avoid possible disruption, ensure the child has been to the toilet before starting the session.

Equipment

- Prepare a series of capsule shells of different sizes containing sugar strands and place in bottles labelled with the sizes. Place some loose sugar strands in a bottle. Keep bottles and labels hidden from the child's view.
- Two cups (one for the child and one for you) and a bottle of water
- Two small trays or containers (eg weighing boats), one on which to place capsules, and one to use if the child spits out a capsule.
- Tissues for mopping up purposes.

Environment

- The room should be quiet, without distractions such as books or toys.
- Have only one other person present (as a witness) and ask them to sit behind the child out of view. Advise them not to intervene at any stage. Ideally, this should not be a parent.
- Sit across the table from the child.

Process

- Explain the purpose of the session to the child in simple terms. Talk enthusiastically and mention good things about taking tablets or capsules, eg avoiding bad-tasting medicine.
- Show the bottle of sugar strands and place a few on the tray. Ask the child to show you they can swallow these.

- Place two of the smallest capsules on the tray. Explain to the child that now you want them to try swallowing the sugar strands inside a capsule. Explain how to swallow a capsule without chewing and demonstrate this:
  - Sit or stand upright.
  - Take a breath.
  - Put the pill in the middle of your tongue.
  - Take a mouthful of water and swallow.
  - Keep your head straight.
- Show the child that you have swallowed the capsule by opening your mouth and sticking out your tongue. Make the process fun, but be firm if necessary.
- Ask the child to show you that they can do the same with the other capsule.
- Get them to show you that their mouth is empty by opening their mouth and sticking out their tongue. Praise the child for their success.
- If the child has been successful, repeat the process with the next size of capsule, again demonstrating how to swallow it if necessary. State that it is the next capsule, not that it is bigger. Give praise and encouragement at each stage.
- If the child has difficulties swallowing a capsule at any stage, get them to spit it out. Encourage them to try again with the same size of capsule.
- If the child is unsuccessful at the second attempt or if they refuse to try again, stop the session. Do not pressure the child because this could create an association between capsule taking and distress. Praise the child for trying hard.
- At the end of the session, if the parents have not been present, bring them in to the room so that the child can demonstrate successful capsule swallowing.
- Give the parents a supply of the largest size swallowed and written instructions on how to take capsules for further practise at home.
- Explain to the child that the medicines they will take could look different to the sample capsules but they should be able to swallow them in the same way.

After the session

- Discuss the child's achievement with medical staff.
- Review current or planned medication to establish whether it can be dispensed as tablets or capsules of a suitable size and shape.
- Bear in mind that uncoated and/or round tablets are harder to swallow than capsules, coated tablets or oval/capsule-shaped tablets.

Medicines for elderly people: introduction

Elderly people are high consumers of medicines—both prescribed and nonprescribed. In the UK, 50% of NHS drug expenditure is consumed by medicines for older people. Much prescribing for elderly people is done as 'repeats' and without regular review this can frequently lead to inappropriate or unnecessary therapy, including prescribing for 'diseases' that are actually ADRs.

In the UK, the NSF for Older People[1] has a specific section on medicines management, with the following primary aims:

- Ensuring older people gain maximum benefit from their medication to maintain or ↑ their quality and duration of life.
- Ensuring older people do not suffer unnecessarily from illness caused by excessive, inappropriate or inadequate consumption of medicines.

Elderly people are at ↑ risk of medication related problems:

- ↑ risk of ADRs (many preventable) caused by polypharmacy, drug interactions and changes in pharmacokinetics and pharmacodynamics.
- Underprescribing of some medicines—eg thrombolysis in MI.
- Nonadherence.
- Repeat medicines not being reviewed leading to unnecessary long-term therapy and stockpiling.
- Difficulty accessing the surgery and/or pharmacy.

---

1 www.dh.gov.uk/PolicyAndGuidance/HealthAndSocialCareTopics/OlderPeoplesServices/fs/en

Medicines for elderly people: pharmacokinetics and pharmacodynamics

Physiological changes that occur with age affect drug handling and sensitivity. Predicting at what age these changes become significant is almost impossible because people 'age' at different rates, depending on environmental, social and other factors. However, the pharmacist should be alert to possible changes in drug handling and sensitivity in any patient >75yrs of age.

Absorption

Ageing rarely has a significant effect on absorption. Delayed gastric emptying ↑ time to peak concentrations (C_{max}) but is rarely clinically significant.

↓ production of gastric acid can lead to ↓ absorption of drugs that require an acid environment for absorption, eg itraconazole, but can slightly ↑ the amount absorbed of drugs that are broken down by gastric acid, eg penicillins.

Bioavailability of levopdopa is ↑ in elderly people, possibly because of ↓ levels of dopa decarboxylase in the gastric mucosa.

↓ regional blood flow might ↓ the rate of absorption of drugs administered by the intramuscular or subcutaneous route, but the total amount absorbed is the same.

Distribution

- Lean body mass ↓ with age, leading to ↑ levels of drugs distributed in the muscle, eg digoxin.
- Adipose tissue ↑ up to the age of 85yrs, leading to ↑ tissue levels and thus prolonged duration of effect of lipid-soluble drugs, eg diazepam. Patients >85yrs tend to lose adipose tissue.
- The ↓ in total body water leads to ↑ in the serum concentration of water-soluble drugs, eg gentamicin and digoxin.
- ↓ serum albumin leads to ↑ levels of free drug for highly protein-bound drugs, eg NSAIDs, sulphonylureas and warfarin. In the acute phase, homeostatic mechanisms usually counteract the ↑ drug effects. ↑ level of free drug also means ↑ amounts for clearance so the effect is rarely significant in the long term.

Metabolizm

Elderly people can have up to a 40% ↓ in hepatic blood flow. Drugs with high first-pass metabolizm can be significantly affected (see p.192). There might be up to a 60% ↓ in metabolizm of some drugs, such as NSAIDs and anticonvulsants, leading to ↑ concentration, duration of action and, possibly accumulation.

Excretion

The natural ageing process between the ages of 20yrs and 80yrs lead to a 30–35% loss of functioning of glomeruli, with a consequent up to 50% loss of normal renal function. Serum creatinine levels might be normal or near normal because of ↓ muscle mass but creatinine clearance will be ↓. Acute illness and dehydration can cause a rapid decline in renal function, which can be exacerbated by the use of potentially nephrotoxic drugs, including high-dose antibacterials. Even a fairly well elderly patient can tolerate a combination of potentially nephrotoxic drugs, eg a diuretic plus an NSAID, but the addition of one more nephrotoxic drug, eg an antibacterial can tip the balance towards renal impairment.

It is advisable to always calculate the creatinine clearance (using the Cockroft and Gault equations; see p.201) for any patient >70yrs who is prescribed renally cleared or potentially nephrotoxic drugs. Remember that drugs such as morphine have active metabolites that are renally cleared. Drugs that rely on excretion into the urine for their effect—notably nitrofurantoin—can be ineffective in elderly people.

Pharmacodynamic changes

As the body ages, there is a natural loss of function at a cellular level. This can lead to ↑ or ↓ drug sensitivity. Changes in receptor–drug interactions can occur, eg there is a ↓ response to both β-adrenoceptor agonists and β-adrenoceptor antagonists.

Homeostatic responses can be blunted in old age—eg postural hypotension is more likely to be caused by blunting of reflex tachycardia, and cardiac failure might result from fluid overload caused by overenthusiastic rehydration or NSAIDs combined with ↓ cardiac output and renal function.

There is ↑ susceptibility to CNS effects of drugs. Even drugs that are not normally associated with CNS effects can cause such symptoms in the elderly, eg histamine H2 receptor antagonists and diuretics. These effects can occur without changes in kinetics, probably because of ↑ CNS penetration or altered drug response. For example, confusion and disorientation are more common in elderly people receiving benzodiazepines, antidepressants and NSAIDs, even at standard doses. In addition, changes in kinetics can lead to CNS effects not usually seen in younger people, eg ↓ renal function can lead to confusion associated with ↑ levels of drugs, such as ciprofloxacin and aciclovir.

Medicines for elderly people: medication review (See also p.56)

Regular medication review is an essential, but often overlooked, aspect of care of the elderly. Both hospital and community pharmacists are ideally placed to do this. Ideally, elderly patients should have their medication reviewed on admission to hospital, and in the community all patients >75yrs should have their drugs reviewed at least annually. Prioritize those at highest risk of medication-related problems:

- Elderly patients taking four or more drugs.
- Elderly patients recently discharged from hospital.
- Elderly patients taking 'high-risk' medicines:
  - Hypnotics—drowsiness and falls.
  - Diuretics—dehydration, renal failure and confusion caused by hypokalaemia.
  - NSAIDs—fluid retention and GI bleeds.
  - Antihypertensives—falls resulting from postural hypotension.
  - Digoxin—nausea and vomiting, confusion could be missed as signs of toxicity.
  - Warfarin—bruising and bleeding.

Other factors that can ↑ the risk of medication-related problems are as follows:

- Social—lack of home support.
- Physical—poor vision, hearing and dexterity.
- Mental—confusion, depression and difficulty understanding instructions.

Elderly patients are often high users of over-the-counter medicines and the pharmacist should be alert to this. Much over-the-counter drugs can:

- Be unnecessary.
- ↑ the risk of drug interactions.
- ↑ the risk of additive side effects.
- Be an indicator for ADRs to other medicines, eg high antacid consumption could point to NSAID-induced gastric irritation.

Medication reviews should include partners and carers (formal and informal) if possible and the results should be fed back to the GP and other relevant healthcare workers. If patients are attending the clinic for a review, they should be asked to bring all medications with them ('brown bag review'). This enables the pharmacist to check for the following:

- Stockpiling.
- Out of date medicines.
- Problems with reading or interpretation of medicine labels.
- Strategies for self-administration, eg marking containers or transferring medicines to other containers.
- Problems with manipulation, eg opening bottle caps or using technologically difficult products, such as inhalers or eye drops.
- Use of over-the-counter or herbal medicines.

The NO TEARS tool is useful model both for medication review and when considering initiating a new drug[1]:

- Need and indication:
  - Is the drug really necessary?
  - Is it being used to treat an adverse effect?
  - Can it be stopped?
- Open questions:
  - Ask nondirected questions about the medication:
    —Any problems?
    —Tell me how/when you take these medicines?
- Tests and monitoring:
  - Ensure that appropriate monitoring is being done both for desired effect and checking for ADRs.
  - Where possible ensure tests, such as TDM and INR are done beforehand so that the results can be used to inform the review.
  - Check adherence.
- Evidence and guidelines:
  - Ensure that treatment is evidence-based and complies with up-to-date local and national guidelines.
- ADRs:
  - Ask about ADRs.
  - Check whether a medicine is being used to treat side effects and, if possible, stop or change the causative drug.
- Risk reduction and prevention:
  - Pay special attention to 'high-risk' drugs, are they really necessary?
  - Could the dose be reduced?
  - If initiating a drug, start at the lowest dose and cautiously titrate according to the response.
- Simplification and switches:
  - Could a change of drug or formulation simplify the regimen or make self-administration easier?

1 Lewis T (2004). Using the NO TEARS tool for medication review. *British Medical Journal*, **329**: 434.

Dealing with injecting drug users in hospital

Injecting drug users and people who misuse other drugs, including alcohol, can present behavioural, in addition to medical, challenges on admission to hospital. An awareness of the issues involved is important but equally healthcare staff should not assume that all drug misusers are 'difficult' patients. Drugs of misuse include the following:

- Opioids
- Benzodiazepines
- Other prescription or over-the-counter drugs—eg anticholinergics
- Cocaine
- Cannabis
- Alcohol.

Managing behaviour

- Don't assume that all drug misusers will misbehave. Treat the patient with respect, as you would any other patient. A suspicious or negative manner from the healthcare professional is more likely to generate negative behaviour from the patient.
- Remove temptation—ensure that all drug cupboards and trolleys are locked and drug deliveries are put away immediately.
- Use a firm, no-nonsense approach. Guidelines or a contract for acceptable behaviour might be helpful(See p.92).
- Liaise with local addiction teams for advice and support.

Patients who misuse drugs on the ward

Healthcare professionals should be aware that patients (or their visitors) might misuse drugs on the ward. Indicators for this are as follows:

- Large numbers of visitors and/or visitors at odd times.
- Signs of intoxication or a behaviour change, often after receiving visitors or temporarily leaving the ward.
- Actual evidence (eg empty syringe).

Management depends on local policy, but this type of behaviour should not be tolerated. A senior doctor or nurse will normally be the member of staff who addresses this issue with the patient. Other healthcare staff should ensure that their dealings with the patient are consistent with agreed management policies. A suggested approach is as follows:

- Do not condone or tolerate the behaviour, make it clear that it is unacceptable.
- Give a warning that the behaviour will not be tolerated and the patient will be discharged if it is repeated.
- Consider limiting the number of visitors and the time during which they can visit.
- Involve hospital security or the police, especially if the safety of other patients or healthcare staff is compromised.
- Liaise with senior managers/the hospital legal advisers to ensure that action taken is within the law.

Handling illegal drugs

Pharmacists could be asked to take possession of illegal drugs that ward staff have taken from a patient. This might include schedule 1 drugs, which normally require a license for possession. However, UK law allows pharmacists to take possession of illegal (including schedule 1) drugs for the following purposes:

- Destruction of the drug.
- Handing the drug over to the police.

In this situation, it can be difficult to maintain the patient's rights and confidentiality while remaining within the law.

If a sufficiently large quantity is involved, such that it is clear that the drug is not just for personal use, it might be deemed that the public interest outweighs patient confidentiality and the should be police called. The decision to involve the police should only be taken after consultation with senior management and legal advisers.

If the quantity involved is small and clearly for personal use, the drugs should be destroyed. The patient's authority is required to remove and destroy the drug, and if they refuse to hand it over, consideration should be given to discharging the patient or involving the police. Returning the drug to the patient is not an option because this would make the pharmacist guilty of unlawful supply of a controlled drug.

Managing patients who are opioid dependent

Patients who are maintained on opioid replacement therapy (eg methadone or buprenorphine) in the community should have this continued in hospital:

- Verify the dose independently – eg by contacting the GP, addictions service or community pharmacist.
- Notify the community pharmacist of the patient's admission (to ensure the patient doesn't 'double up' by obtaining supplies from the community, in addition to the hospital supply) and discharge (to ensure community supply is restarted).
- Liaise with the GP and addictions service to ensure a consistent approach.
- As a rule, it is best to avoid providing more than one or two doses of replacement therapy on discharge. Liaise with the GP/community pharmacist to ensure a valid prescription is available for therapy to be continued in the community after discharge.
- Avoid prescribing other opioids if at all possible, especially short-acting opioids (eg pethidine).
- Benzodiazepines should only be prescribed if medically indicated (eg for alcohol withdrawal). If night sedation is required, prescribe in accordance with local addictions service guidance.
- If a dose adjustment of the replacement therapy is required (eg because of drug interactions), liaise with the local addictions service.

Patients dependent on opioids who are not on replacement therapy require careful management:

- Methadone or buprenorphine should only be prescribed if there are objective signs of withdrawal (Table 11.4).

- The dose should be titrated according to objective withdrawal symptoms, not according to the patient's reported use of street opioids.
- A suggested regimen is as follows:

  Day 1
  - Objective signs of withdrawal—methadone, 20mg single dose ('stat').
  - Further signs of withdrawal—methadone, 10mg single dose, can be repeated after 4h.
  - Maximum dose of methadone in the first 24h is usually 40–50mg.

  Day 2 onwards
  - Total dose given in the first 24h should be prescribed as a single daily dose.
  - Up to two additional doses of methadone (10mg) can be given every 24h, if further objective signs of withdrawal occur. Rewrite the maintenance dose each day to include additional doses until dose titration is achieved.
  - A dose of methadone 80mg daily is usually considered the maximum maintenance dose, but some centres use higher doses.
- At all times, doses should only be ↑ if there are objective signs of withdrawal. Bear in mind that methadone has a long half-life, so it takes several days to reach steady-state concentrations.
- Additional doses should not be prescribed 'as required' (prn)—the patient should be assessed each time by a doctor and any extra doses (if needed) prescribed as a single dose.
- If the patient wishes to continue replacement therapy after discharge, they should be referred to the local addictions service as soon as possible.
- Patients who do not wish to continue replacement therapy, might require a rapid reduction of the therapy before discharge. Note that these patients will usually return to using street opioids on discharge, thus the risk of withdrawal is minimal.

It is advisable for hospitals to produce written guidelines on opioid-replacement therapy in consultation with the local addictions service. This ensures continuity of care and can also be a great help to junior doctors, who may be pressurized by patients to prescribe replacement therapy inappropriately.

Managing alcohol withdrawal

See p.576.

Management of concurrent illness

In general, concurrent illnesses in patients who misuse drugs should be managed in the same way as for any other patient. However, the following points should be considered:
- Avoid opioids, benzodiazepines and other drugs that could be misused.
- Be aware that enzyme inducers and inhibitors can affect methadone levels.
- If the patient has a chaotic lifestyle, avoid drugs with a narrow therapeutic index—eg daily low molecular weight heparin is preferable to warfarin for DVT.

Table 11.4 Withdrawal scale from opiates

Methadone is indicated if score ≥ 7

Objective signs

Sweating		
	None	0 ☐
	Clammy	1 ☐
	Sweaty	2 ☐
	Running sweat	3 ☐

Retching		
	None	0 ☐
	Mild	1 ☐
	Moderate	2 ☐
	Vomit and retching	3 ☐

Gooseflesh		
	None	0 ☐
	Some	1 ☐
	Moderate	2 ☐
	Severe, with piloerection and shivers	3 ☐

Lacrymation		
	None	0 ☐
	Watery eyes; no tears	1 ☐
	Some tears	2 ☐
	Crying	3 ☐

Score /12

Record values of:

Pulse (record value). ———   Below 80–0 ☐
                                                    Over 80 ☐

BP (record value). ———

Pain control

Pain should be managed in the same way as for any other patient. Many doctors assume that patients on opioid-replacement therapy require less analgesia and the patient might insist they require extra analgesia because of tolerance. If the patient is experiencing pain, it is clear that the replacement therapy is not blocking all opioid receptors and analgesia is required. Ideally, opioids—both weak and strong—should be avoided. If an opioid is required, a long-acting opioid is preferred. Tramadol has no advantage over codeine in this setting.

Because buprenorphine is a partial antagonist, this can present a specific problem in patients who require opioid analgesia (eg postoperatively). It might appropriate to convert the patient to an equivalent dose of morphine before surgery. The local addiction service should be contacted for advice.

Discharge prescriptions for opioid-replacement therapy

Injecting drug users who are stabilized with methadone (IV or oral) or buprenorphine (Subutex®) might require a supply on discharge from hospital. It is usually not advisable to give more than a 24–48h discharge supply, especially if the patient usually gets their supply on a daily basis from the community pharmacist. Sometimes, there can be a delay before a prescription for a community pharmacy supply can be arranged, (eg at weekends or on bank holidays). On these occasions, it might be appropriate to use a prescription issued by the hospital, which can be dispensed in the community (FP10[HP] in the UK).

Things to consider
• Could an alternative arrangement be made—eg could the patient attend the ward/out-patient clinic for a supply?
• In the UK, only Home Office-registered doctors can prescribe diamorphine, cocaine or dipipanone to injecting drug users, but any doctor can prescribe any other replacement therapy.
• Close liaison with the local addiction service/GP/community pharmacist is important to ensure continuity of care

Writing the prescription (guidelines below refer to UK law)
• Normal writing rules for controlled drug prescriptions apply.
• FP10(HP) prescriptions cannot be used for instalment prescribing. If a daily pick up is required, a separate prescription must be written for each day.
• FP10(MDA)[1] prescriptions can be used by any doctor to write installment prescriptions. The prescription must specify the total quantity required, the amount of the instalments to be dispensed and the intervals to be observed between installments.
• A maximum of 14 days' supply of schedule 2 controlled drugs can be prescribed by instalments for the treatment of substance misuse.
• FP10 prescriptions have a potential street value and may be sold to other injecting drug users. Consider posting or delivering the prescription to the community pharmacy, rather than handing it to the patient. Check normal practice with the local addiction service/GP.

---

1 HBP(A), HBP or GP10 in Scotland, WP10 (MDA) or WP10 (HP) Ad in Wales.

Surgical patient and nil-by-mouth (NBM) issues

It is imperative that a comprehensive DHx is undertaken for all patients admitted to hospital for surgery.

The DHx should include regular, if needed and recently stopped or withheld medications.

Over-the-counter and herbal products need to be documented.

- Medicines used to control life-threatening conditions should be continued.
- Optimize the treatment of chronic diseases before admission for surgery—eg for asthma and COPD.
- For surgical emergencies, eg abdominal aortic aneurism (AAA), it might not be possible to optimize drug therapy preoperatively and the pharmacist needs to highlight any possible complications relating to a recently administered drugs that otherwise should have been stopped or dose-modified.

In general, few drugs need to be stopped before surgery.

NBM period

- Patients are at risk of aspirating their stomach contents during general anaesthesia. They are, ∴ usually prevented from eating within 6h of surgery. However, clear fluids leave the stomach within 2h of ingestion and thus free clear fluids that enable a patient to take routine medication are allowed up to 2h presurgery.
- After surgery, oral medicines can be restarted at their previous pre-operative dose as soon as the patient can swallow small amounts of fluid.
- If a patient is likely to be NBM for a long time (eg surgeon's plan and PONV) the drug can be given; by an alternative route—eg rectal, transdermal, parenteral or feeding tube delivery.
- Drugs with a long half-life (eg levothyroxine) or long duration of action (eg antidepressants) shouldn't cause a problem if they have to be omitted for several days.

When reviewing a patients medication during the NBM period

The risks and benefits must be considered when deciding to continue or suspend medication. For example, the consequences of stopping long-term therapy for conditions, such as osteoporosis or osteoarthritis in the NBM period might be considered nonproblematic in the majority of patients.

To avoid interrupting appropriate long-term therapies, oral medicines can be administered with sips of clear oral fluid in the NBM period.

The anaesthetist should be contacted if there is any doubt about a patients specific medication plan—eg if a drug is known to have potential interaction with anaesthetic agents.

There are a few significant interactions between drugs used during surgery and routine medications that require the drugs not to be administered concurrently. This is usually managed by the anaesthetist, by their choice of anaesthetic technique.

Significant interactions are as follows:
- Enflurane can precipitate seizure activity in patients taking tricyclic antidepressants.
- Pethidine can precipitate fatal 'excitatory' reactions in patients taking monoamine oxidase inhibitors and can cause serotonin syndrome in patients taking SSRIs.
- The effects of suxamethonium can be prolonged by neostigmine.

Controversial therapy for surgical patients

Hormone-replacement therapy (HRT)

Women on HRT had an ↑ risk of developing venous thromboembolism (VTE) after major surgery compared with controls. The MHRA advise that there is no need to stop HRT unless patients have other predisposing risk factors for VTE, such patients require suitable thromboprophylaxis.

For patients with predisposing risk factors, HRT should be stopped 4wks before major surgery.

COCs

Again, there is an ↑ risk of VTE in patients having therapy with COCs. Therapy should be discontinued 4wks before major elective surgery and all leg surgery. However, the risk and consequences of pregnancy versus VTE must be discussed with patients.

COCs should be restarted at the first menses that occurs at least two weeks after full mobilization.

Tamoxifen

Patients on tamoxifen therapy have higher risk of VTE after surgery. However, tamoxifen treatment for breast cancer should be continued during surgery unless directed by the patient's oncologist, and close monitoring of VTE symptoms for 3months postsurgery should be planned.

Patients having tamoxifen treatment for fertility should have treatment suspended 6wks before major surgery.

Methotrexate

Fluid restriction, hypovolaemia and renal hypoperfusion can result in ↓ clearance; it is advisable to suspend methotrexate for 2days before surgery and check renal function before recommencing therapy.

Monoamine oxidase inhibitors

Monoamine oxidase inhibitors can result in hypertensive crisis if used concurrently with interacting drugs (eg pethidine, dextromethorphan and pentazocine). They are usually withdrawn 2wks before surgery; however, the risk of psychiatric relapse must be considered. If necessary, monoamineoxidase inhibitors can be substituted with a short-acting forms, such as moclobemide (which can be withheld on the morning of surgery). If withdrawal is not possible, avoid pethidine and indirectly acting sympathomimetics— use isoprenaline instead. Phentolamine can be used to ↓ BP in the event of a hypertensive crisis.

Corticosteroids

Stress caused by surgery is associated with an ↑ cortisol production. Prolonged corticosteroid therapy 'especially at high doses', can cause adrenal atrophy, an impaired stress response and risk of hypoadrenal crisis, manifesting in circulatory collapse and shock.

The risk of HPA (hypothalmic pituary adrenal) axis suppression should be considered if patients have been on steroids for 1–2wks before surgery or within the last 6 months. The dose and duration of steroids determines the risk, in addition to the type of surgery.

Therefore, these patients will require IV hydrocortisone cover. A usual dose is 50–100mg of hydrocortisone given preoperatively, intraoperatively (if necessary) and every 6–8h for 2–3 days after surgery. Normal preoperative steroid cover should be restarted 2 days after surgery (no gradual dose reduction is needed from postoperative cover).

Lithium

Lithium prolongs the action of depolarizing and nondepolarizing muscle relaxants. Ideally, stop therapy 24–72h before major surgery, but therapy can continue during minor surgery. If it is not possible to stop therapy, ensure adequate fluid intake during and after surgery. Monitor U&E regularly; measure lithium blood levels, if necessary.

Diuretics

Omit K^+ sparing diuretics on the morning of surgery because ↓ kidney perfusion in the immediate postoperative period can predispose to hyperkalaemia. Thiazide and loop diuretics need not be omitted. Any electrolyte imbalance should be corrected before surgery.

β-blockers

In patients with hypertension, anesthesia and surgery can provoke tachycardia and ↑ BP. β-blockers can help to suppress these effects and are, therefore, usually continued perioperatively.

Antiplatelet drugs

Aspirin/clopidogrel should be stopped when the risks of postoperative bleeding are high or if the consequences of, even minor, bleeding are significant (eg retinal and intracranial bleeding). This must be balanced against the risk of precipitating thromboembolic complications if these drugs are stopped, particularly in patients with unstable angina. If low-dose aspirin or clopidogrel are stopped, this is generally 7–10 days before surgery to enable recovery of adequate platelet function. It is not usually necessary to stop dipyridamole before surgery, but if complete absence of antiplatelet effect is desired, it should be stopped 24h before surgery.

Anti-Parkinson's drugs

There is a small risk of arrhythmias or hypertension during anaesthesia in patients with Parkinson's disease, however, anaesthesia can worsen symptoms of Parkinson's disease after surgery and uncontrolled symptoms ↓ mobility and impede recovery. These drugs should, 6, be continued wherever possible. Procyclidine can be given by injection to relieve rigidity and tremor if the patient is unable to take oral medication after surgery.

Antipsychotics and anxiolytics

Generally these agents are continued to avoid relapse of the condition. Antipsychotics can ↓ anaesthetic requirements and potentiate arrhythmias. However, clozapine should be stopped 24h before surgery. ∴, if the patient is on the morning list, do not give medication on the day before surgery, in addition to the day of surgery itself. There are no withdrawal problems associated with doing this. If the patient is unable to take clozapine for >2 days because of being NBM, the drug must be gradually re-titrated up from the starting dose (12.5mg once or twice daily)

Oral hypoglycaemics

For major surgery, most patients with type 2 diabetes benefit from IV insulin therapy, especially if a prolonged NBM period is expected or if the stress from surgery has led to unacceptable hyperglycaemia.

However, the following guidance can offer suitable guidance for your patient management:

- Glibenclamide—switch to a sulphonylurea with a shorter half-life 3 days before surgery or switch to soluble insulin.
- Gliclazide/glipizide/tolbutamide—omit therapy on the day of surgery.
- Metformin—to ↓ the risk of lactic acidosis, withdraw the drug 48–72h before surgery and re-stabilize 48h after surgery.

Pharmaceutical calculations

Concentrations

Pharmaceutical preparations consist of a number of different ingredients in a vehicle; ingredients could be solid, liquid or gas.

'Concentration' is an expression of the ratio of the amount of an ingredient to the amount of product.

Concentrations can be expressed in several ways:
- Solutions of solids in liquids, denoted by w/v.
- Solutions of liquids in liquids, denoted by v/v.
- Admixtures of liquids in solids (v/w) or solids combined with solids (w/w).

Concentrations are expressions of ratios and are written in different formats that can cause confusion. Formats traditionally used are as follows:
- Amount strengths.
- Ratio strengths.
- PPM.
- Percentage strength.

Amount strengths

A preparation contains 900mg of sodium chloride dissolved in water to make a final volume of 100mL. The concentration of this solution can be written as an amount strength in units of 900mg/100mL, 9mg/mL, 0.9g/100mL or 9g/L.

Ratio strengths

Convention states that when ratio strength represents a solid in a liquid, involving units of weight and volume, the weight is expressed in grammes and the volume in millilitres.

A 1 in 50 sodium chloride in water perparation is a solid in a liquid (w/v) ratio strength. This means that the solution contains 1g of sodium chloride made up to 50mL with water.

A 14 in 100 sulphuric acid in water preparation is a liquid in a liquid (v/v) ratio strength, ie 14mL of sulphuric acid in 86mL of water.

Ppm

This expression is used when the ratio of ingredient to product is very small, by convention 1ppm weight in volume is 1g in 1 000 000mL. 1ppm weight in weight is 1mg per 1 000 000mg or 1g per 1 000 000g. In volume, it is 1mL in 1 000 000mL or 1L in 1 000 000L.

Percentage strength

'Percentage' in pharmaceutical calculations is quantified as the amount of ingredient in 100 parts of the product.

% w/v, by convention, indicates number of grammes of ingredient in 100mL of product. ∴ 900mg of sodium chloride made up to 100mL with water can be expressed as 0.9g in 100mL and the percentage strength is 0.9% w/v.

A 1 in 1000 adrenaline injection is equivalent to 0.1% w/v or, by convention, 1g of adrenaline made up to 1000mL with water.

A 1 in 10 000 adrenaline injection equivalent to 0.01% w/v or by convention, 1g of adrenaline made up to 10 000mL with water.

Calculations

For example, how many millilitres of a 1 in 50 w/v solution are required to make 500mL of a 0.02% solution?

By convention, 1 in 50 means 1g in 50mL and 0.02% w/v means 0.02g in 100mL. Let the number of millilitres of the 1 in 50 solution be y and let the amount of ingredient in grammes in 500mL of 0.02% solution be x. The amount of ingredient in grammes in ymL of a 1 in 50 solution will also be x.

Setting up proportional sets

For 1 in 50:

| Ingredient (g) | 1 | x | 1g |
| Product (mL) | 50 | y | to 50mL |

For 500mL of 0.02%:

| Ingredient (g) | 0.02 | X | 0.02g |
| Product (mL) | 100 | 500 | to 100mL |

By 'spotting' $x = 0.1$, substitute into the first pair of proportional sets:

For 1 in 50

| Ingredient (g) | 1 | 0.1 | 1g |
| Product (mL) | 50 | Y | to 50mL |

By 'spotting' $y = 5$

∴, 5mL of a 1 in 50 w/v solution is required to make 500mL of a 0.02% w/v solution.

Or alternatively:

How many grammes in 500mL of 0.02% solution?

$0.02\% = 0.02$g in 100mL

in 500mL $= 0.02 \times 5$

$= 0.1$g

1 in 50 solution, by convention 1g in 50mL

Then, to calculate the volume containing 0.1g, 1/10 of 1g or 1/10 of 50mL = 5mL

Moles and millimoles

The atomic and molecular weights of a drug can be used as methods of defining the amount of drug. The substance can be atoms, molecules or ions; a mole is the weight expressed in gramme. The mole is the SI base unit for the amount of a substance; eg the atomic weight of iron is 56 and 1mol of iron weighs 56g.

The molecular weight of sodium chloride is 58.5g and consists of one sodium ion and one chloride ion in a molecule of sodium chloride:
- 1mol sodium ion weighs 23g.
- 1mol chloride ion weighs 35.5g.

In the same way that the system of weights and volumes have multiples and subdivisions (eg milli, micro and nano), so the mole has similar subdivisions and multiples:
- 1mol contains 1000 millimoles (mmol)
- 1mmol contains 1000 micromoles (mcmol)
- 1mcmol contains 1000 nanomoles (nmol)
- 1nmol contains 1000 picomoles (pmol)

Amount of substance concentration

In clinical chemistry, laboratory results are usually written in terms of mol/L (or mmol/L or mcmol/L).

Example

How many mmol of sodium chloride are there in a litre of sodium chloride 0.9% w/v?
First calculate the weight of sodium chloride in a litre:
0.9g in 100mL
= 0.9g×10 in 1000mL
= 9g in 1000mL
 For the molecule sodium chloride: 1mole = 58.5g
  58.5g = 1000mmol
9/58.5 = x/1000
    x = 9000/58.5
    x = 153mmoL

Or alternatively,
To calculate the number of millimoles contained in 1g of substance, use the following formula:

$$mmol = \frac{1000 \times number\ of\ specified\ units\ in\ one\ unit\ (atom,\ molecule\ or\ ion)}{atomic,\ molecular\ or\ ionic\ weight}$$

Number of mmol of sodium in 1g of sodium chloride (molecular weight = 58.5)

$$mmol = \frac{1000 \times 1}{58.5}$$
$$=17mmol\ in\ 1g\ or\ 153mmol\ in\ 9g$$

For $CaCl_2$, $2H_2O$ (molecular weight = 147)

mmol of calcium in 1g $CaCl_2$, $2H_2O = \dfrac{1000 \times 1}{147} = 6.8mmol$

mmol of chloride in 1g $CaCl_2$, $2H_2O = \dfrac{1000 \times 2}{147} = 13.6mmol$

mmol of water in 1g $CaCl_2$, $2H_2O = \dfrac{1000 \times 2}{147} = 13.6mmol$

ie each g of $CaCl_2$, $2H_2O$ represents 6.8mmol of Calcium, 13.6mmol of Chloride, and 13.6mmol of water of crystallization.

Practical issues involving pharmaceutical calculations

• Always work from a written master copy.

Calculate the amounts of ingredients for 200mL Chloral Mixture BP 1988

Ingredients	Master formula	Scaled quantities
Chloral hydrate	1g	20g
Syrup	2mL	40mL
Water	To 10mL	To 200mL

• Use double checks: 1 is 1/10 of 10 and 20 is 1/10 of 200.
• Don't forget your units: 1g = 1000mg = 1 000 000mcg.

Preparing dilutions

• Ensure correct choice of diluent.
• Calculate dilution factor.
• Correctly express the concentration of the diluted product on the label.

Example 1 Calculate the amount of benzalkonium chloride solution BP 2004 needed to prepare a 150mL of a solution of benzalkonium chloride 10% w/v. Benzalkonium chloride solution BP 2004 is a 50% w/v concentration.
Calculation of dilution factor:

Method 1
$$\frac{\text{Strength of concentrate}}{\text{Strength of dilute solution}} = \text{Dilution factor}$$

Strength of concentrate $\frac{50\% \text{ w/v}}{10\% \text{ w/v}}$ = 5 times
Strength of dilute solution
To prepare dilute solution $\frac{\text{Final volume}}{\text{Dilution factor}}$
150/5 = 30mL of concentrate solution

The diluted solution is obtained by using 30mL of BP solution and diluting with 120mL of water.

Method 2
Product of volume and concentration
$V_c \times C_c = V_d \times C_d$ where,
$V_c \times 50 = 150 \times 10$
$V_c = 150/5$
$V_c = 30$mL

V_c = volume of concentrated solution
C_c = concentration of concentrate
V_d = volume of diluted solution
C_d = concentration of diluted solution

Example 2

Calculate the quantity of potassium permanganate 0.25% w/v solution that is required to produce 100mL of a 0.0125% w/v solution of potassium permanganate.

Calculation of dilution factor

$Vc \times Cc = Vd \times Cd$

Vc = volume of concentrated solution	= Unknown
Cc = concentration of concentrate	= 0.25%
Vd = volume of diluted solution	= 100mL
Cd = concentration of diluted solution	= 0.0125%

$Vc \times 0.25\% = 100mL \times 0.0125\%$

$Vc = 1.25/0.25$

$= 5mL$

Dilution instructions

5mL of potassium permanganate solution 0.25% w/v must be diluted to 100mL with water to produce a 0.0125% w/v solution.

Pharmaceutical calculations involving drug administration

Calculations

- Calculations usually involve fairly straightforward theory, but difficulties can arise as a result of interruptions, tiredness or lack of experience.
- In preparing infusions, the mathematics normally involve translating units such as mcg/kg body weight/min into a practical number of mL of diluted infusion solution/h.

Examples

A patient requires a parenteral loading dose of 0.5mg of digoxin. Digoxin is available as an injection containing 250 mcg/mL. How many millilitres of injection will supply the required dose?

First convert mg to mcg:

0.5mg to mcg = 500mcg

Setting up a proportional set

Weight of digoxin (mg)   250 500
Volume of injection (mL)   1 y

250 multiplied by 2 gives 500, so 1 is multiplied by 2 to give $y = 2$

Because the injection contains 250mcg in 1mL, a 500mcg dose will be provided in 2mL.

ITU prepare dobutamine as a standard concentration of 250mg in 50mL 5% dextrose solution. You need to confirm that the prescribed 5mcg/kg/body weight/min dose for a 70kg patient is correctly delivered by the volumetric hourly rate set by the nurse.

Standard concentration=250mg in 50mL (patient 70kg)

To calculate the hour rate: = 5mcg × kg body weight × min
= 5 × 70 × 60(min)
= 21 000mcg/hr

Concentration of dobutamine = 250mg in 50mL
(convert to mcg)   = 250 × 1000 (mcg) in 50mL
= 250 000mcg in 50mL
= 5000mcg in 1mL

Volume per hour requires 21 000mcg to be administered = $\dfrac{21\,000\text{mcg/h}}{5000\text{mcg/mL}}$

= 4.2mL/h

Pharmaceutical care

The concept of pharmaceutical care

Pharmaceutical care was probably first defined by Mikeal in 1975 as 'the care that a given patient requires and receives, which assures safe and rational drug use'.[1] Hepler, in 1988, described pharmaceutical care as 'a covenantal relationship between a patient and a practitioner in which the pharmacist performs drug use control functions governed by the awareness of and commitment to the patients interest'.[2] The term has caught the imagination of pharmacists and is frequently applied indiscriminately to describe pharmacy activities.

Definition

The generally accepted definition by Hepler and Strand states 'Pharmaceutical care is the responsible provision of drug therapy for the purpose of achieving definite outcomes that improve a patients quality of life'.[3] This definition built on another earlier one describing pharmaceutical care as 'a practice in which the practitioner takes responsibility for a patients drug-related needs and is held accountable for this commitment'.[4] Early in these debates, the issue of drug-related morbidity was seen as a major problem and, in part, led to the final definitions outlined above.

Pharmaceutical care differs from traditional drug treatment because it is an explicitly outcome-orientated co-operative, systematic approach to providing drug therapy directed not only at clinical outcomes, but also at activities of daily life and other dimensions of health-related quality of life. Historically, pharmacists have used a variety of methods to improve drug therapy, including formularies drug-use reviews, prescriber education and clinical pharmacy, but these have all been drug focused or prescription focused.

Pharmaceutical care involves the process through which a pharmacist co-operates with a patient and other professionals in designing, implementing and maintaining a therapeutic plan that will produce specific outcomes for the patient. This, in turn, involves three major functions:
- Identifying potential and actual drug-related problems.
- Resolving actual drug-related problems.
- Preventing drug-related problems.

1 Mikeal RL, Brown TR, Lazarus HL, Vinson MC (1975). Quality of pharmaceutical care in hospitals. *American Journal of Hospital Pharmacy* **32(6)**: 567–74.
2 Hepler CD (1988). Unresolved issues in the future of pharmacy. *American Journal of Hospital Pharmacy* **45(5)**: 1071–81.
3 Hepler CD, Strand LM (1990). Opportunities and responsibilities in pharmaceutical care. *American Journal of Hospital Pharmacy* **47(3)**: 533–43.
4 Strand LM (1984). Re-visioning the professions. *Journal of the American Pharmacy Association* 100–258.

Core elements of pharmaceutical care

The pharmacist

- Collects and documents relevant information in a systematic, structured manner for the purpose of determining whether the patient is experiencing potential or actual drug-related problems.
- Identifies and lists the drug-related problems the patient is experiencing or is at risk of experiencing.
- Establishes and lists the desired therapeutic outcomes for each drug-related problem identified.
- Considers and ranks all the therapeutic interventions that might be expected to produce the desired therapeutic outcomes for each problem.
- Decides which therapeutic alternative to select and records the dosage regimen for each medication for each patient.
- Formulates and documents a pharmacotherapeutic monitoring plan to verify that the drug-related decisions implemented have resulted in the outcomes desired and not in undesirable ADRs or toxicities.[1]

All must be in place for a comprehensive pharmaceutical care service. The only variable that affects the level of service is the patient's needs. This is assessed by determining the patient's risk factors. Patients who are considered at low risk might only require minimal intervention, where as high-risk patients, by definition, require a higher level of pharmaceutical care.

Identifying risk in clinical practice

Risk factors fall into three distinct areas:

- Patients clinical characteristics—these include physical and readily determined characteristics, such as age, gender, ethnicity, pregnancy status, immune status, kidney, liver and cardiac functions, nutritional status, and patient expectations.
- The patient's disease—some assessment of the rate and extent of harm caused by the disease and the patient's perception of these factors.
- The patient's pharmacotherapy—the risk is determined by an assessment of the toxicity of the drug therapy, the ADR profile, the route and techniques of administration, and the patient's perception of these three elements.

1 Strand LM (1991). Pharmaceutical care: challenge of implementation. ASHP Annual Meeting **48**: PI–28.

Medication problem checklist

The following list covers the range of potential medication problems that could be encountered by pharmacists seeking to deliver pharmaceutical care:

- Medications without medical indications.
- Medical conditions for which there are no medications prescribed.
- Medications prescribed inappropriately for a particular medical condition.
- Inappropriate medication dose, dosage form, schedule, route of administration or method of administration.
- Therapeutic duplication.
- Prescribing of medications to which the patient is allergic.
- Actual and potential ADEs.
- Actual and potential adverse clinically significant drug–drug, drug–disease, drug–nutrient and drug–laboratory test interactions.
- Interference with medical therapy by social or recreational drug use.
- Failure to receive the full benefit of prescribed medication therapy.
- Problems arising from the financial impact of medication therapy on the patient.
- Lack of understanding of the medication therapy by the patient.
- Failure of the patient to adhere to the medication regimen.

There have been a number of attempts to formulate these problems into an easily remembered checklist. One of these is called PRIME, which is an acronym for **P**harmaceutical-**R**isks to patients, **I**nterventions **M**ismatch between medications and indications and **E**fficiency issues. Table 13.1. The key message behind these detailed checklists is that pharmacists must move from a prescription focus to a patient focus.

Table 13.1 PRIME pharmacotherapy problem types

Pharmaceutical—assess for incorrect factors, as follows:

- Dosage
- Form
- Route
- Timing
- Duration
- Frequency.

Risks to patients—assess for risks, as follows:

- Known contraindication
- Medication allergy
- Drug-induced problem
- Improper use (ie risk if misused)
- Common/serious ADEs
- Medication-error considerations.

Interactions—assess for the following:

- Drug–drug
- Drug–disease/condition
- Drug–food
- Drug–laboratory test.

Mismatch between medications and indications/conditions—assess for the following:

- Medication used without indication
- Indications/condition untreated.

Efficacy issues—assess for the following:

- Suboptimal selection of pharmacotherapy for indications
- Minimal or no evidence of therapeutic effectiveness
- Suboptimal pharmacotherapy (taking/receiving medications incorrectly)—eg patient preference considerations (undesirable prior experiences with medications or, does not believe it works)
- Medications availability considerations (eg no access to medications)
- Compliance/administration considerations (eg inability to pay or unable to administer correctly or at all).

Pharmaceutical care economics

Clinical pharmacy services can be perceived as expensive by hospital managers. The reality is that clinical pharmacy can significantly improve patient outcomes and ↓ drug budgets. These data are presented as a sample of what is available in the wider pharmacy literature and can be used to improve facilities and funding.

Clinical pharmacy interventions ↓ costs. Bond[1] in a large annual pharmacy staff survey, showed that each whole-time pharmacist ↓ the drug budget by approximately US $22 000/ hospital and that each US dollar spent on a pharmacist resulted in savings of just under US $50 in the drug budget. The same survey, in a different report,[2] also showed that although there was no association between number of medical staff and hospital mortality rates, pharmacists were one group demonstrating ↓ mortality rates as staffing levels ↑. The authors were unable to identify reasons for this finding but surmised that preventing adverse events could be significant. In yet another report on the same data the authors claim that hospitals that provide the services outlined in the Table 13.2 within their pharmacy are associated with a reduction in deaths.

An Australian trial on fee for service[3] demonstrated savings in the intervention group. This was a randomized controlled trial of four parallel groups of community pharmacies conducted in 1996.

The numbers in each group are small, but the authors claim that it was based on sufficient differences in intervention rates. The basic education covered drug information, attendance on hospital-ward rounds, basic therapeutics and problem solving. The advanced course included a weekend university-based course, covering complex medication reviews, attendance on ward rounds, advanced therapeutics, multiple co-existing disease states and problem solving. The cost was A $1500/ person.

Outcomes were based on cost savings or healthcare costs avoided based on healthcare costs increased charges in medication costs, pharmacy times and telephone calls.

1 Bond CA, Raehl CL, Franke T (1999). Clinical pharmacy services, pharmacist staffing, and drug costs in United States hospitals. *Pharmacotherapy* **19(12)**: 1354–62.
2 Bond CA, Raehl CL, Pitterle ME, Franke T (1999). Health care professional staffing, hospital characteristics and hospital mortality rates. *Pharmacotherapy* **19(2)**: 130–8.
3 Benrimoj SI, Langford JH, Berry G, Collins RL, Stewart K *et al.* (2000). Economic impact of increased clinical intervention rated in community pharmacy. *Pharmacoeconomics* **18(5)**: 459–68.

Table 13.2

Service	Reduction in mortality
Clinical research service	195 deaths/hospital/yr
DI services	41 deaths/hospital/yr
Drug-administration histories	128 deaths/hospital/yr
Pharmacist on CPR team	18 deaths/hospital/yr

The savings were as follows (except in group D which showed on ↑ in costs):

- Group C   Professional fee + advanced education $85/1000 prescriptions
- Group B   Professional fee + basic education $26/1000 prescriptions
- Group A   No fee or education $14/1000 prescriptions
- Group D   Professional fee + no education $1/1000 prescriptions

The study is particularly interesting because a fee for services alone did not ↓ costs; the most effective contribution was a fee plus advanced education.

Staffing

This information is provided to help clinical pharmacists make a case for establishing additional clinical services. There is good evidence that ↑ clinical pharmacy time has a major, positive affect on budgets.

Work by Bond and Raehl[1,2] was referred to in the monograph on pharmaceutical care.[3] These authors have been responsible for regular useful publications in the USA. Bond and Raehl are based at the Texas Tech University Health Services Centre. Although the work is hospital-based, it does give an indication of the investment being made. The National Clinical Pharmacy Services study is seen as the largest hospital-based pharmacy database in the USA. The work involved a postal questionnaire to >3500 acute-care hospitals that have >50 beds. The percentages of patients receiving clinical pharmacy services was calculated for each hospital during a 10yr period from 1989–1998. Pharmacists numbers ↑ by 23%, pharmacy technicians numbers ↑ by 43% and pharmacy clerk numbers ↑ by 25%. This is in contrast to a rise in total hospital personnel of 55%. This represented an ↑ from 4.2(±2.6) pharmacists/100 occupied beds to 5.35(±2.7) pharmacists/100 occupied beds in 1995—An ↑ of 5% per annum[4].

Although 71% of hospitals surveyed stated that pharmacists had the authority to document pharmaceutical care in patient's notes, in practice this happens in only 31% of hospitals. When the levels of pharmaceutical care were analysed according to the training of the hospital, it was found that 64% of hospitals training PharmD students provided pharmaceutical care, which fell to 42% of hospitals who trained graduates and 33% of nonpharmacy teaching hospitals.[5] By 1998, 52% of hospitals provided some level of pharmaceutical care and time spent had ↑ to a mean of 25mins/patient/day.[3]

The authors analysed the total cost of care in relation to clinical pharmacy services for earlier (1992) data in a population of 1016 hospitals. Although the study was designed to show relationships rather than cause and effect, there is a strong hint that establishing additional clinical pharmacists is associated with a ↓ total care cost; conversely, an ↑ in the number of dispensing pharmacists is associated with a ↑ total cost of care.

1 Bond CA, Raehl CL, Franke T (1999). Clinical pharmacy services, pharmacist staffing, and drug costs in United States Hospitals. *Pharmacotherapy* **19(12)**: 1354–62.
2 Bond CA, Raehl CL, Pitterle ME, Franke T (1999). Health care professional staffing, hospital characteristics and hospital mortality rates. *Pharmacotherapy* **19(2)**: 130–8.
3 Raehl CL, Bond CA (2000). (1998). National Clinical Pharmacy Services Study. *Pharmacotherapy* **20(4)**: 436–60.
4 Bond CA, Raehl CL, Pitterle ME (1999). Staffing and the cost of clinical and hospital pharmacy service in United States hospitals. *Pharmacotherapy* **19(6)**: 767–81.
5 Raehl CL, Bond CA , Pitterle ME (1998). Clinical pharmacy services in hospital educating pharmacy students. *Pharmacotheraphy* **18(5)**: 1093–102.

Standards for research

Pharmaceutical care is an obvious research area for pharmacists, but much of the publications in this area have been of poor quality. Two checklists are presented here in to aid those who read pharmaceutical-care literature and for those who undertake research into pharmaceutical care.

A review of pharmaceutical care by Kennie et al[1]. led to the authors to make 15 recommendations' which are aimed at improving the quality of further research:

- Pharmacists must exercise discipline when using the term 'pharmaceutical care'.
- Database systems should take measures to ensure that pharmaceutical-care research literature can be correctly and easily extracted.
- A standard reporting method should be adopted that clearly describes the pharmaceutical-care process in the research methodology.
- Randomized controlled studies should be conducted to measure the affect of the provision of pharmaceutical care.
- Pharmaceutical-care research should contain a clear description of the pharmacy practice setting and patient demographics.
- Consistent methods for data collection for different practice sites should be created and validated.
- Informed consent should be obtained for all patients involved in pharmaceutical research, and the procedure should be stated.
- A pharmacist's qualifications and/or certification in providing pharmaceutical care should be addressed and described.
- Pharmaceutical-care research should not only emphasise the evaluation of patient outcomes, but must also first evaluate the structures that exist for the provision of pharmaceutical care.
- The three aspects of evaluation (ie structure, process and outcome) should be linked when assessing the quality of pharmaceutical care.
- The economic impact of pharmaceutical care should be evaluated.
- Standards for pharmaceutical-care research should be developed and accepted by the profession.
- Further pharmaceutical-care research needs to be conducted, with an emphasis on community based pharmacy.
- A pharmaceutical-care research network should be developed to co-ordinate efforts and identify areas where research is required.
- Research should be conducted to determine the feasibility and extent of implementing pharmaceutical care in various practice sites.

The authors concluded that few studies have evaluated the provision of pharmaceutical care in a defined population, and that the volume of research is painfully low.

1 Kennie NR, Schuster BG, Einarson TR (1998). Critical analysis of the pharmaceutical care research literature. *Annals of Pharmacotherapy* **32(1)**: 17–26.

Plumridge *et al.*[2] stated that research into patient perceptions and the patient–pharmacist relationship are needed, because these are critical success factors for pharmaceutical care. Patient understanding and involvement in the process are essential. Furthermore, reliable information is required about patients' willingness to pay for pharmaceutical care. Currently, a dilemma exists because pharmacists want to charge for services but cannot demonstrate improvements on clinical, economic or quality-of-life outcomes.

When research is undertaken, the pharmaceutical-care process used should be such that the study results can be critically analysed and the process replicated as necessary.

The authors made 13 recommendations for future research, which overlap with the previous list above but are worth listing, as follows:

- The paucity of published studies on the economic value of pharmaceutical care reinforces the requirement for additional, well-conducted research in appropriate practice settings to address the high cost of drug-related morbidity and mortality. Descriptive reports, or inadequately conducted studies, of the pharmaceutical-care process do little to advance our present knowledge.
- Studies should use, and be refereed on, the correct definition of pharmaceutical care. If this is not done, the confusion that already exists with other pharmaceutical interventions will be exacerbated.
- The quality of pharmaceutical care requires the development of systems for documenting delivery processes and outcomes. Systems for documenting patient satisfaction are also required.
- Variable study design and lack of standardization in reporting causes difficulties in comparing study results. Uniformity is desirable for comparative purposes and to enable valid conclusions to be made.
- Comparative groups must be more fully described and consistent with intervention groups. Patients should be randomized.
- Evidence that external factors affecting outcomes have been controlled is desirable.
- Practice settings should be fully described to enable readers to understand the processes used, facilitate replication and further develop future pharmaceutical-care practice.
- All relevant direct and indirect costs should be considered. When this is achieved, attempts to use appropriate pharmacoeconomic methods (eg cost-effectiveness and cost–benefit analyses) can be considered. These will probably require specialist expertise.
- Structure and process should be described and appropriate outcome measures used. Process measures, intermediate outcomes indicators and outcomes need to be correctly identified because these terms are often confused by researchers. If feasible, the link between structure, process and outcomes should be evaluated.
- Outcomes must be identified in terms of the feasible effect of pharmaceutical care because certain outcomes can present difficulty in measurement (eg outcomes requiring years to observe, such as the treatment of osteoporosis).

2 Plumridge RJ, Wojnar Horton RE (1998). A review of the pharmacoeconomics of pharmaceutical care. *Pharmacoeconomics*. **14(2)**: 175–89.

- Research is needed to determine the value that specific interventions have on health outcomes so effect is optimized. This includes identifying structures and processes that improve specific health outcomes and types of outcomes that are most effected by pharmaceutical-care programmes.
- Each study should attempt to address relevant pharmacoeconomic parameters, including clinical, economic and quality of life.
- The potential for assessing opportunity costs, especially because healthcare resources are in cost-containment mode, should be considered. This is important in determining the best way of implementing pharmaceutical care as practice is evolving.

Medicines management

Medicines management

Medicines management is made up of two components:
- Clinical and cost-effective use of medicines.
- The safe and secure handling of medicines.

Each hospital should have a strategic plan for medicines management, which reflects the following:
- The strategic direction for the local health economy.
- Priorities of the local population.
- Targets relating to NSFs and implementation of National Institute for Health and Clinical Excellence (NICE) guidance.
- Communication strategy for the dissemination of information.

Hospitals should ensure the following systems are in place to ensure effective medicines management:
- Drug and therapeutics committee (or equivalent).
- Targeting clinical-pharmacy activity to patients requiring early assessment following hospital admission.
- Patients should have a complete DHx review within 24h of hospital admission.
- Acute medical admissions should be prioritized, and if possible, seen by a pharmacist.
- PODs should be used if they have been reviewed and considered suitable for continued use.
- As appropriate, all patients should be given the option of self-administering their own medicines while in hospital.
- Dispensing for discharge (or one-stop dispensing) systems should be in place to ensure that patients receive their discharge medication in sufficient quantity and in a timely manner, with the appropriate patient information leaflet.

The multidisciplinary team should be trained on medicines management:
- All doctors, nurses and pharmacists and other relevant healthcare professionals should receive training on medicines management as part of their induction program, including the legislative and GCP aspects of controls assurance (in particular, the safe and secure handling of medicines) and clinical and cost-effective use of medicines.
- Medicines management systems and policies should be incorporated into ongoing clinical training programmes.
- Information technology system support should be available to provide healthcare staff with accurate information on the use of medicines.
- The risk of medication errors occurring should be minimized.

Medicines management policies and procedures should be in place to minimize the risk of medication errors occurring during the medication process, ie for prescribing, dispensing and administration.

Further reading

Department of Health (2003). *A Vision for Pharmacy in the new NHS*. London.
Audit Commission (2001). *A Spoonful of Sugar*. London.
Smith J (2004). *Building a Safer NHS for Patients: Improving Medication Safety*. Department of Health: London.

Evaluating new drugs

New drugs appear on the market all the time and healthcare professionals are constantly bombarded with promotional material from the pharmaceutical industry. The pharmaceutical industry's business is to sell drugs—otherwise, it would not survive—but promotional material should be reviewed with a critical eye.

Just because a drug has received regulatory approval, does not necessarily mean that it is a clinically significant advance, because regulatory authorities evaluate quality, safety and efficacy not therapeutic value. Assessments of the value of new drugs from Canada, France and USA have shown that, at best, only one-third offer some additional clinical benefit and as few as 3% are a major therapeutic advance.[1]

Premarketing trials are often placebo controlled, so they don't give comparative data. Ideally, the trial should compare the new drug with an established reference treatment. Even if the trial compares the new drug with a reference treatment, it might be too small or short to provide meaningful data—in particular, rare ADRs or differences in response in subgroups of patients are unlikely to be identified.

Much of the data presented by the pharmaceutical industry is disease-orientated rather than patient-orientated, and this can make a difference to the patient outcome. For example, disease-orientated evidence (DOE) demonstrates that cyclo-oxygenase 2 NSAIDs cause fewer endoscopically detected ulcers than standard NSAIDs; however, many of these ulcers would not be clinically significant. A more relevant evaluation is to determine the difference between cyclo-oxygenase 2 NSAIDs and standard NSAIDs in causing symptomatic or bleeding ulcers. This latter approach is known as 'patient-orientated evidence that matters' (POEM) and is more relevant to clinical practice.

The STEPS acronym is a useful tool for evaluating new drugs:[2]
• Safety—evaluate the safety of the new drug versus a standard reference preparation, ideally using comparison studies that reflect the real life situation. Pharmaceutical companies often highlight differences in ADRs that are relatively trivial or rare. Check especially for ADRs that would place the patient at particular risk, notably the following:
  • Liver, kidney or bone-marrow toxicity.
  • Cardiovascular events.
  • CNS events—eg fits.
  • Significant skin or hypersensitivity reactions—eg Stevens Johnson syndrome.
  • GI bleeding.
  • Congenital abnormalities.
Look at the frequency of these events versus the significance of the disease. A 5% risk of hepatotoxicity in a life-threatening disease is a more acceptable level of risk than if the disease is self-limiting.

1 Lexchin J (2004). Are new drugs as good as they claim to be? *Australian Prescriber* **27**: 2–3.
2 Preskorn SH (1994). Antidepressant drug selection: criteria and options. *Journal of Clinical Psychiatry* **55**(suppl A): 6–22, 23–4, 98–100.

- Tolerability—are side effects likely to affect adherence? Look at drop-out rates in clinical trials, if there is a high drop-out rate because of ADRs versus the reference drug, this makes the new drug of less therapeutic value. If patients don't take the drug, it won't work!
- Effectiveness—look at head to head trials of the new drug versus the reference drug, rather than comparing different trials. Ask 'does this new drug work as well or better than the reference drug?'. The NNT is the best way of assessing therapeutic value. If the NNT of the new drug is the same or lower than the reference drug, it is worth considering.
- Price—consider all the costs associated with the new drug versus the reference, not just the purchase price. This might include the following:
  - Administration cost—eg IV giving sets.
  - Monitoring costs.
  - Additional time/travel if patient has to attend more frequently at the start of therapy.
- Simplicity of use—is it relatively easy for the patient to use the drug? This would include considering the following:
  - Dosage schedule.
  - Number of tablets.
  - Liquid versus tablets.
  - Parenteral versus enteral administration.
  - Special storage requirements—eg refrigeration.

Table 14.1 WHO criteria for drugs selection[1]

- On the WHO essential-drug list.
- Relevance to pattern of prevalent disease.
- Proven efficacy and safety.
- Evidence of performance in different settings.
- Adequate quality, bioavailability, and safety.
- Favourable cost–benefit ratio, in terms of total treatment cost.
- Preference for drugs that are well known or familiar to use and locally manufactured.
- Single compounds.

---

1 World Health Organization (1988). *How to develop and implement a national drug policy.* Second edition. http://whqlibdoc.who.int/publications/924154547X.pdf

How to write a drug protocol

Drug protocols are evidence-based documents that specify the indications for which a drug treatment can be prescribed within defined clinical settings. They help to ensure that drugs are used cost-effectively and safely within the hospital setting.

The need for a drug protocol is usually highlighted for an area by the multidisciplinary team. Initially, the evidence base must be established. Literature searches, protocols from other hospitals, and information on local practice are used as the basis for the protocol.

Ensure that local practice is followed to implement new drug protocols. This might include approval by a hospital committee, such as a drugs and therapeutics committee.

A drug protocol should include the following:
- Drug name—international-approved name and trade name.
- Formulation.
- Dose.
- Frequency of administration.
- Administration details.
- Side effects and their treatment.
- Dose reductions required for changes in organ function—eg impaired renal or liver function.
- Drug interactions.
- Indications for use.
- Place in therapy—eg if another option should be tried first (especially if use is restricted).
- Restrictions of use.
- Cost.
- References.

Unlicensed use of medicines

- The product licence of a medication defines the therapeutic purpose for which the product can be used.
- Unlicensed medicines have not been formally assessed through the licensing process for safety, quality and efficacy. The risks associated with their use might not have been evaluated.
- If a prescriber uses a licensed medicine for an unlicensed indication, this is outside its product licence.
- The same principles apply to unlicensed medicines as for licensed medicines used for unlicensed indications (off-label), eg in paediatrics (see Medicines for children, p.222).
- Medicines that are not covered by a product licence include the following:
  - Medicines prepared by a manufacturer but not on sale in this country. A specialist importer can obtain these.
  - Medicines prepared for a specified patient in accordance with a prescriber's instructions. This includes any form of extemporaneous dispensing.
  - Unlicensed medicines obtained from a hospital or a commercial supplier with a special manufacturing licence. These medicines are often known as 'specials'.
  - Repacked medicines—the product licence regulates the container in which a medicine is sold. If a medicine is removed from its original container and repacked, it technically becomes an unlicensed product.
- Implications for the prescriber, pharmacist and nurses of prescribing, dispensing and administering unlicensed medicines are as follows:
  - Prescribers need to be aware of the license status of medicines they prescribe. The responsibility of prescribing unlicensed medicines lies with the prescriber. The manufacturer takes no responsibility for any safety or efficacy of unlicensed medicines.
  - A pharmacist shares the responsibility with the prescriber, as the product purchaser, or if the pharmacist's actions or omissions have contributed to any harm.
  - Pharmacists should ensure the prescriber is aware that they are prescribing an unlicensed drug, or a drug outside its licence.
  - Nurses are responsible for administering medication that is administered outside of its licence and must ensure the relevant hospital policies have been adhered to.
- A hospital should have a clear written policy for the 'use of unlicensed medicines', outlining the responsibilities of all those involved in the prescribing, purchase, supply and administration of this category of medicines. It should be a summary document, supported by standard operating procedures and making reference to existing documents and sources of information. The drugs and therapeutics committee, or equivalent, should approve this.

- The use of unlicensed medicines in a hospital needs to be controlled and monitored. A risk assessment should be undertaken before an unlicensed medicine, or medicine outside its licence, is prescribed. This is often done through the drugs and therapeutics committee, or equivalent.
- Written notification, signed by the prescriber and returned to the pharmacy department, is usually used. This usually includes the patient details, the name of the product and its specification, reason for using an unlicensed medicine, and the prescriber's name and signature. The manufacturer, date ordered, quantity ordered and batch number received are usually recorded in the pharmacy department. Check what documentation is used in your local hospital.
- Some hospitals require that informed consent is obtained from patients for some unlicensed medicines to be supplied, eg thalidomide.
- Prescribing a medicine by a route for which it is not licensed is unlicensed but is often 'accepted practice', eg cyclizine.

Further reading

Department of Health (2003). *A Vision for Pharmacy in the new NHS.* DoH: London.

Parkinson R, Beaney A, Phillips M (2004). Guidance for the purchase and supply of unlicensed medicinal products notes for prescribers and pharmacists, 3rd edn. NHS Pharmaceutical Quality Assurance Committee. www.quinfozone.nhs.uk

Drug and therapeutics committees

Each hospital has a drug and therapeutics committee, or an equivalent committee. This committee is responsible for ensuring that the introduction of new drugs to the hospital formulary is cost-effective, safe and has an acceptable evidence base. Before new drugs are bought by the pharmacy department and used in the hospital, they need to be approved by the drug and therapeutics committee using the principles of EBM. The ↑ cost of new drugs being licensed causes financial pressures to hospitals, which leads to some prioritization of drugs available for use.

Generally, the membership of a drug and therapeutics committee comprises representatives from the following disciplines:
- Medical staff—including medical director, surgeon, anaesthetist, clinical pharmacologist and paediatrician.
- Nurse (chief nurse or nominee).
- Pharmacist—chief pharmacist and medicines management/formulary pharmacist.
- Finance (director or nominee).
- Commissioner.
- Primary care prescribing lead.
- Specialists—eg paediatrics, oncology, or clinical pharmacology.
- Public health.
- Medical microbiologist.
- Patient representative/lay member.
- Management.
- Administration.
- Executive board member (if not one of the above).
- Other members are co-opted, as needed.

The drug and therapeutics committee should have terms of reference and membership list. In addition to making decisions on the introduction of new medicines into a hospital according to assessment of the clinical evidence, a drug and therapeutics committee can also have a role in the following areas:
- Maintenance and updating of a hospital formulary.
- Review of medicines expenditure.
- Horizon scanning of medicines to be licensed or those with national approval .
- Prioritization of new drugs.
- Overseeing safe medication-practice systems, including maintaining policies and procedures for medicines, overseeing education and training for safe medication practice and analysing medication error incident reports.

Evidence that is used by drug and therapeutics committee includes the following:
- Results of clinical trials.
- Scientific evidence.
- Cost-effectiveness.
- Safety.
- Effect of adopting a new drug.

- Pre-existing prescribing.
- Decisions of drug and therapeutics committees in other hospitals.
- Restrictions of use of a new drug.

Drug and therapeutics committees should meet regularly (monthly or bimonthly). Decisions made at the committee meetings are made available through minutes, newsletters, e-mail or intranets.

Further reading

Fullerton DS, Atherly DS (2004). Formularies, therapeutics, and outcomes: new opportunities. *Medicine Care.* **42(4 Suppl):**III39–44.

Jenkings KN, Barber N (2004). What constitutes evidence in hospital new drug decision making? *Social Science Medicine.* **58(9):**1757–66.

Martin DK, Hollenberg D, MacRae S, *et al.* (2003). Priority setting in a hospital drug formulary: a qualitative case study and evaluation. *Health Policy* **66(3):**295–303.

Schumock GT, Walton SM, Park HY, *et.al.* (2004). Factors that influence prescribing decisions. *Annals Pharmacotherapy* **38(4):**557–62.

Department of Health. *A Vision for Pharmacy in the new NHS* (2003). DoH: London. www.doh.gov.uk

Patient group directions (PGDs)

Definition

- Written instruction for the sale, supply and/or administration of a named medicine for a defined clinical condition.
- PGDs allow a range of specified healthcare professionals to supply and/or administer a medicine including PODs directly to a patient with an identified clinical condition, without them necessarily seeing a prescriber. The healthcare professional working within the PGD is responsible for assessing that the patient fits the criteria set out in the PGD.
- Implementing PGDs might be appropriate both in circumstances where groups of patients might not have been previously identified (eg minor injuries and first-contact services) and in services where assessment and treatment follows a clearly predictable pattern (eg immunization and family planning).
- In general, a PGD is not meant to be a long-term means of managing a patient's clinical condition. This is best achieved by a healthcare professional prescribing for an individual patient on a one-to-one basis.
- Legal requirements and guidance on PGDs are set out in the circular HSC 2000/026.

Health professionals allowed to use PGDs

Nurses, midwifes, health visitors, optometrists, pharmacists, chiropodists, radiographers, othoptists, physiotherapists and ambulance paramedics.

The pharmacist's role in PGDs

- Apart from developing practice using a PGD, pharmacists are expected to be involved in various aspects of PGDs.
- Development of a PGD for other healthcare professionals.
- Responsibility to ensure that only fully competent, qualified and trained professionals operate within PGDs.
- Organization of arrangements for the security, storage and labelling of PGD medicines; such medicines would normally be expected to be supplied prepackaged, and *robust reconciliation system for stock use is established.*
- Checking that the use of the medicine outlined in a specific PGD is consistent with the summary of product characteristics, although off-licence use could be considered in exceptional circumstances, providing it is justified by current best-clinical practice.

Further reading

A practical guide and framework of competencies for all professionals using Patient Group Directions. www.npc.co.uk/publications/pgd/pgd.pdf
National Electronic Library for Medicines. www.nelm.nhs.uk/pgd/default.aspx
Department of Health website (UK) has PGDs for drugs and chemical and biological counter measures. www.dh.gov.uk

Supplementary prescribing

Supplementary prescribing

Pharmacists in the UK can train to become supplementary prescribers. It is mandatory that specific supplementary prescribing training is undertaken at a designated university, followed by a period of supervised practice.

Definition

Supplementary prescribing is a 'voluntary partnership between an independent prescriber (doctor or dentist) and a supplementary prescriber to implement an agreed patient-specific clinical management plan with the patient's agreement.'

There are some key principles that underpin supplementary prescribing. These principles emphasise the importance of the prescribing partners. The prescribing partners include the independent prescriber, supplementary prescriber and patient:

- The independent prescriber is responsible for the assessment and diagnosis of patients, and deciding on the clinical management required, which includes prescribing.
- The supplementary prescriber is responsible for prescribing for patients who have been clinically assessed by the independent prescriber, according to an agreed patient-specific clinical management plan.
- The patient must be treated as a partner in their care and be involved at all stages of decision making, including the decision for part of their care to be delivered by supplementary prescribing.

The criteria that are set in regulations for lawful supplementary prescribing include the following:

- The independent prescriber must be a doctor (or dentist).
- The supplementary prescriber must be a registered nurse, midwife or a pharmacist.
- The patient must be involved in the decision for a supplementary prescriber to be involved in their care. The patient must be provided with written information and informed consent must be obtained from the patient before supplementary prescribing starts.
- There must be a written clinical management plan relating to a named patient and to that patient's specific conditions. Both the independent and supplementary prescribers must record agreement to the plan before supplementary prescribing begins.
- The independent and supplementary prescribers must share access to, consult and use the same common patient record.

There are no legal restrictions on the clinical conditions that supplementary prescribers can treat, and there is no specific formulary or list of medicines for supplementary prescribing. The independent and supplementary prescribers decide when supplementary prescribing is appropriate and when the clinical management plan is drawn up (Figure 14.1). The medicines to be prescribed by the supplementary prescriber must be prescribed by an independent prescriber at NHS's expense and referred to in the patient's clinical management plan. Some of the areas where supplementary prescribing might be of most benefit include the treatment of long-term medical conditions, such as asthma, coronary heart disease or patients requiring anti-coagulation.

Hospital name and department
Clinical management plan

Name of patient:
Patient medication sensitivities/allergies:
Patient identification (eg ID number or, date of birth):
Independent prescriber(s): Name and profession
Supplementary prescriber(s): Name and profession

Condition(s) to be treated:
Might be specific indications or broader terms and might also include treating side effects of specified drugs/classes of drug (eg treatment of HIV and related opportunistic infections/complications or treatment of side effects of antiretrovirals and other drugs used in the treatment of HIV).

Aim of treatment:

Medicines that could be prescribed by supplementary prescriber:
    Preparation
    Drug names and preparations
    Can also be drug classes (eg antiretrovirals)
    Indication—doesn't have to be very specific
    Dose schedule—doesn't have to be very specific (eg could say 'as *BNF*')

Specific indications for referral back to the independent prescriber:

Guidelines or protocols supporting the clinical management plan:

Frequency of review and monitoring by:
Supplementary prescriber
Supplementary prescriber and independent prescriber

Process for reporting ADRs:

Shared record to be used by independent prescriber and supplementary prescriber:
Agreed by independent prescriber(s): (signature and name)

Agreed by supplementary prescriber(s): (signature and name)

Date agreed with patient/carer:

Fig. 14.1 Example of a clinical management plan for supplementary prescribers

Supplementary prescribers are able to prescribe:
- All general sales list (GSL), pharmacy medicines, appliances and devices, foods and other borderline substances approved by the advisory committee on borderline substances.
- All POMs.
- Controlled drugs .
- Medicines for use outside of their licensed indications (ie 'off-label' prescribing), 'black-triangle' drugs and drugs marked 'less suitable for prescribing' in the *BNF*.
- Unlicensed drugs that are part of a clinical trial, which has a clinical trial certificate or exemption.

Benefits of supplementary prescribing include the following:
- Quicker access to medicines for patients.
- ↑ efficiency.
- ↓ in doctor's workload.
- Improved use of skill mix.

The supplementary prescriber should not be required to enter into a prescribing partnership that entails them prescribing any medicine that they do not feel competent to prescribe. It is recommended that pharmacists prescribe generically if possible, except where this would not be clinically appropriate or if there is no approved generic name.

Further reading

Department of Health supplementary prescribing. www.doh.gov.uk/PolicyAndGuidance/

Community (FP10) prescription use in hospitals

Hospital out-patient departments can use community (FP10) prescriptions, according to local policy. In the UK, these are prescriptions that can be written by hospital doctors and dispensed by a community pharmacy, ↓ workload of busy pharmacy departments.

Who is it appropriate to use them for?

- Patients who are mobile and can easily get to a community pharmacy.
- Patients requiring an item that cannot be easily obtained by the hospital pharmacy.
- Patients who don't have time or would rather not wait in the hospital pharmacy.
- Patients on hospital transport who are unable to wait in the hospital pharmacy.

Who is it inappropriate to use them for?

- Patients requiring expensive items, unless they are part of a shared-care arrangement.
- Patients on clinical trials.
- Patients on drugs that are only available from hospitals.
- Patients requiring items that can be purchased without a prescription.
- Patients on complex therapy who may need counselling, but might miss out if they don't attend the hospital pharmacy.

Things to remember

- These prescriptions incur a dispensing fee for each item prescribed.
- Prescriptions are removed from the hospital and dispensed by community pharmacists and, as such, could be vulnerable to loss or tampering.
- The pharmacist who dispenses the prescription might not be familiar with prescribing habits or handwriting.
- It is very difficult for the dispensing pharmacist to contact the doctor in the event of error, omission or illegible prescribing.
- The hospital is charged the commercial costs, in addition to the dispensing fees for the items prescribed.
- The hospital is reimbursed for any prescription charge, so for cheaper items, they can be cheaper or issued without charge.
- Drugs supplied are value-added-tax (VAT) exempt; hence, some drug supply might be cost-effective to prescribe on FP10 prescriptions.

Electronic prescribing

Electronic prescribing systems are available commercially and are fully implemented by some hospitals, often linked to a patient-management system. All prescribing in secondary care, within the UK must be undertaken electronically by 2008.

Some systems ensure a paper-free environment, because an electronic prescription is used for patient care, electronic signatures are used for drug administration and electronic transfer is used for ordering drugs from the pharmacy. Fully implemented electronic systems can mean that all patient records are electronic.

Electronic prescribing systems are often intelligent and flag areas of drug interaction, incorrect dosing, other prescribing errors, additional information required for safe drug administration and formulary issues. These systems require input and maintenance by pharmacy and information technology teams.

High-risk areas, such as chemotherapy prescribing, should be implemented as a high priority. Most cancer hospitals and networks are working towards electronic prescribing systems for oral and injectable chemotherapy to minimize the risks associated with the prescribing and administration of these drugs.

Pharmacy staff using an electronic prescribing system require training in its use before working with the system. These systems have various levels of security, depending on the role of the professional in the use of the system. It is essential that there is good security for any electronic prescribing system, with frequent back-ups, and a system must be in place in case of system failure. Standard operating procedures should be in place for all aspects of the system.

The benefits of electronic prescribing include the following:
- Safer use of medicines.
- ↓ of medication errors.
- Improved quality and safety of prescribing.
- Improved safety of prescribing medication to patients with drug allergies.
- Prescriptions are legible.
- Accessibility of information between primary care and secondary care.
- Improved patient compliance with protocols.
- Management of formulary compliance.
- Supports decision making when prescribing.
- Implementation of policy decisions.
- Improved use of staff time.
- Pharmacy early identification of new scripts for screening and supply.
- Audit trail of transactions.
- Drug-usage reports for individual patients.
- Aids clinical audit.

Further reading

Smith J (2004). *Building a safer NHS for patients: improving medication safety*. London: Department of Health.

Incident reporting

- Each hospital should have a policy in place for the reporting of incidents. An incident reporting policy often covers all incidents, including adverse events, hazards and near misses of an adverse event or hazard. Such a policy applies to all hospital staff. An induction programme to a hospital usually covers details of any local policy.
- An incident-reporting programme identifies, assesses and manages risks that could compromise or threaten the quality of patient services or staff working in safe environment, as part of the overall management of risk. It is a confidential process, and all staff should complete the appropriate documentation if they are involved in, or aware of, an incident.
- An 'incident' is usually defined as an event or circumstance that could have, or did, lead to unintended or unexpected harm, loss or damage. Incidents might involve actual or potential injury, damage, loss, fire, theft, violence, abuse, accidents, ill health and infection.
- It is necessary for incidents to be reported to ensure that the hospital can analyse the data for trends, causes and costs. Action plans can then be developed to minimize future similar incidents. Reporting of incidents is also a mechanism for staff to input into change of practice and procedures. Incident reporting follows a 'no-blame' culture.
- Medication incidents must be reported through this mechanism to ensure that there can be a review of trends, a root-cause analysis, arrangements for improvement and follow-up audit. This is a requirement of medicines management in hospitals.
- The type of incident that a pharmacist can report includes medication errors and failure of a system or process that affects patient care.
- In addition to reporting an incident, a pharmacist must also deal with an incident by communicating with the relevant members of staff involved (see p.66).

Further reading

Department of Health (2003). *A Vision for Pharmacy in the new NHS*. DoH: London.

Medical representatives

- Medical representatives provide information to healthcare practitioners, but their prime function is to promote and sell their products and services.
- Medical representatives should provide their service according to The Association of the British Pharmaceutical Industry (ABPI) code of practice (or similar). If the code of practice is breached, medical representatives can be reported to the director of the Prescription Medicines Code of Practice Authority (PMCPA).
- Most hospitals have a policy for dealing with medical representatives—check the local policy.
- Some hospitals do not allow medical representatives to leave samples. Check the policy for the local hospital before accepting trial samples from medical representatives.
- It is GCP for medical representatives to make an appointment before meeting with a member of staff. Some hospital policies restrict the grades of staff that are allowed to meet with medical representatives.
- Medical representatives are not allowed to promote unlicensed indications for their products or products that have not yet been licensed; however, they are allowed to answer specific questions on unlicensed use (see p.278).
- Hospital drug prices are confidential to the hospital and under no circumstance must they be revealed to a medical representative.
- Most hospitals limit the level of hospitality provided by representatives. For example, it is reasonable for representatives to provide food for a working lunch, but not expensive meals at a restaurant.

Further reading

Guidance notes for health professionals, understanding the ABPI code of practice for the pharmaceutical industry and controls on the promotion of prescription medicines in the UK. www.abpi.org.uk

Overseas visitors

- The term 'overseas visitor' is used for patients who have fallen ill unexpectedly while visiting the UK and who, consequently, require standard NHS emergency care.
- People who do not normally live in the UK are not automatically entitled to use the NHS free of charge.
- Patients who are eligible for full NHS treatment include the following:
  - Anyone legally living in the UK for ≥12 months.
  - Permanent residents.
  - Students in the UK for >6 months.
  - Refugees or asylum seekers who have made an application to remain in the UK and are waiting for a decision on their immigration status.
  - People detained by the immigration authorities.
  - People from countries with a reciprocal agreement—eg European Union residents.
- Patients who are not eligible for full NHS treatment include the following:
  - Students on courses in the UK for <6 months.
  - Refugees or asylum seekers who have not yet submitted applications to the home office.
  - Those who have had an asylum application turned down and exhausted the appeals process.
  - Illegal immigrants.
- The NHS hospital is legally responsible for establishing whether patients are not normally resident in the UK.
- If patients are not eligible for free NHS care, the hospital must charge the patient for the costs of the NHS care.
- When the patient is charged is dependent on the urgency of the treatment needed:
  - For immediately necessary treatment, treatment must not be delayed or withheld while the patient's chargeable status is being established.
  - For urgent and nonurgent treatment, patients should pay a deposit equivalent to the estimated full cost of treatment in advance.
  - Any surplus can be returned to the patient on completion of the treatment.
- Treatment that is available to overseas patients free of charge is as follows:
  - Accident and emergency (A&E) visits. (However, treatment in other departments following an A&E visit, eg X-ray, is charged.)
  - Emergency or immediately necessary treatment.
  - Treatment of sexually transmitted diseases (except HIV).
  - Treatment of diseases that are a threat to public health, eg tuberculosis (TB) and acute treatment of all infectious diseases.
  - Family planning.
  - Compulsory psychiatric treatment.
- If an overseas visitor chooses to be treated privately, they are classed as an 'international private patient'. These patients are treated as private patients (see p.298).

Further reading

Department of Health (2004). Implementing the overseas visitors hospital charging regulations. London.

Department of Health—overseas visitors. www.doh.gov.uk/overseasvisitors

Pollard AJ, Savulescu J (2004). Eligibility of overseas visitors and people of uncertain residential status for NHS treatment. *British Medical Journal* **329**: 346–9.

Private patients

In the UK, patients can choose to have treatment either from the NHS, or privately. Private patients usually have private health insurance, which covers some, or all, of the costs of private treatment. Patients can be treated privately either in a private hospital or in NHS hospitals. Private patients treated in NHS hospitals are discussed in this section:

- NHS hospitals either have specific wards for private patients or private patients are treated on the same ward as NHS patients, often in a side room.
- Patients who are treated privately either have private health insurance or are paying themselves.
- Before receiving treatment, the private health insurance company must confirm what they will cover, according to the patient's insurance policy.
- Patients' drugs must be charged accurately to the private health insurance companies, to ensure that the NHS generates income from using NHS facilities to treat these patients.
- If a patient is having private treatment, this should be annotated in some way on the patient notes or identification labels.
- Any prescription for a private patient must be annotated as 'private patient' to ensure that the pharmacy department can ensure the appropriate charging for the drugs.
- Private patients do not have to pay NHS prescriptions charges.
- Charging and systems can vary for in-patients and out-patients.
- An on-cost is usually added to the drug price when charging for private-patient drugs.
- Clinical pharmacists' input into patient care for drug review and counselling might be appropriate.
- Check what systems are in place for private-patients' drugs in your hospital.
- Usually patients cannot be 'private' for one part of the treatment and NHS for another part.
- Patients can choose to change from being a private patient to an NHS patient between consultations.

Professional supervision skills

- Start with goals or an action plan for the member of staff you are supervising.
  - These should be SMART—ie **S**pecific, **M**easurable, **A**chievable, **R**elevant and **T**imescale.
  - Effective goals have five parts:
    —Intentions
    —Outcomes
    —Methods and resources
    —Midpoints and deadlines
    —Action plans.
- Prioritize the workload with your staff.
- Set timelines.
- Time management—ensure time is managed effectively.
- Listen effectively to your member of staff.
- Review and monitor action plans and progress at regular intervals.
- Support and coach, as necessary.
- Be available to discuss ways forward with the member of staff.
- Communicate the 'bigger picture', so that staff understand why tasks are being undertaken.
- Be honest.

Tips on day-to-day supervision

- Some of the above skills should be used on a daily basis to help with day-to-day supervision.
- Be aware of the workload to be covered that day and the staff available to undertake the work.
- If necessary, prioritize the day's work with the staff.
- Be available to trouble shoot.
- Support the staff with the urgent and important work, if necessary.

National Service Frameworks (NSFs)

NSFs are national standards for specified clinical areas, to ensure equality of NHS services throughout the UK.

NSFs were developed by the Department of Health, with the help of external reference groups. These groups are made up of health professionals, service users and carers, health service managers, partner agencies and other advocates. Usually, there is one new framework developed each year.

NSFs:
- Establish national standards and promote specific service models.
- Identify key interventions for a defined service or care group.
- Put in place strategies to support implementation.
- Establish ways to ensure progress within an agreed timescale.
- Are a measure to ↑ quality and ↓ variations in service within the NHS.
- Drive the delivery of the NHS modernization agenda.

NSFs developed since April 1998 include the following:
- Coronary heart disease
- Cancer
- Paediatric intensive care
- Mental health
- Older people
- Diabetes
- Long-term conditions—eg neurological
- Renal services
- Children.

Opportunities for pharmacy

Some NSFs specifically mention pharmacy or medicine-related issues:
- Become familiar with the framework standards, and consider how to contribute to the achievement of the standards.
- A pharmacist should be involved with the local implementation team responsible for the development and delivery of a service plan and identifying what has to be done to implement the NSF.
- Decide on the services that can be initiated and the relevant links to the NSF standards.
- Identify links to the local delivery plan and other local priorities.
- Participate with an existing or developing service where possible.
- Identify the opportunities for pharmacy.
- Consult with other stakeholders who can influence the development of a proposed service.
- Identify training needs to provide a new service.
- Identify the outcomes proposed—are they realistic and measurable?
- Develop a business case, which refers to the NSF, local priorities and needs, and includes integration into local services.

Further reading

Department of Health–policy and guidance: NSF. www.doh.gov.uk/Policy And Guidance

Stanley J (2004). Benchmarking the role of pharmacists in implementing NSFs. *Pharmacy Management* **20(1)**: 2–5.

Appraisal

An appraisal meeting provides a formal opportunity for managers and staff to meet and discuss job performance, achievements against objectives previously set, future work objectives and priorities, career aspirations, and training and development needs. This process should ensure that staff are clear about what they are trying to achieve and why, and managers are clear on the progress being made by everyone in their department.

Definitions

'*Appraisal*' is a dynamic, ongoing process of performance management through objectives and staff development.

'*Performance management*' is a system to align the work of individuals as closely as possible to the work of the organization.

The appraisal process

- Appraisal supports effective performance and personal development.
- Appraisals should take place annually, according to the local hospital policy.
- The line manager usually conducts the appraisal.
- Both the appraiser and the appraisee should prepare for the annual appraisal meeting. It is good practice to have at least 2wks' notice to enable an individual to have time to prepare.
- In preparation for the annual appraisal, the appraisee should list their strengths and weaknesses, achievements, and performance highs and lows for the previous 12 months.
- The annual appraisal should be conducted to ensure an open, two-way discussion, and usually lasts for ~2h.
- During the appraisal, the following areas are usually covered:
  - Introduction and purpose of an appraisal.
  - Review of the objectives set at the last appraisal, a discussion of which ones are met and resolving difficulties with those that have not been met.
  - Review of an individual's work over the past year.
  - Outline and agree future objectives.
  - Review of individuals current knowledge and skills.
  - Prioritization of areas requiring development to improve effectiveness at work.
  - Agree a personal development plan for the next year.
  - Discussion of how an individual's objectives fit within the team and organization's objectives.
  - Discussion on how the organization/line manager can help the appraisee achieve their objectives.
  - Constructive feedback on performance.
  - Recognition of an individual's performance.
  - Discussion of any of the appraisee's concerns.
  - Review of job description and plans to update it accordingly.
- There should be a paper record kept of the appraisal, which is signed by the appraisee and the appraiser.
- Review of performance should be continuous, and any concerns should be raised throughout the year and not left to the annual appraisal.

Further reading
Naisby A (ed) (2002). *Appraisal and performance management*. London: Spiro Press.

Confidentiality

Pharmacists and pharmacy staff are expected to maintain the confidentiality of any patient or customer they have contact with during the course of their professional duties. Information that should remain confidential includes the following:

- Patient's identity and address.
- Diagnosis.
- Details of prescribed and nonprescribed medicines.

Pharmacists must also ensure that at any written or electronic patient information is stored and disposed of securely and that electronic systems are password protected.

To avoid unintentional disclosure, it is important to develop good habits when dealing with patient information:

- Discussing a patient with colleagues is often necessary for patient care or training purposes, but be cautious about revealing names or other patient identifiers.
- Do not discuss patients in public areas—eg the lifts or front of the shop.
- If talking about your work to family or friends, only talk about patients in very general terms.
- Ensure written information (eg patient handover lists and, prescriptions) is not left lying where other patients or the public can see it.
- If discussing medication with a patient, try to do this in a reasonably private area. If hospital in-patients have visitors, ask if the patient would like you to return when they have gone.
- Ensure that computers have passwords and always log off at the end of a session.

Disclosure of information

In certain situations, pharmacists might have to disclose confidential information. The UK pharmacy code of ethics allows this in the following circumstances:

- With patient consent or parent/guardian/carer consent for a child or adult not competent to give consent themselves. Information about adolescent patients should not normally be revealed without their consent.
- If required by law or statute.
- If necessary to prevent serious injury or damage to the health of the patient, a third party or the public health.

The RPSGB has published a fact sheet on confidentiality, which includes guidance on disclosure of information.[1]

In addition, advice on disclosure of information if necessary to protect children and vulnerable adults can be found on the website below.[2]

---

1 RPSGB. ww.rpsgb.org/pdfs/factsheet12.pdf
2 The Pharmaceutical Journal. www.pharmj.com/pdf/society/pj_20050806_childprotectionguidance.pdf

Confidentiality when a friend, relative or colleague is a patient

Pharmacists and pharmacy staff can be put in a difficult position in this situation, especially if others know that the patient is in their care. Well-meaning questions about the patient's welfare might be difficult to deal with without causing offence.

- Explain to the patient what level of involvement you have in their care and that you would have access to their medical notes and ask whether they would prefer that another pharmacist deals with their care (although this might not always be feasible).
- If at all possible, discuss the situation with the patient and ask them what information they are willing for you to reveal to other friends, family or colleagues.
- If the patient is unwilling for you to reveal any information, or if you are unable to discuss with the patient, any enquiries should be dealt with by politely explaining that you cannot provide information about the patient. Bear in mind, however, that simply making this statement potentially discloses the fact that the individual is known to you as a patient.
- Try to avoid compromising your integrity by denying all knowledge of the patient, but in some situations this might be necessary.
- Inform the medical team that the patients is known to you socially.
- Personal information known to you because of your relationship to the patient should not be revealed to medical or nursing colleagues without the patient's consent.
- The patient might use your relationship to ask you to provide medical information that you would not normally reveal. Provide only the same information as you would to any other patient.
- If a colleague is a patient, be especially sensitive to any aspect of care that could breach confidentiality. As appropriate, you might need to consider the following:
  - Avoid writing your colleague's name on ward order sheets.
  - Use an agreed alias for labelling of medicines.
  - Label, dispense and deliver medicines yourself.
  - Keep any written records separate from others to which other pharmacy staff have access.

Gene therapy

The development of genetically modified viruses and advances in cloning and sequencing the human genome have offered the opportunity to treat a wide variety of diseases using 'gene therapy'. The term 'gene therapy' applies to any clinical therapeutic procedure in which genes are intentionally introduced into human cells. Gene therapy clinical trials have been undertaken in cystic fibrosis, cancer, cardiac disease, HIV and inherited genetic disorders. Preparation of gene therapy products is a pharmaceutical preparation process that should be carried out under the control of a pharmacist in suitable facilities, to minimize the risk of microbiological contamination and medication errors.

Gene therapy can be divided into two main categories: gene replacement or addition. Gene replacement tends to be used for monogenic diseases, in which a single 'faulty' gene can be replaced with a normal gene. For example, an abnormal cystic fibrosis transmembrane conductance regulator (CFTR) gene can be replaced in cystic fibrosis. Currently, the majority of gene-therapy clinical trials use a gene-addition strategy for cancer, whereby a gene or genes can be 'added' to a cell to provide a new function, eg tumour-suppresser genes to cancer cells.

For gene therapy to be successful, a therapeutic gene must be delivered to the nucleus of a target cell, where it can be expressed as a therapeutic protein. Genes are delivered to target cells by vectors, in a process called 'gene transfer'. The greatest challenge to gene therapy is finding a vector that can transfer therapeutic genes to target cells specifically and efficiently. Gene transfer vectors can be broadly divided into nonviral and viral systems. Nonviral vectors, such as liposomes, have limited efficiency. Genetically modified viruses have proved to be the most efficient way of delivering DNA. Viruses are merely genetic information protected by a protein coat. They have a unique ability to enter (infect) a cell delivering viral genes to the nucleus using the host-cell machinery to express those viral genes. A variety of viruses have been used as vectors, including retroviruses, herpes viruses and adenoviruses. Many viral vectors have been genetically modified so that they cannot form new viral particles and so are termed 'replication-deficient' or 'replication-defective'. Replication-deficient viruses have had the viral genes required for replication and the pathogenic host response removed. This prevents the virus replicating and the potential for the therapeutic virus to reverse back to a pathogenic virus. The deleted genes are replaced by a therapeutic gene, thus allowing the delivery and expression of the therapeutic gene without subsequent spread of the virus to surrounding cells. Future gene-therapy vectors will be able to replicate under genetically specified conditions.

There are potential infectious hazards with gene therapy, which include possible transmission of the vector to hospital personnel. ∴, gene therapy products should be manipulated in pharmacy aseptic units, because of the uncertain effects of specific genes on normal human cells, potential for operator sensitization on repeated exposure and potentially infective nature of some products. Consideration has to be given to protect both the product and the staff handling these agents. Some gene-therapy agents might require handling in negative-pressure isolators in separate, specific aseptic facilities.

A risk assessment should be made for each product, with input from the lead investigator or trust biological safety officer, because they should have a good understanding of molecular biology and virology.

Further reading

Stoner NS, Logan P, Bateman R. (2006). Appendix 6—Gene Therapy. In Beaney AM *Quality Assurance of Aseptic Preparation Services*, 4th edition, Pharmaceutical Press: London

Brooks G (ed) (2002). *Gene therapy, the use of DNA as a drug*. London: pharmaceutical Press.

Gene therapy advisory committee (GTAC). www.advisorybodies.doh.gov.uk/genetic/gtac

The UK Health and Safety Executive (2000). *A guide to the genetically modified organisms (contained use) regulations*. HSE Books.

Searle PF, Spiers I, Simpson J, James ND (2002). Cancer gene therapy: from science to clinical trials. *Drug Delivery Systems and Sciences* **2(1):** 5–13.

Simpson J, Stoner NS (2003). Implications of gene therapy to pharmacists. *Pharmaceutical Journal* **271(7259):** 127–30.

Stoner NS, Gibson RN, Edwards J (2003). Health and safety considerations for the administration of gene therapy within the clinical Setting. *Journal of Oncology Pharmacy Practice* **9:** 29–35.

Standards of business conduct for clinical pharmacists

Declaration of interests has become an integral part of professional life and pharmacists are not exempt from showing that they are independent and unbiased. In addition, clinical pharmacists have access to valuable confidential data and can influence purchasing decisions that can have a major effect on a particular company's products. It is important, ∴, that pharmacists are aware of relevant guidelines. In the UK, Department of Health guidelines have been produced on these issues and it is prudent to have a local policy desired from this or similar guidance.

The Department of Health guidelines cover the standards of conduct expected of all NHS staff, where their private interests could conflict with their public duties, and the steps that NHS employers should take to safeguard themselves and the NHS against conflict of interest.

Details can be found in HSG 93(5) and in code of conduct for NHS managers, 2002; both are available on the DH website[1]. Some key relevant issues are listed below:

- Avoid conflict of interest between private and NHS interests. It is a well-established principle that public sector bodies, which include the NHS, must be impartial and honest in the conduct of their business, and that their employees should remain beyond suspicion.
- NHS staff are expected to ensure that the interest of patients is paramount at all times, be impartial and honest in the conduct of their official business and use the public funds entrusted to them to the best advantage of the service, always ensuring value for money.
- It is also the responsibility of staff to ensure that they do not abuse their official position for personal gain or to benefit their family or friends.
- Modest hospitality, provided it is normal and reasonable in the circumstances (eg lunches in the course of working visits), are acceptable, although it should be similar to the scale of hospitality that the NHS, as an employer, would probably offer. Anything else should be declined.
- Casual gifts can be offered by contractors or others, eg at Christmas time. Such gifts should nevertheless be politely, but firmly, declined. Articles of low intrinsic value, such as diaries or calendars, or small tokens of gratitude from patients or their relatives, need not necessarily be refused.
- NHS employers need to be aware of all cases in which an employee or his/her close relative or associate has a significant financial interest in a business.
- Individual staff must not seek or accept preferential rates or benefits in kind for private transactions carried out with companies with which they have had, or might have, official dealings on behalf of their NHS employer.

1 Department of Health. www.dh.gov.uk. Accessed August 2006.

- All staff who are in contact with suppliers and contractors, in particular those who are authorized to sign purchase orders or place contracts for goods, are expected to adhere to professional standards of the kind set out in the ethical code of the Institute of Purchasing and Supply (IPS).
- Fair and open competition between prospective contractors or suppliers for NHS contracts is a requirement of NHS standing orders and of EC directives on public purchasing for works and supplies.
- NHS employers should ensure that no special favour is shown to current or former employees in awarding contracts to private or other businesses run by them.
- NHS employees are advised not to engage in outside employment that could conflict with their NHS work, or be detrimental to it.
- Acceptance by staff of commercial sponsorship for attendance at relevant conferences and courses is acceptable, but only if the employee seeks permission in advance and the employer is satisfied that acceptance will not compromise purchasing decisions in any way.
- Pharmaceutical companies, for example, might offer to sponsor, wholly or partially, a post for an employing authority. NHS employers should not enter into such arrangements, unless it has been made abundantly clear to the company concerned that the sponsorship will have no effect on purchasing decisions within the authority.
- Staff should be particularly careful of using, or making public, internal information of a 'commercial in-confidence' nature, if its use would prejudice the principle of a purchasing system based on fair competition.

Finally, many employers maintain a record of interests and pharmacists should co-operate with such practices.

Disposal of medicines

Your hospital will have a waste management policy that details general themes, including dealing with pharmaceutical waste such as cytotoxics.

Medicine supplied by the hospital department

All out-of-date medicines and any nonstock drugs that are no longer required are usually returned to pharmacy who will either return the medication into stock or arrange for destruction (as appropriate). Procedures for return of medication into stock and destruction of medication should be in place.

Transportation of returns to pharmacy

- By dedicated pharmacy box/container—unused or expired products.
- By ward/department personnel—controlled drugs, including PODs, fridge items and hazardous, harmful or toxic pharmaceuticals.

Medicines brought into hospital by patients

Medicines brought by the patient into hospital are the property of the patient and should only be sent to pharmacy for destruction with the prior agreement from the patient or his/her agent. It is GCP to record the details of PODs sent to the pharmacy for destruction.

Disposal of pharmaceuticals within the pharmacy

Black-lid yellow-burn bins should be used for all pharmaceutical waste, including cytotoxic agents and antibiotic products.

Bins must be subsequently labelled, stating 'pharmaceutical waste for incineration'.

Disposal of pharmaceuticals at ward level

Black-lid yellow-burn bins should be used for all empty and partially used pharmaceutical containers, including liquids and injectables. Giving sets used for administration should also be disposed of using the same burn bin.

Radioactive waste

Radioactive waste is governed by the environment radiochemical inspectorate, who issue organizations with certificates of authorization that regulate the routes of disposal, limits of disposal and type of radioactive material disposed of.

Disposal and destruction of controlled drugs by wards, units and departments

A controlled drug ceases to be classified as a controlled drug after it has been rendered irretrievable, ie all controlled drugs that are disposed of should be unrecognizable as a controlled drug (Misuse of Drugs Act, 1971).

Controlled drugs that can be destroyed on the ward

Part contents of ampoules of controlled drugs, broken ampoules of controlled drugs, leftover syringe contents or individual doses of controlled drugs that are prepared but not administered to a patient must be destroyed on the ward/unit/department.

Destruction can be conducted by the registered nurse/registered operating department practitioner with whom the administration lies and a second person who can be a registered nurse, doctor, pharmacist, registered operating department practitioner (or a final year student nurse at the discretion of the ward sister/charge nurse for the ward/unit/department); the second person must witness the disposal, in addition to countersigning the ward controlled drug record book[1].

Controlled drugs destroyed on the ward must be emptied out of the ampoule (if an injection), crushed (if a tablet or suppository) or opened (if a sachet or capsule) into an in-use sharps bin. This must be witnessed by a second person, as detailed above. Controlled drugs must not be put down the sink.

Controlled drugs that must be returned to pharmacy

All other controlled drugs, eg expired stocks, PODs and excess stock, must be notified to the pharmacist responsible for the ward/unit/department; these controlled drugs must not be destroyed on the ward[1].

The pharmacist must return the controlled drugs to the pharmacy to either the pharmacy controlled drug record book for destruction (in the case of expired stock) or the pharmacy controlled drug record book (in the case of excess stock of controlled drugs, which can be entered back into pharmacy stock).

Departments who do not receive a pharmacy visiting service must either arrange for a pharmacist to come to the ward or agree a mutually convenient time for the nurse to take their controlled drugs and the controlled drug record book to the pharmacy, where a pharmacist will sign for their return.

Records of destruction

In both cases above, an entry must be made in the ward controlled drug record book or the patients' own controlled drugs record book on the appropriate page for the drug in question, specifying 'destruction' or 'return to pharmacy', the quantity involved, the new stock balance and the signatures of the two persons involved.

Prefilled PCA/PCEA/epidural syringes and opiate infusions

Part contents of opiate infusions/PCA/PCEA/epidural syringes that were initially set up and issued in theatres but no longer needed must be destroyed on the ward where the patient resides.

Opiate infusions/PCA/PCEA/epidural syringes containing residual unused injections must be emptied into an in-use sharps bin, in addition to the empty syringe. Empty bags can be disposed of in a clinical waste bag according to procedure for disposing of empty infusion bags. This must be witnessed by a second person. One of the two witnesses should be the nurse looking after the patient.

1 Royal Pharmaceutical Society of Great Britain (2005). The Safe and Secure Handling of Medicines: A Team Approach. Available at www.rpsgb.org/pdfs/safsechandmeds.pdf

Research

Audit and research

Research on humans should be subject to ethical committee review. Sometimes, there is a blurred distinction between audit and research. Pharmacists need to consider projects carefully and ensure they comply with local requirements. The following help to distinguish research from audit:

Audit (which might not need to go to ethics committee review)
- Measures the process and outcome of care.
- Is not randomized.
- Is usually initiated and conducted by those providing the clinical service.
- Involves review of recorded data by those entitled to have access to such data.
- Is not material gathered with a view to publication.

Research (which should go to ethics committee review if it involves patients or volunteers)
- Randomized studies.
- Data collection if outside personnel can access sensitive information about patients.
- Interventions involving contact with patients by a health professional previously unknown to them.
- Questionnaires asking for personal data or sensitive sociodemographic details.
- If there is an intention to publish data as research.
- If pharmaceutical data is collected (other than postmarketing surveillance).
- If patients or volunteers have any procedure additional to normal medical care.
- If samples of any sort are taken additional to normal medical care.

Personal bibliographic databases

Personal bibliographic databases are simply structured database files with some useful features that enable references to be quickly stored, retrieved or inserted into word-processed documents. The basic layout of the database is designed to handle information published in various formats (eg journal articles or books) and the fields are set up to hold that information. There are additional fields that include sections for key words and reference numbers. The simplest use of the database is to manually add information into the fields in a logical sequence. The data is held as records that can then be searched using a variety of options, such as author, date of publication or keywords. It is then a simple task to assign a number to the record that matches a number added to a stored original article, eg in numerical order of the collection, and subsequently to retrieve the hard copy of a reference by searching for key words, for example. Databases of many thousands of papers can be built up in this way and single articles identified in seconds. For example, a single reference in a ProCite® database of 20 000 records can be found in <5 seconds.

There are some useful additions that make this type of software particularly valuable. Firstly, searches that were carried out electronically using a database, such as MEDLINE, can be downloaded directly into the personal bibliographic database using a linking software package, such as Bibliolinks. Translators are available for most of the commonly used databases and this facility enables a database of useful information to be created quickly without rekeying the information. The full record is usually imported, including the abstract, thus extending the search possibilities within the personal database.

Secondly, all the software packages have the means for either simple or complex searches. In ProCite® the following options are available:

To search a database, it is possible to build a 'search expression' in the text box. You can type the text or use the 'Fields', 'Operators' and 'Terms' buttons to help build your search expression. For example, you could enter: AUTHOR = Smith and KEYWORDS = Asthma.

It is possible to search by date, or a range of dates. You can save your search expression with the 'Expressions' button, so you can perform the same search again after more records are entered. Or, you can save the list of records that results from your current search by highlighting them and using the 'Group' menu to save them to a 'Group'.

The third key feature is the ability to link a manuscript to the database to generate a reference list. This task, which is usually time consuming and tedious, is quickly performed because the word-processing package interacts to find the references mentioned, marks the text in the appropriate way (eg superscript number) and produces the reference list. Various styles of reference are available, so if your manuscript in (eg Vancouver style) is rejected by your favourite journal, it can be submitted to another journal that might require Harvard formatting, for example, with ease.

Author Analytic (01): Carroll, D.// Jadad, A.// King, V.// Wiffen, P.//
Glynn, C.// McQuay, H.

Article Title (04): Single-dose, randomized, double-blind, double-
dummy cross-over comparison of extradural and i.v. clonidine in
chronic pain
Journal Title (03): Br J Anaesth
Date of Publication (20): 1993
Volume Identification (22): 71
Issue Identification (24): 5
Page(s): 665-9
ISSN (40): 0007-0912
Notes (42): HC

Abstract (43): We studied 10 patients with chronic back pain who
had claimed benefit with a previous extradural dose of clonidine 150
micrograms combined with local anaesthetic. We compared a single
dose of clonidine 150 micrograms given by either the extradural or i.v.
route in a double-blind, randomized, double-dummy and cross-over
fashion, with 80% power to detect a difference in the analgesic effect of
the two routes. Pain intensity, pain relief, adverse effects, mood, sedation and vital signs were assessed by a nurse observer. I.v. clonidine
produced significantly ($P < 0.04$) greater analgesia than extradural
clonidine in one of the five analgesic outcome measures. Clonidine
given by either route produced statistically significant sedation and
significant decreases in arterial pressure and heart rate. In this study,
extradural clonidine had no significant clinical advantages compared
with i.v. clonidine; clonidine 150 micrograms by either route produced
a high incidence of adverse effects.

Keywords (45): Yes/Chronic non-malignant pain/Pharmacolgical
intervention/Adult/Aged/Analgesia, Epidural/Clonidine administration
and dosage/Clonidine adverse effects/Double Blind Method/Injections,
Intravenous/Middle Age/Pain Measurement/Back Pain drug therapy/
Clonidine therapeutic use/Comparative Study/Female/Human/Male/
Support, Non U.S. Gov't

Fig. 15.1 Example from ProCite

The reference appears as follows when presented in Vancouver format:
Carroll D, Jadad A, King V, Wiffen P, Glynn C, McQuay H. Single-dose, randomized, double-blind, double-dummy cross-over comparison of extradural and i.v. clonidine in chronic pain. Br J Anaesth 1993; **71(5)**: 665–9.

It is beyond the scope of this book to recommend a particular package, but a number of packages are available, including Reference Manager®, ProCite®, Idealist® and EndNote®. Other less well-known packages include Papyrus®, Citation 8® and RefWorks®.

Writing a research proposal

Structure of a research proposal
- Title of project
- Purpose of the project
- Background of project
- Central research question(s)
- Research design
- Data analysis
- Timetable
- Research staff required
- Resources required
- Proposed budget
- References.

Title of project
- Descriptive
- Clear
- Succinct
- Use recognizable key words
- Comprehendible (to nonspecialists)
- Should not imply an expected outcome.

Examples
- 'A randomized controlled trial of amitriptyline in chronic pain.'
- 'A controlled evaluation of advice giving for low back pain.'
- 'A descriptive study of the needs of patients on an orthopaedic surgery ward.'

Purpose of the project
- Why undertake the project?
- For whose benefit?
- Academic potential/contribution?
- Clinical potential/contribution?
- Patient potential/contribution?
- What gaps are likely to be filled?

Background of project
- Literature review
- Critical appraisal of literature/evidence
- Establish scientific adequacy of evidence
- Establish clinical and social adequacy of evidence
- Identify positive evidence and the potential to support, replicate or challenge it
- Identify negative evidence and the potential to support, replicate or challenge it
- Identify uncertain evidence and the potential to clarify, support or reject it
- Identify lack of evidence and potential to remedy this
- Justify central research questions.

Central research questions
- Clear
- Specific
- Distinctive
- Comprehendible (to self and others)
- Answerable
- Feasible (scientifically and financially)

Research design
- Type of design:
  - Randomized controlled trial
  - Matched comparison
  - Cohort study
  - Single case study
  - Descriptive/ethnographic
- Sampling frame
- Sample selection criteria
- Baseline and follow-up strategy
- Measures/data to be collected (process/outcome/satisfaction/costs)
- Access to data arrangements (Data Protection Act might apply)
- Ethical considerations (research often requires approval from an ethics committee or equivalent body (see p.316).

Data analysis
- How data will be stored?
  - Manually and computerized
  - Coded
  - Entered
  - Confidentiality and anonymity
- How data will be retrieved from computer?
- How data will be manipulated?
  - Descriptive versus inductive
  - Univarite/bivarite/multivariate analysis
  - Tests of significance
  - Qualitative data handling
- Which statistical/epidemiological package?
  - (eg SPSS/EpiInfo/NUDIST)
- Data-presentation strategy
  - Report writing strategy:
    (eg report/journal publications/book)

Timetable
- Preparation time
- Start/baseline data collection
- Follow-up data collection
- End-of-data collection
- Data-retrieval time
- Data manipulation and analysis
- Report preparation, writing and dissemination
- Do not under estimate time involved be realistic keep to schedule.

Research staff required
- Self
- Research assistants
- Interviewers
- Secretarial/administrative support
- Data entry, retrieval and handling staff
- Consultancies (specialist advice/support).

Resources required
- Staff
- Accommodation (office space and storage space)
- Equipment:
  - Computer hardware/software
  - Telephones/fax/E-mail
  - Furniture/filing cabinets/storage
  - Audio/video recording machinery
  - Specialist/technical equipment
- Laboratory time/access
- Books, journals and, library services
- Printing and stationery
- Postage
- Travel—both staff and reimbursement for participants in the study
- Overheads (staff and agency).

References
Provide supporting references in a standard format, such as Vancouver (see p.326).

Citations in documents and articles for publication

There are a variety of styles used to cite publications in the medical literature. The commonly used ones are listed here with examples.

Harvard style
- Journal/book articles—In the text:
  - Davies and Mehan (1988) have argued …
- Journal/book articles—in the references:
  - Davies, P.T. and Mehan, H. (1988). Professional and family understanding of impaired communication. *British Journal of Disorders of Communication*. **23**, 141–151.
- Books—in the text:
  - Davies (1983) has argued that …
- Books—in the references:
  - Davies, PT (1983). *Alcohol Problems and Alcohol Control in Europe*. London. Croom Helm.

Vancouver style
- Articles in journals in references:
  - List all authors (up to six).
  - Onghena P, Van Houdenhove B (1992). Antidepressant induced analgesia in chronic pain: a meta analysis of 39 placebo controlled studies. *Pain* **49**: 205–219.
- Books in references:
  - Colson JH, Armour WJ (1986). *Sports injuries and their treatment*. 2nd rev ed. London: S Paul.
- Both types usually linked to the text with superscript numbers.
- For further details about reference styles, see the BMA website[1].

---

1 BMA. www.bma.org.uk/ap.nsf/Content/LIBReferenceStyles. Accessed August 2006.

Therapy-related issues

Diarrhoea

Description and causes

'Diarrhoea' is a term generally understood to mean an ↑ frequency of bowel movement relative to normal for an individual patient.

The normal bowel habit in western society lies somewhere in the range between two bowel actions/wk and three bowel actions/day.

The mechanisms that result in diarrhoea are varied and include ↑ secretion or ↓ absorption of fluid and electrolytes by cells of the intestinal mucosa and exudation resulting from inflammation of the intestinal mucosa.

Diarrhoea is a nonspecific symptom that is a manifestation of a wide range of GI disorders, including inflammatory bowel disease, irritable bowel syndrome, GI malignancy, a variety of malabsorption syndromes, and acute or subacute intestinal infections and infestations.

Diarrhoea can be an unwanted effect of almost any drug, particularly those listed below.

Medications commonly causing diarrhoea

- Acarbose and metformin.
- Alcohol.
- Antibiotics: clindamycin, erythromycin, rifampicin and, cefuroxime.
- Colchicine.
- Cytotoxic agents.
- Food and drug additives.
- Sorbitol, mannitol, fructose and lactose (lactose intolerance).
- Laxatives (including surreptitious use).
- Magnesium-containing antacids.
- NSAIDs.

All patients presenting with diarrhoea should be questioned about the relationship between symptoms and changes in medications.

If an underlying cause of diarrhoea can be identified, management is directed at that the cause rather than at the symptom of diarrhoea.

Treatment

Chronic diarrhoea

The treatment of chronic diarrhoea depends on controlling the underlying disease.

Acute diarrhoea

Fluid and electrolyte therapy

Even in the presence of severe diarrhoea, water and salt continue to be absorbed by active glucose-enhanced sodium absorption in the small intestine. Oral replacement solutions are effective if they contain balanced quantities of sodium, potassium, glucose and water; glucose is necessary to promote electrolyte absorption.

Proprietary soft drinks and fruit juices might be inadequate treatment for individuals in whom dehydration poses a significant risk, eg the elderly and patients with renal disease.

In adults, an oral rehydration solution should be considered for patients with mild-to-moderate dehydration (loss of <6% of body weight). Solutions should be made up freshly according to manufacturers' recommendations, refrigerated and replaced every 24h.

Several proprietary rehydration products are available and made up according to brand recommendations. The recommended range of concentrations for rehydration solutions for use are as follows:

- Sodium 50–60mmol/L.
- Potassium 20–35mmol/L.
- Glucose 80–120mmol/L.

For adults, encourage 2–3 L of rehydration solution orally to be taken over 24h. This will provide ~90–180mmol of sodium and 40–60mmol of potassium.

Once rehydration is complete, further dehydration is prevented by encouraging the patient to drink normal volumes of an appropriate fluid and by replacing continuing losses with an oral rehydration product.

Drug therapy

Antimotility drugs might be of symptomatic benefit in adults with mild or moderate acute diarrhoea. Their most valuable role is in short-term control of symptoms during periods of maximum social inconvenience, eg travel and work. They are contraindicated in patients with severe diarrhoea, if there is a possibility of invasive organisms and in patients with severe inflammatory bowel disease or dilated or obstructed bowel. However, antimotility drugs are also sometimes useful for control of symptoms if treatment of the underlying cause is ineffective or if the cause is unknown.

Antimotility drugs are never indicated for management of acute diarrhoea in infants and children.

If an antimotility drug is considered appropriate, it is reasonable to use one of the following regionens:

- Loperamide 4mg orally initially, followed by 2mg orally after each unformed stool (maximum of 16mg/daily).
- Diphenoxylate+atropine 5+0.05 mg orally three to four times daily initially (↓ dose as soon as symptoms improve).
- Codeine phosphate, 30–60mg orally up to four times daily.

Adsorbents, such as kaolin and activated charcoal, have not been shown to be of value in the treatment of acute diarrhoea. They could interfere with absorption of other drugs and should not be used.

Antibiotics are rarely indicated in uncomplicated infective diarrhoea, except to treat properly diagnosed enteric infections, such as dysentery and antibiotic-associated colitis.

Constipation in adults

Description and causes of constipation in adults

Defined as a ↓ frequency of defaecation.

The *normal* frequency of bowel motions in western countries varies from three times/day to twice/wk.

A person might complain of constipation for the following reasons:
- Defaecation occurs less frequently than usual.
- Stools are harder than usual.
- Defaecation causes straining.
- Sense of incomplete evacuation.

There are a large number of causes of constipation, ranging from common dietary problems to mechanical obstruction, including the adverse effects of many commonly used drugs. One of the most common causes is a low-residue diet.

Some medications commonly causing constipation

- Aluminium and calcium-containing antacids.
- Anticholinergic agents (eg tricyclic antidepressants, antipsychotics and antispasmodics, antiParkinson agents).
- Clozapine, olanzapine, risperidone and quetiapine.
- Iron preparations.
- Opioids.
- Verapamil.

Changing or stopping these drugs might be all that is required to restore normal bowel function.

Most of the factors predisposing to constipation are potentially magnified or compounded in the older patient. In this group particularly, prolonged constipation can lead to faecal impaction, causing urinary and faecal overflow incontinence. It is an avoidable cause of hospital admission.

Treatment of constipation in adults

Patients, especially if ambulant and otherwise healthy, should be encouraged to control their bowel activity by attention to diet and exercise. The diet should contain adequate amounts of fibre and fluid.

Physical exercise has been shown to ↓ intestinal transit time and is believed to stimulate regular bowel movements.

If these measures are ineffective, intermittent or regular use of a laxative might be necessary (Table 16.1). The duration of treatment with laxatives should be limited to the shortest time possible. The undesirability of long-term laxative use should be explained to the patient.

Diet

The major lifestyle factor leading to constipation is inadequate dietary fibre intake. Dietary fibre consists of plant complex carbohydrates that escape digestion in the small intestine and are only partly broken down by bacterial enzymes in the large intestine. The ingestion of dietary fibre ↑ stool bulk by ↑ both solid residue and stool water content. This results in ↓ intestinal transit time and ↓water absorption in the large bowel, resulting in stools that are softer, wetter and easier to pass.

The recommended amount of dietary fibre is 30g/day. The fibre content of the diet should be built up gradually to avoid adverse effects, such as bloating or flatulence. Patients should be encouraged to choose a wide variety of fibre sources, eg wholegrain or wholemeal products (breads, cereals, pastas and rice), fruits and vegetables, legumes, seeds and nuts, rather than adding a few very high fibre foods, eg unprocessed bran, to the diet. Ensure fluid intake is encouraged.

Drug therapy

First-line therapy

If dietary management is not sufficient, bulk-forming agents are the laxatives of choice for mildly constipated individuals. Provided good fluid intake is maintained, use the following agents:

Oral bulk-forming agents

The effect of bulk-forming laxatives is usually apparent within 24h, but 2–3 days of medication might be required to achieve the full effect.

Second-line therapy

- Osmotic laxative–lactulose syrup, 10–30mL orally twice or three times daily. Lactulose syrup contains free lactose and galactose and, ∴, it should be used with caution in patients with diabetes mellitus and is contraindicated in galactosaemia. The laxative can take 48h to work, so it must be take regularly.
- Stimulant laxative–senna, 7.5mg, or bisacodyl, 5mg, one or two tablets daily (interchangably). The agents used for second-line therapy can also be used as first-line therapy in acute illness or for hospitalized patients.
- Although stool-softening agents, such as docusate salts, are often used in the treatment of constipation, they have limited effectiveness as monotherapy.

Third-line therapy

If constipation is resistant to the above measures, there should be a re-evaluation of the underlying cause(s), including impaction. For further therapy, use one of the following regimens:
- Magnesium sulphate, 5–15g (5–15mL) orally in water daily.
- A stimulant agent, eg senna 30mg or bisacodyl 20mg orally daily at night.

And, if required, consider the following regimens:
- Glycerin suppository rectally (allow to remain for 15–30min)
- Phosphate enema rectally.

Magnesium salts should not be used in pregnant women or patients with impaired renal function.

Fourth-line therapy

In a minority of patients the above measures are unsuccessful and repeated enemas, polyethylene glycol (eg Movicol®, sodium phosphates or sodium picosulphate bowel preparations) and/or manual evacuation might be required, sometimes after admission to hospital.

Movicol, 1–3 sachets daily in divided doses usually for ≤2wks; each sachet should be dissolved in 125mL of water.

Opioid-induced constipation

When an opioid is first prescribed, co-danthrusate (one or two) at night should be added as a prophylactic measure. (Sometimes the dosage must be ↑ to two twice daily acutely, then reduced to one or two at night)

If the patient is already constipated, ↑ the dosage to co-danthrusate two capsules at night; adjust the dose according to response, up to a maximum of three capsules three times daily.

If the maximum dose is ineffective, ↓ the dose by 50% and add an osmotic laxative, eg lactulose, 20–30mL twice daily or Movicol® one sachet twice daily.

Table 16.1 Laxative choice

Bulk-forming laxatives

Constituent(s), form and preparation	Dose (adult dose, unless otherwise specified)	Time to onset
Note: it is recommended that bulk-forming agents be taken with adequate fluid.		
Ispaghula granules (Fybogel®, Regulan®, Isogel®)	1 sachet or 1 teaspoonful, twice daily Child 6–12yrs: 50% adult dose	Usually 24h, 2–3 days for full effect
Sterculia (Normacol® granules)	1–2 heaped 5mL spoonful twice daily Child 6–12yrs: 50% adult dose	Usually 24h, 2–3 days for full effect
Osmotic laxatives		
Lactulose syrup	15–30mL daily, in one or two doses initially Child, <1yr: 5mL; child, 1–6yrs: 10mL; child, 7–14yrs: 15mL daily, initially	1–2 days
Magnesium sulphate mixture	5–15mL in 250mL of water	1h
Polyethylene glycol powder (Movicol®)	1–3 sachets in 125mL water daily	1h
Phosphate enemas	See product information	2–5mins
Stool-softening laxatives		
Docusate tablets	200mg twice daily	1–3 days

Table 16.1 (*Contd.*)

Stimulant laxatives

Constituent(s), form and preparation	Dose (adult dose, unless otherwise specified)	Time to onset
Bisacodyl, 5mg tablets	1–2 tablets daily	6–12h
Bisacodyl, 10mg suppositories	1 suppository daily	15–60mins
Senna, 7.5mg tablets (Senokot®)	2–4 tablets daily child, >6 years: 50% adult dose	6–12h
Co-danthrusate (opioid-induced constipation)	1–3 capsules at night	6–12h

Lubricant laxatives

Glycerol/glycerin suppositories	1 suppository, as required	15–30mins
Liquid paraffin oral emulsion	10–30mL at night	8–12h

Note: prolonged use of liquid paraffin oral emulsion can cause deficiency of fat soluble vitamins and is associated with lipoid pneumonia.

Bulk-forming combined with stimulant laxatives

Note: it is recommended that bulk-forming agents be taken with adequate fluid.

Frangula+sterculia granules (Normacol Plus™)	1–2 heaped teaspoonsfuls once or twice daily	6–12h

Management of nausea and vomiting

Nausea and vomiting are common and distressing symptoms, which can lead to the following chinical conditions:
- Poor hydration and nutrition.
- Weight loss.
- Depression.
- ↑ length of stay.
- Poor adherence to oral medicines.

Causes of nausea and vomiting
- Chemical
  - Exogenous—eg microbial toxins and drugs.
  - Endogenous—eg uraemia and hypercalcaemia.
- CNS
  - Emotional and anxiety.
  - CNS lesions.
  - Vestibular.
  - ↑ intracranial pressure.
- Obstructive
  - Constipation
  - Gastrointestinal tumours

Factors that can ↑ the risk or severity of nausea and vomiting include the following:
- ♀.
- Tendency to nausea and vomiting—eg motion sickness and drug intolerance.
- Nonsmoker.
- History of migraine.
- Pain.
- Anxiety.

Management of nausea and vomiting requires accurate diagnosis of the cause and knowledge of control pathways and the ways in which anti-emetics work.

Four steps to managing nausea and vomiting
- Identify cause—this is not always easy because nausea and vomiting are often multifactorial, but it is important because antiemetics are not equally effective against all types of nausea and vomiting. Take an accurate and detailed history, including prescribed and over-the-counter drugs.
- Remove or correct cause if possible—eg stop NSAIDs and prescribe laxatives if constipated.
- Treat according to cause—start an appropriate treatment according to the diagnosis (Table 16.2). About 10% of cases require more than one drug. These should preferably be from different groups (but anticholinergics antagonize the prokinetic effect of metoclopramide and domperidone). Parenteral administration is frequently more appropriate than oral. See table for recommended drugs.

- Specialist advice should be sought for patients with chemotherapy induced (p.468) or radiotherapy-induced nausea and vomiting or bowel obstruction.
- Review frequently and regularly—if nausea and vomiting persist, change from oral to parenteral administration, ↑ dose or try drugs from a different therapeutic class. Allow a 24h trial of each intervention before trying another option.

Postoperative nausea and vomiting (PONV)

PONV is a highly undesirable complication of surgery, which can occur in up to 50% of cases. In addition to the consequences described above, severe retching and vomiting postoperatively can put tension on suture lines, cause haematomas below surgical flaps and ↑ postoperative pain.

Additional risk factors for PONV are as follows:
- Use of inhalation anaesthetics.
- Duration of anaesthesia.
- Use of opioids.
- Use of nitrous oxide.
- Abdominal surgery, notably laparoscopic procedures.
- Perioperative dehydration.

For nonemergency surgery, good preoperative care can ↓ the risk of PONV:
- Identify risk factors and correct or minimize wherever possible.
- Assess unavoidable risk factors:
  - If one risk factor or less, no prophylaxis is required.
  - If two or more, risk factors are present give prophylactic antiemetics preoperatively.
  - For patients at high risk of PONV, give two antiemetics from different classes preoperatively.

If the patient experiences PONV despite prophylaxis, give an additional antiemetic from a different class.

Table 16.2

Cause	First-line drug group	First-line treatment	Second-line treatment	Other treatment
Obstruction	Anticholinergic*/ antihistamine	Cyclizine	Hyoscine	Dexamethasone Antihistamine Laxatives
Gastric stasis	Prokinetic	Metoclopramide**	Domperidone	Antacid Dexamethasone
Gastritis	Prokinetic	Metoclopramide**	Cyclizine Domperidone	Antacid Ranitidine Proton-pump inhibitor
Chemical	Dopamine antagonists	Prochlorperazine Haloperidol	Levomepromazine Granisetron/ ondansetron /tropisetron Nabilone	Dexamethasone Acupressure (eg Sea Band)
CNS	Antihistamine/ anticholinergic	Cyclizine	Hyoscine	Dexamethasone
Psychological Emotional	Anxiolytic	Diazepam	Midazolam Levomepromazine Lorazepam	Reassurance

* Note anticholinergic side effects can ↑ obstruction.
** At high doses, metoclopramide acts as a 5-HT₃ antagonist.

Drug points
- Avoid metoclopramide in younger (≤20-year-old) patients, especially ♀, because of ↑ risk of dystonic reactions.
- Domperidone does not cross the blood brain–barrier and so is a suitable alternative to metoclopramide in young (♀) patients.
- Long-term metoclopramide, prochlorperazine and haloperidol can cause extrapyramidal side effects in older patients.
- Levomepromazine should be administered in low doses and titrated cautiously because it is sedative and hypotensive at higher doses.
- Anticholinergics antagonize the prokinetic effect of metoclopramide and domperidone.
- Anticholinergics can cause a 'high' in some patients; avoid in patients with a current or past history of drug misuse.
- Tolerance to opioid-induced nausea and vomiting usually develops after 7–10 days. A prophylactic antiemetic should be used initially and the continued need reviewed after 7–10 days.

Angina

Definition

Angina is defined and diagnosed by clinical criteria. Cardiac pain is retrosternal, intense and gripping, constricting or suffocating, and diffuse rather than sharp.

Pain can radiate to one or both arms, the neck, jaw or teeth. It can, however, be difficult to distinguish/angina from severe dyspepsia, so other signs need to be considered to help differential diagnosis, such as whether pain comes on acutely following exertion and is relieved within a few minutes by resting or sublingual nitrates.

The underlying pathology is usually, but not always, coronary atherosclerosis. Smoking, hyperlipidaemia, hypertension, obesity and diabetes mellitus are risk factors that accelerate coronary atherosclerosis.

Types of angina

Stable angina is induced by effort and relieved by rest.
- Unstable angina (crescendo) is angina of ↑ frequency or severity, which occurs at minimal exertion and ↑ with ↑ risk of MI.
- Decubitus angina as precipitated by lying flat.
- Variant (Prinzmetal's) angina is caused by coronary artery spasm.

In stable angina, the problem is chronic atherosclerotic obstruction which is slowly progressive, although the onset of symptoms is often sudden. Severe obstructive coronary atherosclerosis restricts myocardial blood flow, whereas exercise or emotional stress creates a demand for more blood flow, which cannot be achieved because of the obstruction.

Anginal pain signals temporary myocardial ischaemia, which subsides promptly with rest because the ↑ demand subsides.

Not all patients experience typical chest pain. Some experience atypical pain, shortness of breath or light headedness.

Aims of treatment

- To relieve or prevent pain.
- To slow progression of atherosclerosis.
- To improve prognosis.

Assess the occurrence of pain in relation to the patient's lifestyle. Drug therapy should be initiated immediately, and risk factors should be assessed.

Attention to good drug adherence/concordance is important, and potential obstacles to this should be considered.

Advice should be given regarding regular moderate exercise and avoidance of heavy, sudden and unaccustomed exertion and acute emotional stress if practicable.

Acute attack

The patient should stop activities as soon as pain is felt. To shorten the attack, use one of the following regimens:
- GTN spray, 400mcg metered-dose sublingually—repeat the dose once after 5mins if pain persists (maximum of two metered doses).

- GTN tablet, 500mcg sublingually; repeat every 3–5mins up to a maximum of 1500mcg. (It is important that patients are made aware of the limited 8wk shelf-life of opened containers.)

Note: avoid nitrates if the patient has used sildenafil (Viagra®) in the previous 24h or tadalafil (Cialis®) or vardenafil (Levitra®) in the previous 5days.

The patient should sit or lie down, particularly when first using GTN, because of the possibility of hypotension.

If pain persists after three tablets taken over 15mins or two sprays at 5mins intervals, the patient should be advised to call an ambulance for transfer to the nearest hospital.

Continuing therapy

The aims of continuing therapy are to ↓ myocardial ischaemia, hence ↑ effort tolerance, and to prevent the development of acute coronary syndrome, arrhythmia and death. Antiplatelet therapy ↓ the incidence of ischaemia at rest and the risk of MI or death. β-blockers enhance effort tolerance by ↓ the onset of myocardial ischaemia. Either of the following regimens can be used for continuing theapy:

- Aspirin, 75–300mg oral daily.
- Clopidogrel 75mg daily (if intolerant of aspirin).
- The above therapies are given in addition to one of the following regimens:
- Atenolol, 25–100mg oral daily.
- Metoprolol, 25–100mg oral twice daily.

Nitrates can be used prophylactically before exertion that is likely to provoke angina.

For patients in whom a β-blocker alone does not prevent angina, add a dihydropyridine calcium-channel blocker and/or a nitrate and/or nicorandil, as follows:

- Amlodipine, 2.5–10mg oral daily or nifedipine controlled-release 30–60mg oral daily.
- Isosorbide mononitrate, 30–120mg oral daily in divided doses or GTN, 5–15mg transdermally (apply for a maximum of 16h in a 24h period).
- Nicorandil, 5mg oral twice daily, ↑ after a week to 10–20mg twice daily.

For patients in whom there is a contraindication to a β-blocker, substitute a calcium-channel blocker, preferably a long-acting nondihydropyridine and/or a nitrate and/or nicorandil, as follows:

- Diltiazem, 30–120mg oral three times daily; diltiazem controlled-release, 180–360mg oral daily; verapamil, 40–120mg oral twice or three times daily; verapamil sustained-release, 160–480mg oral daily;or amlodipine, 5–10mg oral daily.
- Isosorbide mononitrate, 30–120mg oral daily in divided doses or GTN 5–15 mg transdermally (apply for a maximum of 16h in a 24h period).
- Nicorandil, 5mg oral twice daily, ↑ after a week to 10–20mg twice daily.

Choice of calcium-channel blockers

When calcium-channel blockers are used without a β-blocker, the agents of choice are verapamil or diltiazem which slow the heart rate. In general, verapamil should not be administered in combination with β-blockers because of the risk of severe bradycardia, and diltiazem should be administered with caution in combination with a β-blocker for the same reason. Dihydropyridine calcium-channel blockers can be administered in combination with beta-blockers.

Amlodipine, which has a very long half-life, and the once-daily form of nifedipine, can be used alone for angina—but caution should be exercised because of the possibility of ↑ sympathetic tone and heart rate 2° to arteriolar dilatation.

Tolerance to nitrate therapy

Tolerance to all forms of nitrate therapy develops rapidly. Sustained-release isosorbide mononitrate administered once daily, and a GTN patch worn for <16h/day avoid this complication by allowing a nitrate-free period. The commonly used regimen of isosorbide dinitrate three or four times daily results in rapid development of tolerance.

In patients who have a low ischaemic threshold, rebound ischaemia can develop during the drug-free interval when the GTN patch is not worn. This problem might be less common during the low-drug-concentration period with sustained-release isosorbide mononitrate, which might, ∴, be useful for patients with a very low ischaemic threshold.

It should be noted that a combination of long-acting nitrate regimens (eg sustained-release isosorbide mononitrate plus transdermal GTN) results in the rapid development of tolerance and should be avoided.

Heart failure

Heart failure is mainly a disease of the elderly. It can be predominantly left ventricular, with pulmonary congestion and dyspnoea, or predominantly right ventricular, with ↑ venous pressure, peripheral oedema and hepatic congestion. Usually both forms co-exist in the classical syndrome of congestive or biventricular heart failure.

Heart failure is generally a consequence of myocardial damage, leading to ↓ systolic function. Underlying causes and/or precipitating factors include the following:
- Hypertension.
- Coronary artery disease.
- Valvular heart disease.
- Hypertrophic cardiomyopathy.
- Hyperthyroidism can cause heart failure, particularly in association with rapid atrial fibrillation (AF).
- Alcohol abuse.
- Pericardial effusion.
- Obstructive sleep apnoea.

Non-drug interventions

Physical activity
Patients should be encouraged to be active if symptoms are absent or mild. However, bed rest might have a marked diuretic effect and, in general, patients should be rested if symptoms are severe. When confined to bed, they should receive heparin prophylaxis.

Weight reduction
Obesity is a risk factor for heart failure and left ventricular hypertrophy. Weight reduction should be advised for obese patients.

Sodium restriction
The use of diuretics avoids the need for strict sodium restriction in many patients with heart failure. However, excessive salt ingestion can precipitate or exacerbate heart failure and a no-added-salt diet (60–100mmol/day) should be recommended. More severe salt restriction might be necessary in patients with severe heart failure.

Water restriction
In patients with severe heart failure the ability to excrete a free water load is diminished. The combination of ↓ sodium intake, potent diuretics and continued water intake often leads to dilutional hyponatraemia. Liberalizing salt intake or ↓ diuretic dosage is usually inappropriate, because these patients are often still oedematous. Water intake should be limited to ≤1.5L/day in patients with hyponatraemia, particularly those in whom the serum sodium concentration falls below 130mmol/L.

O_2
Patients with acute pulmonary oedema are hypoxaemic and require O_2. Carbon dioxide (CO_2) retention is usually not a problem, except in patients with cor pulmonale or very severe pulmonary oedema.

Pleurocentesis and, pericardiocentesis

Occasionally, patients with heart failure have significant pleural effusions, which might require pleural aspiration. Pericardial aspiration should be performed in patients who have compromised circulatory function resulting from pericardial effusion and cardiac tamponade.

Drug interventions for mild-to-moderate heart failure

Optimization of therapy can take several months and requires close monitoring of symptoms, fluid status, renal function and electrolyte levels.

ACE inhibitors improve prognosis in all grades of heart failure and should be used as initial therapy in all patients.

Angiotensin II receptor antagonists offer a potential alternative therapy in patients who are intolerant of ACE inhibitors, except if there are contraindications to either class of drug.

ACE inhibitor therapy

Virtually all patients with clinical heart failure should receive an ACE inhibitor as initial therapy (Table 16.3). Asymptomatic patients should also receive an ACE inhibitor if there is significant left ventricular dysfunction (ie left ventricular ejection fraction is <40%).

Most symptoms and signs of heart failure are caused by retention of salt and water and the consequent ↑ in cardiac filling pressures. Diuretics should be added to ACE inhibitor therapy to help control congestive symptoms and signs. If the patient's response to ACE inhibitor monotherapy is inadequate, add a diuretic and/or ↑ the dose of ACE inhibitors. Virtually all patients with clinical heart failure require combination therapy with an ACE inhibitor and a diuretic.

Table 16.3 Dosing regimens for ACE inhibitors in heart failure

Drug	Initial dose	Maintenance range
Captopril	6.25mg twice daily	50mg three times daily
Enalapril	2.5mg daily	20mg daily in one to two divided doses; maximum 40mg
Lisinopril	2.5mg daily	20–40mg daily
Perindopril	2mg daily	4–8mg daily
Ramipril	1.25mg daily	5–10mg daily

Angiotensin II receptor antagonists

Some patients are unable to tolerate ACE inhibitors because of adverse effects, such as cough or skin rashes. In these patients, the new angiotensin II receptor antagonists should be used to provide an alternative mechanism of inhibiting the renin–angiotensin system. However, if a patient has experienced angioedema with an ACE inhibitors, angiotensin II receptor anatgonists are also contraindicated. They probably provide the same benefits as ACE inhibitors with regard to control of heart failure and improvement in prognosis. At the time of writing, the angiotensin II receptor antagonists are approved only for the treatment of hypertension.

If progressive worsening of renal function is the principal reason for ceasing an ACE inhibitor, angiotensin II receptor inhibitors are likely to produce the same effect on renal function.

Diuretic therapy

- Diuretics should be added to ACE inhibitor therapy to control congestive symptoms and signs. Close monitoring of weight, renal function and electrolytes is required.
- Loop diuretics are commonly used, particularly for heart failure of moderate severity; thiazides produce a gradual diuresis and are effective for mild heart failure.
- Caution: if thiazide and loop diuretics are combined, there is a considerable synergistic effect and the combination should be reserved for severe heart failure.
- In patients with normal renal function, the combination of ACE inhibitor and diuretic, a k^+-sparing diuretic or k^+ supplement is occasionally needed.
- In patients with renal impairment, if diuretics are used with an ACE inhibitor, k^+-sparing diuretic or k^+ supplementation is usually not necessary and could cause life-threatening hyperkalaemia.
- If hypokalaemia proves difficult to correct, hypomagnesaemia can be present.

β-blocker therapy

Recent clinical trials have demonstrated beneficial effects of β-blockers in patients with systolic heart failure and low ejection fraction, with control of heart failure, left ventricular ejection fraction and prognosis. Benefits of β-blockade, proven in clinical trials, include ↓ in all-cause mortality, sudden death and hospitalization rates for heart failure and reversal of some degree of heart damage. Carvedilol and bisoprolol are currently licensed in the UK for chronic heart failure.[1,2,3]

1 CIBIS-II Investigators (1999). The Cardiac Insufficiency Bisoprolol Study II (CIBIS-II): a randomized trial. *Lancet* **353**: 9–13.
2 MERIT-HF Study Group (1999). Effect of metoprolol CR/XL in chronic heart failure: Metoprolol CR/XL Randomized Intervention Trial in Congestive Heart Failure (MERIT-HF). *Lancet* **353**: 2001–07.
3 Krum H, Roecker EB, Mohacsi P et al. (2003). Carvedilol Prospective Randomized Cumulative Survival (COPERNICUS) Study Group. Effects of initiating carvedilol in patients with severe chronic heart failure: Results from the COPERNICUS Study. *JAMA* **289**: 712–18.

There are two clinical situations in which β-blockers have been used for some time:

- After stabilization of acute heart failure in patients with AF, to control rapid ventricular rate.
- In patients with primarily diastolic heart failure, to improve diastolic filling.

β-blocker therapy in patients with heart failure can be extremely difficult to manage. The initiation and up-titration should be undertaken in consultation with a specialist.

Patients with systolic heart failure are often very sensitive to β-blockers. Major complications include worsening of heart failure, severe hypotension and bradyarrhythmias. These complications are caused by β-blockade, leading to withdrawal of sympathetic nervous system support for the failing heart. These complications may be minimized by the following strategies:

- Starting therapy with extremely low doses.
- ↑ the dose very gradually.
- Monitoring the patient frequently, by weighing daily.
- Adjusting the dose of other medications, such as diuretics and ACE inhibitors to compensate for any tendency to ↑ heart failure.
- Avoiding simultaneous addition of vasodilator drugs.
- Excluding patients with extremely severe heart failure and those whose heart failure is not well controlled on other therapy.

The best advice is to start low and go slow'. Use one of the following regimens:

- Bisoprolol, 1.25mg once daily (the dose can be doubled every 2–4 wks, providing the patient is stable, with the aim of ↑ the dose to 10mg once daily).
- Carvedilol, 3.125mg twice daily (the dose can be doubled every 2–4 weeks, providing the patient is stable, with the aim of ↑ the dose to 25mg oral twice daily).
- Metoprolol, 12.5mg twice daily (the dose can be doubled every 2–4 weeks, providing the patient is stable, with the aim of ↑ the dose to 100mg oral twice daily).

It seems probable that standard β_1-blockers, such as metoprolol provide similar benefits to the newer β-blockers, such as bisoprolol and carvedilol, and might, ∴, be much more cost-effective. However, both bisoprolol and carvedilol offer the advantage of lower strength tablets for initiation of therapy. Moreover, they are the only β-blockers explicitly approved for use in heart failure.

Digoxin therapy

There are two indications for the use of digoxin in patients with heart failure:

- In patients with AF, to control rapid ventricular rate.
- In patients with sinus rhythm (SR), if heart failure is not adequately controlled by optimal doses of ACE inhibitors and loop diuretics.

If the patient has not been taking digoxin, give the following dose regimen:
- Digoxin, 62.5–500mcg oral daily, according to age, plasma creatinine and plasma digoxin level.

In patients with normal renal function, the half-life of digoxin is ≥24h. Following initiation of therapy or change in the digoxin dose, the patient will require ≥5 days (five half-lives) to achieve a steady state. In patients with impaired renal function, the half-life of digoxin might be greatly prolonged. Patients take much longer to reach steady state, and require ↓ in the maintenance dose. Monitoring of digoxin plasma level is recommended.

If the patient requires more rapid digitalization, eg AF with rapid ventricular rate, give the following dose regimen:
- Digoxin, 500mcg to 1mg oral immediately, followed by 250–500mcg oral every 4–6h (up to 1.5–2mg in the first 24h).
- Followed by digoxin, 62.5–500mcg oral daily, according to age, plasma creatinine and plasma digoxin level.

Caution: elderly patients are susceptible to digoxin toxicity, partly because of ↓ renal clearance and partly because their cardiac tissue is more sensitive to drugs action; therefore, loading and maintenance doses need to be lower, generally.

Drug interventions for severe heart failure

Patients with severe symptomatic heart failure should be hospitalized, and require bed rest.

Therapy will include all of the following drug regimens:
• Maximum tolerated dose of an ACE inhibitor orally.
• ↑ dose of furosemide, up to a maximum of 500mg/daily.
• Low-dose spironolactone, 25mg/daily (range, 12.5–50mg/daily).

Low-dose spironolactone, 25mg/daily, when added to therapy with a loop diuretic and an ACE inhibitor, improves prognosis in patients with severe heart failure, without a major risk of hyperkalaemia or dehydration.

In patients with severe refractory oedema owing to severe heart failure, k^+-sparing diuretics, such as amiloride and spironolactone (which are weak diuretics), can facilitate diuresis when used in combination with loop diuretics. They are also much more effective than k^+ supplements in maintaining the serum k^+ level.

All k^+-sparing diuretics can cause severe life-threatening hyperkalaemia, particularly in patients with renal impairment or those taking k^+ supplements or on ACE inhibitor.

The combination of an ACE inhibitor, loop diuretics and spironolactone can cause severe dehydration and/or hyperkalaemia.

If heart failure is poorly controlled, consider adding one of the following three regimens:
• Bendroflumethiazide, 2.5mg oral (use a single dose initially, repeat in 2–7 days, according to diuretic effect).
• Spironolactone ↑ doses to 100–200mg daily.
• One of the following three (only when the patient is stable on optimal doses of ACE inhibitor and combination diuretic therapy)–Bisoprolol, 1.25mg oral once daily (the dose can be doubled every 2–4 wks, providing the patient is stable, with the aim of ↑ the dose to 10mg oral once daily);
• Carvedilol, 3.125mg oral once daily (the dose can be doubled every 2–4 weeks, providing the patient is stable, with the aim of ↑ (the dose to 25mg oral twice daily); or
• Metoprolol, 12.5mg oral once daily (the dose can be doubled every 2–4 wks, providing the patient is stable, with the aim of ↑ the dose to 100mg oral twice daily).

If patient has not been taking digoxin, add digoxin.

If the patient has been taking digoxin, check the trough plasma digoxin level not less than 6h after the latest dose and consider ↑ the maintenance dose to achieve a plasma level in the high therapeutic range, providing there are no symptoms or signs of toxicity.)

If patient is confined to bed, also give prophylactic heparin.

Useful additional therapies in severe heart failure

Nitrates/GTN

Nitrates cause prompt, but temporary, lowering of pulmonary venous pressure. Patients with heart failure associated with hypertension or ischaemia are particularly likely to benefit.

GTN is the preferred IV vasodilator therapy, usually in the setting of an intensive care or coronary care unit. Normally, IV therapy is required for only a short period; prolonged infusion rapidly induces tolerance. Use GTN 10mcg/min IV and ↑ the dose according to the clinical response, but maintain the systolic BP >90mmHg.

Warfarin

Warfarin is recommended for patients who have heart failure with AF and in those with previous systemic embolism and severe left ventricular systolic dysfunction. The INR should be maintained between 2 and 3. The INR might be less stable in the presence of heart failure, making warfarin therapy more difficult to control.

Patients who have underlying ischaemic or hypertensive heart disease and who are not on warfarin should take low-dose aspirin.

Patients with very severe heart failure might benefit temporarily from further intensive measures. These should only be employed if there is some transient exacerbating factor, eg myocardial ischaemia, infection or surgery, or if some remedial measure, eg cardiac transplantation, is planned.

Sodium nitroprusside

Sodium nitroprusside can also be used. It is generally administered with BP monitoring using an arterial line. It is particuarly effective for patients with heart failure associated with severe hypertension. If treatment is continued for >24h, to avoid toxicity monitor thiocyanate and cyanide levels. Use sodium nitroprusside, 0.3mcg/kg body weight/min IV initially and ↑ by 0.3mcg/kg body weight/min every 5–10mins to maintain SBP at ~90mmHg. Do not use for >3days.

Other theropies

Short-term catecholamine inotrope administration can cause temporary improvement. However, therapy with positive inotropic drugs has been associated with ↑ mortality. Use dobutamine, 2.5–10mcg/kg body weight/min IV.

Increasingly, patients presenting with severe heart failure are taking a β-blocker. In these patients, the dose of β-blocker should be ↓ or the drug completely withdrawn. If temporary IV inotropic support is required, the phosphodiesterase inhibitor milrinone can be used and is effective in ↑ contractility even in the presence of β-receptor blockade.

Finally, an intra-aortic balloon pump might occasionally be required, and in younger patients with severe refractory heart failure, cardiac transplantation should be considered. Ventricular-assist devices can provide a bridge to transplantation and, perhaps, even a long-term alternative.

Acute cardiogenic pulmonary oedema

- A medical emergency requiring urgent treatment in hospital. Initially, the patient should receive O_2 4–6L/min through a mask and furosemide, 20–80mg IV (repeated 20mins later, if necessary).
- Larger doses might be required, particularly in patients on pre-existing diuretic therapy or with impaired renal function. If the response to IV furosemide is inadequate, consider morphine, with or without nitrates.
- Morphine, 2.5–10mg IV (use the lower end of the range in the elderly).
- If pulmonary oedema is severe, not responding or associated with ischaemia or significant hypertension, add GTN 10mcg/min IV and ↑ according to clinical response, but maintain systolic BP >100mmHg.
- If the patient is in AF with a rapid ventricular rate and has not been taking digoxin, add digoxin, 500mcg oral or IV and repeat at 4 and 8h, if necessary. Administer digoxin, 500mcg oral the following day, followed by digoxin, 62.5–500mcg oral daily, according to age, plasma creatinine and plasma digoxin level.
- If the patient is not in AF, withhold digoxin until acute pulmonary oedema is controlled, when a maintenance dose of digoxin can be commenced or restarted.
- If pulmonary oedema remains severe and does not respond to treatment, add continuous positive airway pressure ventilation (CPAP) to improve oxygenation.
- If pulmonary oedema is severe and not responding to diuretics and vasodilator therapy, consider adding either of the following regimens:
  - Dobutamine, 2.5–10mcg/kg body weight/min IV.
  - Milrinone, 50mcg/kg body weight IV slowly over 10 minutes, followed by 0.375–0.75mcg/kg body weight/min IV, adjusting the dose according to clinical and haemodynamic responses, up to a maximum of 1.13mg/kg body weight daily.
- See Table 16.4.

Table 16.4 Guidance on selecting antihypertensive therapy with concomitant disease [1]

Drug	Compelling indications	Possible indications	Compelling contraindications	Possible contraindications
Hypertensive patients aged 55 or more, or Black patients of all ages. First line of choice of initial therapy should be either a calcium channel blocker or a thiazide-type diuretic. (Black patients—does not include patients of mixed race or Asian patients.)				
Low-dose thiazides thiazide-like drugs	Heart failure Elderly patients Systolic hypertension	Diabetes mellitus	Gout	Dyslipidaemia Symptomatic Orthostatic hypotension
Calcium-channel blockers	Angina Elderly patients Systolic hypertension	PVD	Heart block	Congestive heart failure
Hypertensive patients under 55. First choice initial therapy should be an ACE inhibitor (or an angiotensin receptor blocker if an ACE inhibitor is not tolerated).				
ACEI	Heart failure Left ventricular dysfunction Acute mycordial infarct Diabetes mellitus		Pregnancy Hyperkalaemia Bilateral renal artery stenosis	

Table 16.4 (Contd.)

Drug	Compelling indications	Possible indications	Compelling contraindications	Possible contraindications
Angiotensin II receptor blockers	ACEI cough Type 2 diabetes	Heart failure	Pregnancy Bilateral renal artery stenosis Hyperkalaemia	

If initial therapy was with a calcium channel blocker or thiazide-type diuretic and a second drug is required, add an ACE inhibitor (or an angiotensin receptor blocker if an ACE inhibitor is not tolerated). If initial therapy was with an ACE inhibitor, add a calcium channel blocker or a thiazide-type diuretic.

Triple therapy: ACE inhibitor, thiazide-type diuretic, calcium channel blocker

If a fourth drug is required, one of the following should be considered: • a higher dose of a thiazide-type diuretic or the addition of another diuretic (careful monitoring is recommended) or • beta-blockers or • selective alpha-blockers.

Drug	Compelling indications	Possible indications	Compelling contraindications	Possible contraindications
Beta-blockers	Angina Acute myocardial infarct Tachyarrhythmias heart failure	Pregnancy Diabetes mellitus	Asthma and COPD Heart block	Dyslipidaemia Athletes and physically active patients PVD
Alpha-blockers	Prostatic hypertrophy	Glucose intolerance Dyslipidaemia	Orthostatic hypotension	

Treatment of hypertension

High BP is characterized by elevated arterial BP and ↑ risk of stroke, MI, renal failure, heart failure or other vascular complications.

High BP is one of many risk factors for cardiovascular disease. Presently, there is a shift from consideration of individual risk factors, such as BP, to overall cardiovascular risk. Normal BP is defined as <130/85mmHg.

BP is ↑ by drugs such as the following:
- NSAIDs (including cyclo-oxygenase-2 inhibitors).
- Corticosteroids.
- Oral contraceptives.
- Topical or oral decongestants.
- Excessive liquorice or salt intake.

Assessment and management of other cardiovascular risk factors, particularly smoking and diabetes mellitus, is an important part of management. These factors can modify substantially the overall cardiovascular risk. Lipids and blood glucose might need checking after changes of therapy, eg initiation of diuretics.

Nonpharmacological measures to reduce both BP and cardiovascular risk should be introduced in all patients with hypertension. These might be the only interventions necessary in some patients.

Effective measures include the following:
- Weight reduction in overweight patients.
- ↓ of heavy chronic or intermittent alcohol intake (defined as >3 units/day in ♀ or >5 units/day in ♂)
- Regular physical activity.
- Moderate sodium restriction (eg no-added-salt diet).
- Management of sleep apnoea.
- Stress reduction.

Obstructive sleep apnoea is a strong independent risk factor for stroke and cardiovascular events. Effective management ↓ BP and can reverse these risks, but this has not been formally demonstrated.

Patients should be vigorously encouraged to stop smoking, and hyperlipidaemia should be managed. Management of cardiovascular risk factors, in addition to good glycaemic control is particularly important in hypertensive patients with diabetes mellitus.

Drug treatment

If the above nonpharmacological measures do not achieve risk factor and BP goals, drug treatment should be commenced.

In patients with no other risk factors, treatment should be commenced at systolic BP levels > 160mmHg and at diastolic BP levels ≥ 95–100mmHg.

See Clinical guideline 34 (NICE) and refer to British Hypertension Society guidelines for when to initiate antihypertensives when risk factors (eg risk of coronary events, diabetes or end-organ damage) are present[1].

---

1 British Hypertersion Society. www.bhsog.org

The six major drug groups used at present are diuretics, β-blockers, ACE inhibitors, angiotensin II receptor antagonists, calcium-channel blockers and α-blockers. The major objective is to achieve satisfactory control of BP and overall cardiovascular risk. In many patients, this requires a combination of antihypertensive medications to achieve therapentic targets.

Overall, the major drug groups have similar efficacy in ↓ BP in most groups of patients (African patients excluded) with mild-to-moderate hypertension.

β-blockers are no longer preferred as a first line therapy, as according to NICE, β-blockers raise a patient's risk of developing diabetes. Recently published update by NICE (www.nice.org.uk).

Target BP

Target BP is <130/85mmHg, but some patients, especially the elderly, might not achieve or tolerate these levels. The achievement of target levels in patients with diabetes mellitus is particularly important.

The optimal outcome is to attain target levels of BP using only one preparation and once-daily dosing. If the initial drug chosen does not achieve target levels, one worthwhile strategy is to consider ↑ the dose or changing to an acceptable substitute until monotherapy is successful or clearly fails. If possible, allow at least a 1 month before changing therapy to allow steady-state effects to occur at each dose level. Alternatively, use an appropriate drug in combination.

Further reading

CG18 Hypertension (persistently high BP) in adults: NICE guideline www.nice.org.uk

Understanding anticoagulation

After injury, three separate mechanisms are activated to ↓/halt bleeding: vasoconstriction, gap plugging by platelets and the coagulation cascade. These mechanisms can be activated inappropriately and predispose patients to stroke.

The endothethial surface cells of blood vessels are involved in the balance between clotting and bleeding by secreting compounds such as von Willebrand factor, tissue plasminogen activator (t-PA) and prostaglandins (eg prostacyclin). The surface cells are also involved in the balance between fibrinolysis and fibrin formation.

Platelet response
- Adhesion
- Secretion
- Aggregation
- Propagation of procoagulant activity.

Regulation of coagulation and fibrinolysis
The coagulation factors consist of 12 plasma proteins that circulate in their inactive form. Coagulation of blood causes a cascading series of proteolytic reactions that result in an active protease, which activates (in an enzymatic way) the next clotting factor, until a fibrin clot is formed.

Coagulation factors
- Vitamin K-dependent factors (II, VII, IX and X).
- Contact activation factors (XI, XII, prekallikrein and high-molecular-weight kininogen).
- Thrombin-sensitive factors (V, VIII, XIII and fibrinogen).

Clotting begins at either an instrinsic or extrinsic pathway, with activation cascading to the common pathway.

Tissue injury releases either of the following factors:
- Tissue factor (extrinsic to blood), which activates the extrinsic pathway through factor VII.
- Subendothelial membrane contact with factor XII initiates intrinsic pathway (intrinsic—all necessary coagulation factors are present in blood).

Fibrinolysis
Formation of a fibrin clot occurs as a result of the coagulation system, the fibrinolytic system opposes coagulation and dissolves the developing clot and restores blood flow. The process starts by the release of t-PA from endothelial cells, and in response to thrombin or venous stasis, t-PA is incorporated into the forming clot by binding to fibrin. t-PA converts inactive plasminogen into plasmin, which digests fibrin and dissolves the clot.

Laboratory tests
Bleeding time
Bleeding time measures the length of time to the cessation of bleeding following a standardized skin cut.

Factors that prolong bleeding time include the following:
- Thromocytopenia.
- Platelet dysfunction.
- Aspirin/NSAIDs.
- SSRIs.

Prothrombin time (PT)

Thromboplastin is added to test the extrinsic system. PT is expressed as a ratio compared with control (INR) and has a normal range or 0.9–1.2. The INR is prolonged by warfarin, vitamin K deficiency and liver disease.

Thrombin time

Thrombin is added to plasma to convert fibrinogen to fibrin (normal range, 10–15s). The thrombin time is ↑ by heparin therapy, disseminated intravascular coagulation (DIC) and fibrinogen deficiency.

Kaolin cephalin clotting time (KCCT; APTT,=PTT partial thromboplastin time)

Kaolin activates the intrinsic system (normal range, 26–34s) KCCT is prolonged by heparin therapy or haemophilia.

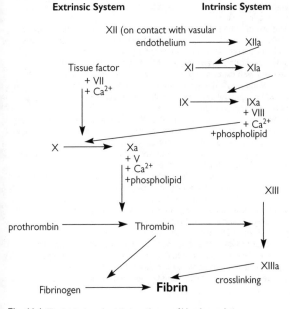

Fig. 16.1 The intrinsic and extrinsic pathways of blood coagulation

Reproduced with permission from Longmore M, Wilkinson IB, and Rajagopalan S (2004). *Oxford Handbook of Clinical Medicine*, 6th edn. Oxford: Oxford University Press.

Clinical use of anticoagulants

Prevention of deep vein thrombosis (DVT)

DVT is a common complication of hospital admission and the need for DVT prevention should be assessed in all inpatients. The risk of developing DVT during hospitalization, immobilization at home or in a nursing home depends on factors related to the individual patient and the features of any predisposing medical illness or surgical procedure performed. Individual patient risk should be assessed (Table 16.5).

Types of prophylaxis

Pharmacological and nonpharmacological methods of prophylaxis are both effective in preventing DVT, and their use in combination is additive.

Pharmacological prophylaxis

- Unfractionated heparin (UFH) is the appropriate cost-effective pharmacological method in most instances.
- Low-molecular-weight heparin (LMWH) has been shown to be clearly superior to UFH in preventing DVT in patients undergoing orthopaedic surgery and should be used in that situation. Its efficacy in other high- and moderate-risk situations is at least that of UFH, and it is ∴ a reasonable alternative.
- The use of LMWH for DVT prophylaxis ↑ the risk of epidural haematoma in patients undergoing epidural anaesthesia. The risk is greatest with co-existent ♀ gender, advanced age, orthopaedic surgery or other antithrombotic therapy (aspirin, NSAIDs or warfarin). LMWH should be used with caution in the presence of an epidural catheter and is contraindicated if the above risk factors are present. Insertion or withdrawal of epidural catheters should not be performed within 12h of LMWH administration.
- Fondaparinux is a selective anti-Xa inhibitor that, unlike UFH and low-molecular-weight heparin, has no antithrombin activity. Fondaparinux is more effective at DVT prevention than LMWH in patients undergoing hip and knee arthroplasty and hip fracture surgery, and is a suitable option for those procedures.
- Aspirin has only a weak effect in preventing venous thrombosis and is not to be considered adequate as sole prophylaxis.
- DVT prophylaxis should continue until the patient is fully ambulant and fit for hospital discharge. In particularly high-risk clinical situations, including hip and knee arthroplasty and oncology surgery, prolonged prophylaxis of 28 days duration should be strongly considered.
- In situations where the slightest risk of local bleeding is unacceptable (eg after neurosurgery, ophthalmic surgery, some plastic surgery, head injury or haemorrhagic stroke) anticoagulant therapy should be avoided and mechanical preventive methods should be used.

Table 16.5 Risk factors associated with development of DVT

Risk category	Medical	Surgical
High	Stroke Age >70yrs Congestive heart failure Shock Cancer History of DVT/ pulmonary embolism Thrombophilia	Orthopaedic surgery on pelvis, hip or lower limb Major surgery, age >60yrs Major surgery, age 40–60yrs with cancer or history of DVT/pulmonary embolism or other risk factors Thrombophilia
Moderate	Immobilized patient with active disease	Major surgery, age 40–60yrs, or other risk factors Minor surgery, age >60yrs, or age 40–60 years and history of DVT/pulmonary embolism or oestrogen therapy, or other risk factors
Low	Minor medical illness	Major surgery, age <40yrs Minor surgery, age <60yrs

Major surgery–any intra-abdominal operation and all other operations lasting >45mins.
Risk factors include deficiency of antithrombin, protein C or protein S, or the presence of antiphospholipid antibodies, activated protein C resistance (eg factor V Leiden mutation) or hyperhomocysteinaemia.

Mechanical prophylaxis

Methods of mechanical prophylaxis include graduated compression stockings providing 16–20mmHg pressure at the ankle, sequential pneumatic compression devices and pneumatic foot compression. These should be applied the evening before surgery and continued until the patient is fully ambulant.

Prophylaxis treatment

The type of prophylaxis recommended depends on the patient's risk category. In all patients, however, it is advisable to avoid dehydration and to commence mobilization as soon as possible.

Effective regimens for prophylaxis include the following:
• UFH, 5000U SC every 8–12h.
• Enoxaparin, 40mg or dalteparin, 5000IU SC daily, or other low molecular weight heparin, commencing ≥ 6h postoperatively, for high-risk cases.
• Enoxaparin, 20mg or dalteparin, 2500IU SC, daily, commencing ≥6h postoperatively, for moderate-risk cases (or for patients with a low body weight or if renal impairment is present).
• Fondaparinux, 2.5mg SC daily, commencing ≥ 6h postoperatively.

Treatment of thromboembolism

The object of treatment for established venous thrombosis is to prevent thrombus extension, pulmonary embolism, the postthrombotic syndrome and recurrent VTE.

The type of therapy employed depends on the anatomical extent of the thrombus (Table 16.6).

Anticoagulation

Before anticoagulant therapy is instituted, blood should be collected for determination of APTT, INR and platelet count. A thrombophilia screen should be considered if there is a family history of VTE, recurrent VTE and, possibly, if there is spontaneous VTE. This should include activated protein C resistance, fasting plasma homocysteine, prothrombin, protein C, protein S, antithrombin III, lupus anticoagulant, blood count and anticardiolipin antibody tests. More specialized testing is occasionally indicated.

LMWH has been shown to be at least as effective and safe as an IV UFH infusion in the initial management of DVT. LMWH has the advantages of not requiring routine laboratory monitoring and enabling management in a hospital out-patient or general practice setting in selected cases, and is now the treatment of choice.

Any of the following regimens are recommended:
- Enoxaparin, 1.5mg/kg body weight SC daily (up to a maximum dose of 150mg daily).
- Dalteparin once daily dose graduated to weight (see *BNF*) or 100 IU/kg body weight SC twice daily (up to a maximum dose of 10 000 IU twice daily).
- Tinzaparin, 175units/kg body weight SC daily.
- In the presence of renal impairment low-molecular-weight heparin requires factor Xa monitoring and possible dose adjustment. (calculated creatinine clearance ≤30mL/min).
  - Oral anticoagulation can be commenced on the same day as low-molecular-weight heparin.
  - A normal loading dose of warfarin is: 15–30mg, divided between 3 days.
- The INR should be monitored daily and the dose adjusted according to the INR, until a therapeutic level is achieved. The initial dose of warfarin should be ↓ in the elderly.
- Low-molecular-weight heparin should be given for a minimum of 5 days and until the INR has been >2 on two consecutive days.
- Warfarin should not be commenced alone (ie without a low-molecular-weight heparin) because this is associated with a high rate of subsequent DVT recurrence.
- The duration of anticoagulation depends on the risk of both recurrent VTE and bleeding.
- One recent study showed a ↓ in DVT recurrence using long-term, low-intensity warfarin (INR 1.5–2.0) following idiopathic DVT. This benefit occurred with no ↑ in major bleeding or other side effects. This is reasonable therapy in this group of patients.

- Graduated compression stockings ↓ the incidence and severity of the post-thrombotic syndrome and should be used in all cases. Stockings should provide 30–40mmHg pressure at the ankle and extend to the level of the knee. Graduated compression stockings should be worn for 18 months and indefinitely if the post-thrombotic syndrome is present; this important therapy is often overlooked. Patients should be encouraged to mobilize as soon as possible.

Table 16.6 Overview of the treatment of deep vein thrombosis

Extent of DVT	Therapy
Proximal veins (the popliteal or more proximal veins)	Anticoagulation and graduated compression stockings
Distal veins	Anticoagulation or ultrasound surveillance program and graduated compression stockings

Treatment of pulmonary embolism

Pulmonary embolism without haemodynamic compromise

The mainstay of treatment is supportive medical care, particularly O_2 and analgesia, and therapeutic anticoagulation; anticoagulation should be commenced in hospital. Anticoagulation using low-molecular-weight heparin and warfarin should be commenced as outlined previously.

Pulmonary embolism with haemodynamic compromise

- Patients with major pulmonary embolism have persisting tachycardia, hypotension, right heart failure and/or severe hypoxaemia. These patients require supportive medical treatment with O_2 at high flow rates. If there is associated severe chest pain analgesia might also be required. Therapeutic anticoagulation is required and thrombolytic therapy can be of benefit in selected cases.
- Anticoagulation with UFH through an infusion should be commenced, because the efficacy of LMWH in this situation is unknown:
- UFN 5000 units IV, as a loading dose, followed by 1250 units/hour by IV infusion and then adjust according to the APTT.
- The APTT should be checked after 4–6h and the dose adjusted if it is not in the therapeutic range. (target range, 60–85); Table 16.7
- When the APTT is in the therapeutic range, the dose should be reviewed daily. The platelet count should be checked three times weekly to detect the important, although uncommon, syndrome of heparin-induced thrombocytopenia.
- In the acute stages of a major thromboembolic episode, there is often relative heparin resistance and the dose requirement can be high. However, this heparin resistance can suddenly reverse, emphasizing the importance of monitoring the APTT closely.
- Warfarin should be commenced within 48h, using the regimen for DVT
- The outcome in the majority of patients with major pulmonary embolism who *receive anticoagulant therapy only* is good. The role for thrombolysis or surgical thrombectomy is limited, but these are reasonable options for patients with ongoing hypotension, right heart failure or severe hypoxaemia and without contraindications. Clinical trials in this area, however, are small and the results inconclusive.
- If thrombolytic therapy is used, use one of the following regimens:
  - Alteplase, 10mg bolus IV, followed by 90mg by IV infusion over 2h (in patients <65kg in weight, the total dose should not exceed 1.5mg/kg body weight).
  - Streptokinase, 250 000 IU IV over 30mins, followed by 100 000IU/hour by IV infusion for 24–72h.
- After the initial haemostatic defect has partly resolved and the with APTT is less than twice the normal (60–85), use the following regimen:
  - UFH 1000 units/hour by IV infusion; subsequently, adjust frequently according to the APTT to ensure therapeutic anticoagulation.
- There is an ↑ risk of bleeding (especially intracranial) with thrombolytic therapy.
- Streptokinase therapy can cause anaphylactic reactions and should not be given to patients who have previously had streptokinase therapy, because of the probable presence of neutralizing antibodies.

Unfractionated heparin dosage adjustment
- Syringe preparation UFH, 25 000 units to 50mL sodium chloride 0.9% in a syringe pump.
- Administer a loading dose of 5000 units (10 000 units in severe pulmonary embolism). Then 15–25 units/kg body weight/hour (equivalent to 1000–2000 units/h; 2.8mL/h = 1400 units/h).

Table 16.7 Heparin dosage adjustment recommendations

APTT(s) Normal 26–34sec	Bolus dose (units)	Pause (mins)	Dose change (units/h)	Rate change for 500 units/mL solution (mL/h)	Next APTT
<50	5000	0	+150	+0.3	4–6h
50–59	0	0	+100	+0.2	4–6h
60–85 target range	0	0	0	0	12h
86–95	0	0	−50	−0.1	12h
96–120	0	30	−100	−0.2	4–6h
>120	0	60	−150	−0.3	4h

Warfarin dosing

Loading dose

A normal loading dose of warfarin is 15–30mg, divided over 3 days.

The individual response is unpredictable and factors that particularly influence first doses should be considered:

- Age and weight—consider ↓ loading dose if patient >60yrs of age or weight <60kg.
- Pathophysiological changes—consider ↓ loading dose in the following condition:
- Liver disease.
- Cardiac failure.
- Nutritional deficiency.
- Drug interactions—check BNF (appendix 1); remember over-the-counter medicines and complementary therapies.

Maintenance dose

The response to the loading dose can be used to predict the maintenance dose. Aim for an INR of 2–4, depending on the indication. A useful, conservative estimate can be calculated using Table 16.9 considerations. Good correlation is obtained provided that the following considerations are adhered to:

- The loading dose has been given correctly.
- The APTT ratio <2.5.

Calculation of an estimate

- Calculate the total loading dose given over the 3 days
- From the column headed by 'cumulative dose', read along the horizontal line corresponding to the INR measured on the fourth day to obtain the predicted maintenance dose (Table 16.9).

For example if the total loading dose is 25mg, the predicted maintenance dose is 4.5mg when the measured INR on day 4 is 2.5.

Monitoring therapy

It is important to take account of trends rather than single results. If a patient has an unusual individual result, consider whether recent changes in behaviour (eg diet) could have affected it. If so, these changes should be 'corrected' rather than the warfarin dose corrected.

Factors that can affect response to warfarin include the following:

- Compliance—including timing of dose.
- Changes in kinetic parameters—eg weight change and, fluid balance.
- Diseases—eg infection, CCF, malabsorption, liver disease, renal impairment and, GI disturbances.
- Changes in social behaviour—eg smoking and, alcohol.
- Diet (green vegetables contain significant amounts of vitamin K).
- Stress.

Drug interactions—consult BNF (appendix 1) or Stockley.

Further reading

Dager W (2003). Initiating warfarin therapy. *Ann Pharmacother*. **37**(6): 905–8.
Fennerty A (1994). Flexible induction dose regimen for warfarin and prediction of maintenance dose. *BMJ* **288**: 1268–70.

Table 16.8 INR targets and durations for anticoagulant therapy

Indication	Target INR and (range)	Duration
Antiphospholipid syndrome syndrome (arterial thrombosis)	3.5 (3.0–4.0)	Consider long term
Antiphospholipid syndrome (venous thrombosis)	2.5 (2.0–3.0)	Consider long term
Arterial thromboembolism	3.5 (3.0–4.0)	Discuss with haematologist
AF	2.5 (2.0–3.0)	Long term
Calf DVT	2.5 (2.0–3.0)	3 months
Cardiomyopathy	2.5 (2.0–3.0)	Long term
Cardioversion	2.5 (2.0–3.0)	3wks before and 4wks after
Mechanical prosthetic heart valve (MHV)	3.5 (3.0–4.0)	Long term
Mural thrombosis	2.5 (2.0–3.0)	3 months
Proximal DVT	2.5 (2.0–3.0)	6 months
Pulmonary embolus	2.5 (2.0–3.0)	6 months
Recurrence of VTE (if no longer on an oral anticoagulants)	2.5 (2.0–3.0)	Consider long term
Recurrence of VTE (while on oral anti-coagulants)	3.5 (3.0–4.0)	Consider long term

Table 16.9

INR	Cumulative warfarin dose (mg)			
	15	20	25	30
2	3.5	4	5	5.5
2.5	3.5	4	4.5	5
3	2.5	3	3.5	3.5
3.5		2.5	3	3
4			3	3
4.5			2.5	3
5			2.5	2.5

Counselling patients treated with warfarin

After the decision had been made to initiate anticoagulation therapy, the ward pharmacist should counsel the patient about the risks associated with warfarin.

Counselling

All patients whether initiated within the hospital setting or the community should ideally be given written information on anticoagulants.

The following points should be covered:
- Dose—how much, how often and how long?
- The colour of tablets corresponding to strength. (Imperative to check the patient's understanding on how to work out which tablet(s) to take to allow for the correct dose; This can be done by getting them to explain what they' would take for a selection of doses.)
- Missed doses—what to do?
- Compliance importance.
- How warfarin works—might need to be simplistic for certain patients (ie makes the blood take longer than usual to clot ↓ the risk of clot extending).
- Need for blood tests.
- Importance of telling or reminding healthcare professionals (dentist, community pharmacist and practice nurse) about their warfarin treatment.
- Signs of over dose/underdose and what to do.
- Avoidance of drug interactions, including over-the-counter medicines and herbal preparations.
- Alcohol and diet.
- Pregnancy (if appropriate).
- Record detail of dose and INR result.
- Follow-up and duration of therapy, including arrangements for further monitoring (eg need to attend GP practice or out-patient clinic).

Patients should be informed that the dose of warfarin might need to be changed from time to time, and that monitoring their blood is necessary for as long as the therapy is administered. The therapeutic range is narrow and varies according to the indication; it is measured as a ratio of a standard PT.

Each patient should have an explanation of intended duration of therapy, indication for therapy, concurrent medical problems, other medication that must be continued and target coagulation laboratory values for the patient's condition. This information also needs to be communicated to the patient's primary care team.

Thereafter, there should be a mechanism to ensure the patient's therapy is monitored in terms of efficacy and risk during the duration of anticoagulation therapy.

Discharged patient should be reviewed within 1 week of discharge. Each condition requires a specific range of INR values. Therefore, adjusting the oral anticoagulant loading dose and maintenance doses is very necessary. Some patients could be particularly sensitive to warfarin—eg the elderly, those with high-risk factors, such as liver disease, heart failure or diabetes mellitus, those who regularly consume of alcohol, those on drug therapy that is known to ↑ or ↓ the effect of oral anticoagulation and those with poor compliance. Knowledge of concomitant medical problems and medication is essential for the safe management of anticoagulation.

Out-patient anticoagulation clinics

Anticoagulation management is a good example of an area in which patient care is undertaken by physicians, nurses and pharmacists. Although an effective anticoagulant, warfarin is limited in its use in clinical practice by its narrow therapeutic index, with a relatively small margin between safety and toxicity, dietary fluctuations in vitamin K, the effects of certain disease states and physiological, genetic, and patient-specific factors (eg compliance with therapy).

The major implications of long-term therapy with anticoagulants are a tendency to bleeding, haemorrhage and other factors, such as interaction between warfarin and other drugs, which make it difficult to maintain anticoagulant control in the therapeutic range.

The anticoagulation clinic provides ongoing monitoring of the PT and INR. Continual recommendations for warfarin dose adjustment, including management of drug interactions involving warfarin and supratherapeutic INRs. The goal is to provide follow-up and dose adjustment adequate to maintain the PT/INR within designated therapeutic ranges specific to the conditions for which the anticoagulation is indicated.

Hospital-based-clinics

Oral anticoagulation monitoring has traditionally taken place in secondary care because of the need for laboratory testing. The need for frequent monitoring and for close patient follow-up introduced the need for co-ordinated warfarin management by means of an organized system of clinical follow-up. Anticoagulation clinics have historically fulfilled this role. The patients attend the hospital for venepuncture; blood is then sent to the laboratory for testing. The pharmacist, doctor or nurse is informed of the results and can then discuss dosage adjustment and arrange a further appointment for blood test and review. The healthcare professional also discusses whether any changes in the patient's diet or recent change in alcohol consumption, for example, might have been the reason for the INR being outside the patient's therapeutic range.

GP-surgery-based-clinics

The development of reliable near-patient testing systems for INR estimation has facilitated the ability to manage patients within primary care. With the introduction of finger-prick testing services, there is no longer a reliance on the hospital pathology laboratory for INR measurement. The GP discusses with patients their compliance and recommends dose and the follow-up date for INR recheck.

Outreach DVT service

In some cases, co-ordination between primary and secondary care is established. Patients attend their local surgery for blood sampling the samples for laboratory analysis are collected and subsequent dosing and patient management is undertaken within the secondary care anticoagulation clinic.

Domiciliary service

This service is only suitable for patients who are on the telephone and whose anticoagulation is reasonably well controlled. The patient's GP sends a district nurse to the patient's home to collect blood samples.

Future of services

- The emergence of novel anticoagulant therapies might have dramatic implications not only for patient management, but also for anticoagulation clinics. Oral direct thrombin inhibitors (DTI) show promise as future agents to improve the field of oral anticoagulation management.
- Ximelagatran, a prodrug of melagatran, is the oral DTI that is in the most advanced phases of clinical development.
- Ximelagatran is awaiting regulatory approval in a number of indications, namely the prevention of stroke in patients with AF, the prevention of blood clots in patients undergoing knee-replacement surgery and the long-term secondary prevention of blood clots following standard treatment.
- Ximelagatran has, in theory, several advantages over warfarin: it has a wider therapeutic index, a predictable dose–response profile (ie it does not require dosing adjustments and monitoring), it is not metabolized through known hepatic microsomal enzymes and it seens to lack CYP450-related drug and food interactions. These advantages make it is easier and more convenient to administer than warfarin therapy.
- The introduction of ximelagatran could lead to a significant drop in the volume of warfarin patients referred to anticoagulation clinics for monitoring. However, because ximelagatran is very expensive compared with warfarin and clinicians have limited clinical experience of its use, anticoagulation services will remain a necessary service for the foreseeable future.

Acute coronary syndrome

- These syndromes are attributable to myocardial ischaemia 2° to coronary obstruction. The syndromes cover a spectrum of conditions ranging from unstable angina to STEMI.
- Unstable angina is a syndrome of chest pain caused by myocardial ischaemia; MI is heart muscle damage caused by prolonged ischaemia. The two conditions share the same pathophysiology, similar symptoms and the same early management.
  - Syndrome depends on the extent of thrombosis, distal platelet and thrombus embolization and resultant myocardial necrosis.
- The acute coronary syndromes are differentiated according to the extent and duration of chest pain, electrocardiogram (ECG) changes and biochemical markers.
- Acute coronary syndromes are differentiated into syndromes associated with the following:
  - ST-segment elevation on the ECG (ST-segment elevation MI; STEMI)
  - Without ST-segment elevation (non-ST-segment elevation MI; NSTEMI), which is associated with either ST-segment depression, T-wave inversion or no changes on the ECG.
- NSTEMI is differentiated from unstable angina by biochemical evidence of myocardial necrosis. The diagnosis of myocardial necrosis is indicated by an ↑ troponin level. Cardiac tropinins are the most sensitive and specific markers of myocardial necrosis. Troponin T better reflects myocardial damage (peaks at 12–24h; elevated for >1 week. If troponin is normal >6h after the onset of pain and the ECG is normal,the risk of MI is small.
- Unstable angina and NSTEMI represent a continuum, and their management is similar.
- Patients presenting with pain at rest or severe exacerbation of stable angina are differentiated into high, low or intermediate risk, depending on various factors.
- Patients with unstable angina are classified according to the highest-risk category of which they exhibit at least one feature.
- High-risk features:
  - Prolonged (>10mins) ongoing chest pain/discomfort.
  - ST-segment elevation or depression (>0.5mm) or deep T-wave inversion in three or more ECG leads.
  - ↑ serum markers of myocardial injury (especially cardiac troponin I or T).
  - Diabetes mellitus.
  - Associated syncope.
  - Associated heart failure, mitral regurgitation or gallop rhythm.
  - Associated haemodynamic instability (systolic BP <90mmHg, cool peripheries and diaphoresis).
- Intermediate-risk features:
  - Prolonged, but resolved, chest pain/discomfort.
  - Nocturnal pain.

- Age >65yrs.
- History of MI or revascularization.
- ECG normal or pathologic Q-waves.
- No significant (<0.5mm) ST-segment deviation, or minor T-wave inversion in <3 ECG leads.
- Low-risk features:
  - ↑ angina frequency or severity.
  - Angina provoked at a lower threshold.
  - New-onset angina >2wks before presentation.
  - Normal ECG and negative serum troponin.
  - No high-risk or intermediate-risk features.

ST-segment elevation myocardial infarction (STEMI)

- If the thrombus that occurs on a ruptured plaque completely occludes the coronary artery so there is no flow beyond it, the result is severe transmural myocardial ischaemia with ST-segment elevation on the ECG.
- This can cause sudden death from ventricular fibrillation.
- If the coronary occlusion is not relieved, MI develops progressively over the next 6–12h.
  The aim of emergency treatment of STEMI is as follows:
  - Prevent and treat cardiac arrest.
  - Relieve pain.
  - Reperfuse the myocardium urgently, to minimize infarct size.
- In STEMI it is important to reopen the artery and re-establish flow as soon as possible. This can be achieved by the administration of thrombolytic therapy or primary percutaneous coronary intervention (PCI).
- Thrombolytic therapy consists of a combination of a fibrinolytic agent, an antiplatelet agent and an antithrombin.
- Reperfusion therapy should be delivered as soon as feasible. Current standards indicate that if thrombolytic therapy is chosen, it should be given within 30mins of arrival in hospital.
- If primary PCI is the selected therapy, the aim should be to have the artery reopened within 60mins of arrival at hospital.
- Early risk-assessment allows categorization in terms of prognosis and choice of treatment. Initial indicators of high risk are ECG evidence of a large infarct, clinical and radiographic evidence of circulatory congestion, hypotension and shock, and serious arrhythmias.

STEMI: prehospital management

- The patient should be advised to call the ambulance directly, rest until it arrives and immediately take aspirin, 300mg (chewed or dissolved before swallowing), if available.
- The patient should also be advised to take a short-acting nitrate, if available:
  - GTN spray, 400mcg sublingually; repeat after 5mins if pain persists (up to a maximum of two metered doses).
  - GTN tablet 500mcg sublingually; repeat every 3–5mins (up to a maximum dose of 1500mcg; three tablets).
- If a doctor is present, add the following for pain relief, if required:
  - Morphine, 2.5–5mg IV; repeat as necessary.

STEMI: immediate and early hospital management

- An ECG should be performed immediately. If on the basis of clinical assessment and ECG, a diagnosis or presumptive diagnosis of STEMI can be made, give the following treatment:
  - Aspirin, 300mg chewed or dissolved before swallowing, (if aspirin has not been given) plus O_2 therapy.

- Patients known to have severe obstructive airway disease could underventilate with O_2 therapy and retain CO_2, becoming drowsy.
- For chest pain, use the following treatment:
  - GTN 500mcg sublingually; repeat after 5mins if pain persists, providing the systolic BP >95mmHg.
- For persisting chest pain, add the following treatment:
  - Morphine, 2.5–5mg IV (repeat as necessary) plus reperfusion therapy.

STEMI: reperfusion therapy

Patient selection for reperfusion therapy

Reperfusion therapy is indicated in the following circumstances:
- Ischaemic/infarction symptoms >20mins. This would include not only chest pain, but also other symptoms of MI, such as chest discomfort or pressure, shortness of breath, pulmonary oedema, sweating, dizziness and light-headedness.
- Patient's symptoms commenced within 12h.
- ST-segment elevation or left bundle branch block on the ECG.
- No contraindications to reperfusion therapy.

Percutaneous coronary intervention (PCI)

PCI is the therapy of choice if it is available in a timely manner. Adjuvant therapy for PCI includes aspirin/clopidogrel and heparin. Some patients need a gycoprotein IIb/IIIa inhibitor. The timing of delivery of the agents is determined by the individual interventionalist.

Fibrinolytic therapy

Fibrinolytic therapy is indicated in the following situation: prolonged ischaemic chest pain that has begun within the previous 12h, in the presence of significant ST-segment elevation or left bundle branch block (presumed new).

The decision whether or not to give fibrinolysis requires analysis of risk versus benefit. Patients likely to gain most benefit from fibrinolytic therapy present early with large MI, usually anterior, especially if there is any evidence of heart failure. Those with small MI, often inferior, benefit less. Elderly patients at higher risk also benefit. After 24h, the chances of benefit are very small and there is ↑ risk of cardiac rupture.

Contraindications to fibrinolytic therapy can be absolute or relative.

Absolute contraindications
- Risk of bleeding:
  - Active bleeding.
  - Recent (<1 month) major surgery or trauma.
- Risk of intracranial haemorrhage.
  - Any history of haemorrhagic stroke or history: schaemic stroke within the past 1yr.
  - Anatomical abnormalities, intracerebral neoplasms, and atriovenoncular malformation.

Relative contraindications
- Risk of bleeding:
  - previous use of anticoagulants or an INR >2.0.

- Noncompressible vascular punctures.
- Prolonged cardiopulmonary resuscitation (>10mins).
- Risk of intracranial haemorrhage:
  - Previous stroke at any time.
  - Previous (TIA). transient ischaemic attack.
- Other:
  - Pregnancy.
  - Severe hypertension that cannot be controlled (>180mmHg systolic BP and/or >110mmHg diastolic BP).

Patients with absolute contraindications should be transferred for a PCI. With relative contraindication, the risks and benefits of treatment must be weighed up.

Use one of the following thrombolytic agents:

- Alteplase, 15mg bolus IV, followed by an IV infusion of 0.75mg/kg body weight over a period of 30mins (up to a maximum of 50mg); then, 0.5mg/kg body weight over a period of 60mins, up to 35mg (the total dose should not exceed 100mg).
- Reteplase, 10 units bolus IV, followed by 10 units 30mins later.
- Streptokinase, 1.5 million IU by IV infusion, over a period of 20–30mins; if systolicBP <80mmHg, the infusion rate should be halved, and if systolicBP <70mmHg, stop the infusion until BP>70mm Hg, and then restart the infusion at half the previous rate.
- Tenecteplase, 500mcg/kg body weight over a period of 30s (up to a maximum dose of 50 mg).

Plasminogen activators, alteplase, reteplase and tenecteplase are superior to streptokinase but considerably more expensive, thus streptokinase is the drug of choice. Because antibodies are produced against strepto-kinase, there is an ↑ risk of allergic reactions if the patient is re-treated within 1yr. Prolonged exposure of antibodies to streptokinase can ↓ the effectiveness of subsequent treatment and streptokinase should not be used again beyond 4 days of the first administration.

The bolus agents' reteplase (double bolus) and tenecteplase (single bolus) have major advantages in terms of convenience and can be used in the prehospital setting, usually by suitably trained paramedic staff.

Recurrence of chest pain with ST-segment elevation is evidence of reocclusion, and, ∴ further thombolysis or urgent angioplasty might be indicated. Hypotension can occur, particularly with streptokinase, and should be treated by raising the foot of the bed and adjusting the infusion rate.

Allergic reactions are common with streptokinase and include bron-chospasm, periorbital swelling, angioedema, urticaria, itching, flushing, nausea, headache and musculoskeletal pain. Delayed hypersensitivity reactions, such as vasculitis and interstitial nephritis, have also been observed. Anaphylactic shock is rare.

For *mild* or *moderate* allergic reactions and fever, use promethazine, 25mg IV and/or hydrocortisone, 100mg IV. For *severe* allergic reactions, immediately discontinue streptokinase and give adrenaline 1 in 10 000 solution, 1mL IV, over a period of 5mins.

Antithrombin therapy

- There is still debate about the use of IV heparin with streptokinase. However, there seems to be a small, but significant, benefit. IV UFH is usually given routinely in conjunction with alteplase, reteplase and tenecteplase. Use UFH 60 units/kg body weight initially (up to a maximum of 4000 units), followed by 12 units/kg body weight/h adjusted according to the APTT.
- The initial APTT should be taken in 3h and adjusted according to local protocol.
- LMWH has been used in conjunction with fibrinolytic agents. It seems to ↓ reinfarction, but at the cost of ↑ bleeding. It is currently undergoing assessment in a large clinical trial. LMWH is not formally approved for use in combination with fibrinolytic agents. Particular care is needed in patients over the age of 75yrs, excess bleeding, including intracranial haemorrhage, has been reported.
- Occasionally, bleeding can occur following treatment with fibrinolytic therapy and heparin. Intracranial haemorrhages are devastating and life threatening. Systemic bleeding and GI bleeding can occur, in which care the following treatments are advised:
  - Reverse heparin with protamine (even if a LMWH has been used). Protamine dosage depends on the level of anticoagulation. Use 1 mg of protamine for every 100 units of UFH.
  - Replace fibrinogen using cryoprecipitate (two bags) or fresh frozen plasma (as required).
  - Give blood, as necessary.

Other therapy

- An IV β-blocker should be considered for patients with persistent pain and tachycardia that is not related to heart failure, those with hypertension and those with a large MI:
  - Atenolol, 5–10mg IV, infusion at a rate of 1mg/min or metoprolol, 5–15mg IV infusion at a rate of 1–2mg/minute.
- Titrate doses to the maximum dose of the recommended range, provided that the systolic BP does not fall below 95mmHg and the heart rate does not fall below 55bpm.
- β-blockers are contraindicated in patients with a significant history of bronchospasm or symptomatic bradycardia.
- The routine use of magnesium in the management of patients with acute MI is not recommended. Electrolyte abnormalities should be corrected appropriately.

STEMI: subsequent management

- On the basis of the probable contribution to clinical decision making, further investigation should be considered. Many patients will undergo coronary angiography. Provided that there are no contraindications, continue with following treatment regimen:
  - Aspirin, 75–300mg oral, daily or (if intolerant of aspirin) clopidogrel, 75mg oral, daily.

β-blocker therapy

- β blockers offer prognostic benefit following MI, especially in high-risk patients such as those with significant left ventricular dysfunction and/or ongoing ischaemia, and should be commenced during hospital admission unless contraindicated. Either of the following regimens is recommended:
    - Atenolol, 25–100mg oral daily.
    - Metoprolol, 25–100mg oral twice daily.
- Titrate doses to the maximum dose in the recommended range, provided that the systolic BP does not fall below 95mmHg and the heart rate does not fall below 55bpm.
- The benefit of β-blocker therapy persists long term, and it should be continued indefinitely in the high-risk patient.
- The usual contraindications to the use of β-blockers apply. Patients with significant left ventricular dysfunction should be observed closely for the development of congestive heart failure.

ACE inhibitor therapy

- ACE inhibitors improve outcome after acute MI. Start ACE inhibitors therapy within 24–48h of acute MI in patients with previous MI, diabetes mellitus, hypertension, anterior location of infarct on ECG, elevated heart rate (>80bpm) and clinical or radiographic evidence of left ventricular failure or significant dysfunction (ejection fraction <45%).
- ACE inhibitors should be continued long term in patients with a low ejection fraction.
- Contraindications to early ACE inhibitor use include haemodynamic instability and hypotension (systolic BP <100mmHg). Complications of early ACE inhibitor therapy include persistent hypotension and renal dysfunction.
- BP should be closely monitored and while the patient is in hospital, renal function and plasma electrolytes should be monitored on alternate days. If the maintenance dose has not been achieved at discharge, the dose must be ↑ more slowly as an out-patient (eg weekly) with renal function and plasma electrolytes determined before each ↑ in dose.
- Angiotensin II receptor antagonists should be reserved (for this indication) for patients who develop a persistent cough with ACE inhibitor therapy.

Statin therapy

Statin therapy reduces premature death, MI and other adverse outcomes, such as stroke and revascularization post-MI. Statin therapy should be continued, or initiated, during hospital admission, no matter what the underlying cholesterol level.

Calcium-channel blocker therapy

The use of calcium-channel blockers should be reserved for patients who have post-MI angina and a contraindication to a β-blocker.

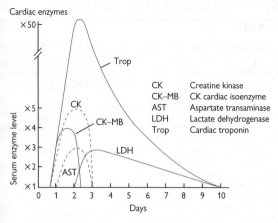

Fig. 16.2 Enzyme changes following acute MI. Reproduced with permission from Longmore M, Wilkinson IB, and Rajagopalan S (2004). *Oxford Handbook of Clinical Medicine*, 6th edn. Oxford: Oxford University Press.

Drug treatment in acute coronary syndromes

Drug treatment of high-risk unstable angina/NSTEMI

- Initial therapy for high-risk patients is hospitalization, with subsequent ECG monitoring and platelet inhibition, antithrombin therapy, use of a β-blocker and, potentially, glycoprotein IIb/IIIa inhibitors and revascularization.
- For pain relief in patients requiring hospital admission, give GTN, 10mcg/min by IV infusion; ↑ by 10mcg/min every 3mins until pain is controlled, providing the systolic BP is >95mmHg. (the dose range for GTN is 10–200mcg/min.)
- Normally, IV GTN is required for only a short period; prolonged infusion rapidly induces tolerance.
- For patients in whom there is a contraindication to β-blockers, a nondihydropyridine calcium-channel blocker can be substituted.for example, use one of the following regimens:
  - Diltiazem, 30–120mg oral, three times daily.
  - Diltiazem controlled-release, 180–360mg oral, daily.
  - Verapamil 40–120mg oral, twice to three times daily.
  - Verapamil sustained-release, 160–480mg oral, daily.
- For patients in whom angina has not been controlled with a β-blocker alone, a dihydropyridine calcium-channel blocker can be added eg nifedipineSR or amlodipine.
- When the pain is nocturnal, long-acting nitrates might be best given at night rather than during the day.
- Isosorbide mononitrate, 20–120mg oral, daily in divided doses.
- Avoid nitrates if the patient has used sildenafil (Viagra®) in the previous 24h or tadalafil (Cialis©) in the previous 2days.
- Pain nearly always settles promptly.
- After initial assessment and management, patients gradually return to the same risk as patients with stable angina.
- Patients who have undergone revascularization procedures involving a coronary stent must be on aspirin and clopidogrel for at least 1 month, and for those receiving the new drug-eluting stents, this should be for a minimum of 3months.

Platelet inhibition

Aspirin, 75–300mg oral, daily and clopidogrel, 75mg oral, daily (initial loading dose of 300mg).

Antithrombin therapy

- UFH or LMWH should be given, in addition to aspirin, to most patients. One of the following regimens is advised:
  - Enoxaparin, 1mg/kg body weight SC, twice daily.
  - Dalteparin, 120IU/kg body weight SC twice daily (up to a maximum of 10 000 units).
  - UFH 5000 units bolus IV, followed by 1000 units/h by IV infusion and then dose adjustment according to the APTT.

- UFH or LMWH should be administered for a minimum of 3days and possibly longer, depending on the clinical response.
- The advantages of LMWH are that it can be given subcutaneously and it has a more predictable effect so constant monitoring is not required. The fact that its effect cannot easily be reversed is, however, a disadvantage for the high-risk patient, who might require urgent intervention. Care should be taken in the elderly and in those with impaired renal function, in whom the dose should be ↓ to once daily.
- For patients on IV UFH, the APTT should be checked initially every 6h, with the target range of 60–80s, and should be checked daily after therapy has been stabilized.

β-blocker
- All patients without contraindications to β-blockade should be commenced on a β-blocker either the following regimens are recommended:
  - Atenolol, 25–100mg oral once daily.
  - Metoprolol, 25–100mg oral twice daily.

Glycoprotein IIb/IIIa inhibitors
- Some glycoprotein IIb/IIIa inhibitors are beneficial in ↓ MI and death in patients with NSTEMI or high-risk unstable angina. They are of particular benefit in patients who have an elevated troponin level and/or who are undergoing PCI. They are recommended for patients who are at high risk and have abnormal ECGs or a positive troponin test.
- Treatment with glycoprotein IIb/IIIa inhibitors occurs in two different clinical situations: patients might be treated in the coronary care unit (with tirofiban only) for a number of hours (up to 9h), before undergoing investigation and PCI, if appropriate; and patients might be treated (with abciximab only) at the time of the procedure.

Treatment in the coronary care unit
A loading dose of tirofiban, 400ng/kg body weight/min administered over a period of 30mins, followed by a maintenance infusion of 100ng/kg body weight/min for up to 108h.

Treatment in the cardiac catheterization laboratory
A loading dose of abciximab, 250mcg/kg body weight bolus before the intervention, followed by a maintenance infusion dose of 125ng/kg body weight/min (up to a maximum of 10mcg/min) administered over the 12h following the PCI.

Revascularization
Revascularization should be considered in all patients who are at high risk. Clinical trials have demonstrated the benefit of an early invasive strategy.

Drug treatment of intermediate-risk unstable angina/NSTEMI

Patients who are deemed to be at intermediate risk are admitted for monitoring and reassessment of clinical status, ECG and biochemical markers. They are then reclassified, depending on the results of these investigations, into high or low risk. If it is thought probable that the patient has coronary artery disease, treatment while undergoing assessment should include aspirin (or clopidogrel) and heparin.

Drug treatment of low-risk unstable angina/NSTEMI

Patients who are low risk need cardiac assessment to rule out coronary disease. This involves stress testing, which could be exercise testing with a ECG, stress echo cardiography or nuclear stress study. Patients proven to have coronary disease should proceed to further investigation and management. Patients should be treated with platelet inhibitors (usually aspirin) while being assessed.

Cardiopulmonary resuscitation

Cardiac arrest in adults: what the pharmacist needs to know
The management of cardiopulmonary arrest can be divided into two categories: basic and advanced life support.

Basic life support

Basic life support is the 'first-responder' phase of the chain of survival. It can be carried out by anyone who has undertaken a basic first-aid course (Fig. 16.3).

Shout for help. Ask someone to call the arrest team and to bring the defibrillator. Note the time.

Before approaching the patient, the first aider should always check it is safe to do so. The patient should then be assessed, eg checking consciousness by calling patients name or shaking (if no response) confirm that an arrest has occurred. This is done by checking the airway, breathing and circulation (ABC).

- Airway
  - Tilt head (if no spine injury) and lift chin/jaw thrust. Clear the mouth.
- Breathing
  - Give two breaths (each inflation should be 2s long), ideally using Ambu system, otherwise give mouth to mouth (unless poisoning is suspected).
- Chest compressions
  - Give 30 compressions to 2 breaths (30:2), cardiopulmonary resuscitation should not be interrupted, except to give shocks or intubate. Use the heel of the hand with straight elbows. Centre over the lower case-third of the sternum, which should be depressed approximately 1inch. Chest compressions work to promote the forward flow of blood.

The most common cause of cardiac arrest is the arrhythmia, ventricular fibrillation. Ventricular fibrillation is known as a 'shockable rhythm' because it responds to defibrillation.

Advanced life support

Advanced life support starts when medical personnel arrive, nominally provided by the cardiac arrest team. Fig. 16.4.

- Basic life support maintained.
- The patient's airway is secured and O_2 is administered.
- IV access is obtained (in hospital, blood is taken for urgent blood-gas analysis and determination of electrolyte levels).

The patient is attached to the cardiac monitor on the defibrillator, to allow diagnosis of the arrhythmia. Further management depends on whether or not the type of arrhythmia present responds to defibrillation.

In addition to ventricular fibrillation, pulseless ventricular tachycardia responds to defibrillation.

Treat ventricular fibrillation/pulseless ventricular tachycardia (VF/VT) with a single shock, followed by immediate resumption of CPR (30 compressions to 2 ventilations). Do not reassess the rhythm or feel for a pulse.

After 2min of CPR, check the rhythm and give another shock (if indicated).
- The recommended initial energy for biphasic defibrillators is 150–200J. Give second and subsequent shocks at 150–360J.
- The recommended energy when using a monophasic defibrillator is 360J for both the initial and subsequent shocks.

Asystole and electromechanical disturbance cannot be corrected using defibrillation. Asystole is the absence of any heart rhythm. Electromechanical disturbance (also known as pulseless electrical activity) is the presence of organized electrical activity that fails to result in mechanical contraction of the heart.

Pharmaceutical aspects of cardiopulmonary resuscitation

Basic cardiopulmonary resuscitation and early defibrillation are the only interventions proven to benefit survival in cardiac arrest. However, drugs have a role and should always be considered.

In hospital, an 'arrest box', containing a variety of drugs, is usually kept with the arrest trolley. Drugs in the arrest box tend to be either minijets, which require some degree of assembly, or, more commonly, prefilled syringes.

Drug administration

- For IV administration, a flush of 20mL of sodium chloride 0.9% solution should be administered after each drug dose to enhance its passage from the peripheral circulation to the central circulation. Alternatively, the dose can be given in tandem with a fast-flowing IV fluid.
- If IV access is unattainable, drugs can be administered down the endotracheal tube. Give twice the IV dose diluted in 10mL of 0.9% sodium chloride, followed by five ventilations to assist absorption.
- Current guidelines recommend the administration of 1mg of (10mL of 1 in 10 000 prefilled syringe) adrenaline IV every 3 to 5mins during resuscitation or 2–3mg via the tracheal tube. IV doses above 1mg are no longer considered to be of benefit and should not be used.
- Atropine is often used in the management of asystole or bradycardia, to block any excessive vagal activity that might be contributing to a ↓ in heart rate. For asystole, a single 3mg IV dose is given. Higher doses have no benefit. Smaller doses (0.5–1mg IV) can be given in bradycardia, up to a maximum total of 3mg.
- Amiodarone is the antiarrhythmic of choice in resistant ventricular fibrillation or pulseless ventricular tachycardia. A dose of 300mg in 20mL glucose 5% solution is given as a slow bolus over a period of at least 3mins. Remember that amiodarone is incompatible with normal saline and bags of dextrose 5% solution should be available to enable prompt setting up of the infusion and for flushing after dose(s).
  A further 150mg can be given, followed by an infusion of 1mg/min for 6h, and then 0.5mg/min for 6h. It is recommended that amiodarone is administered, if possible, using a volumetric control infusion pump rather than drip-counting technique because of the drug's affect on drip size.
    - If amiodarone is not available, lidocaine 1mg/kg may be used as an alternative, but do not give lidocaine if amiodarone has already been given. Do not exceed a total dose of 3mg/kg during the first hour.

- Magnesium is the agent of choice in torsades de pointes, a type of arrhythmia that is often drug-induced. It can also be useful in resistant arrhythmias, especially if they are associated with hypomagnesaemia (more common in patients taking diuretics). A bolus of 8mmol is usually given.
- Sodium bicarbonate: giving sodium bicarbonate routinely during cardiac arrest and CPR is not recommended. Give sodium bicarbonate (50mmol) if cardiac arrest is associated with hyperkelaemia or tricyclic antidepressant overdose. Repeat the dose according to the clinical condition of the patient and the results of repeated blood gas analysis. Should only be administered after arterial blood gas analysis where the pH has fallen below 7.1. A 50mmol (50mL of the 8.4% solution) dose would normally be given as a slow IV bolus.
- Calcium chloride, 10mL of the 10% (equivalent of 6.8mmol of calcium) preparation is administered in suspected or actual calcium-channel blocker overdose or in magnesium-induced heart block.
- After successful resuscitation, perform the following:
- 12-lead ECG, CXR, U&Es, glucose, blood gases, the blood count FBC, creatinine kinase/troponin levels are requested.
- Transfer to coronary care unit.
- Monitor vital signs.
- Communication to relatives.

Resuscitation is generally stopped after 20mins if there is refractory asystole or electromechanical dissociation.

Suggested contents of the adult emergency drug box used in pre-arrest and arrest situations:
- 5 x adrenaline, 1 in 10 000 solution, 1mg in 10mL prefilled syringe (Aurum pre-assembled syringe).
- 1 x atropine, 3mg in 10mL pre-filled syringe (Aurum pre-assembled syringe).
- 1 x amiodarone 300mg in 10mL pre-filled syringe (Aurum pre-assembled syringe).
- 1 x 5% dextrose, 50mL to flush amiodarone.

Suggested contents of back-up emergency box, containing the following drugs:-
- 6 x adenosine, 6mg in 2mL vial.
- 5 x adrenaline, 1 in 1000 solution, 1mg in 1mL ampoule.
- 2 x amiodarone, 150mg in 3mL ampoule.
- 6 x atropine, 500mg in pre-filled syringe (minijet).
- 1 x calcium chloride, 6.8mmol in 10mL (10%) pre-filled syringe (Aurum pre-assembled syringe).
- 1 x 50% glucose solution 50mL vial.
- 1 x magnesium sulphate, 10mmol in 5mL (50% solution) pre-filled syringe (minijet).
- 1 x sodium bicarbonate, 8.4% in 50mL pre-filled minijet.

It is envisaged that back-up emergency boxes are normally issued to the wards and departments with manual defibrillators.

Note: minijets are prefilled syringes designed for rapid use.

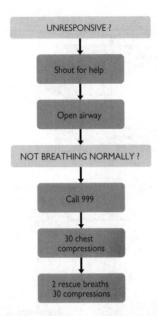

UNRESPONSIVE ?

↓

Shout for help

↓

Open airway

↓

NOT BREATHING NORMALLY ?

↓

Call 999

↓

30 chest compressions

↓

2 rescue breaths 30 compressions

Managing the airway
- You open the airway by tilting the head and lifting the chin—but only do this if there is no question of spinal trauma.
- Use a close-fitting mask if available, held in place by thumbs pressing downwards either side of the mouthpiece; palms against cheeks.

Chest compressions
- Cardiopulmonary resuscitation (CPR) involves compressive force over the lower sternum with the heal of the hands placed one on top of the other, directing the weight of your body through your vertical, straight, arms.
- Depth of compression: ~4cm.
- Rate of compressions: 100/min.

Fig. 16.3 UK adult basic life support algorithm. Reproduced with permission from the Resuscitation Council (UK)

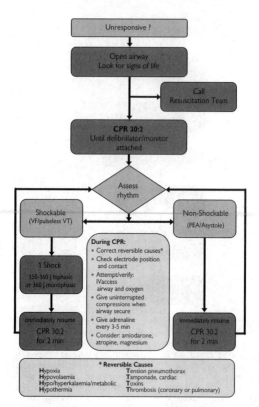

Fig. 16.4 UK adult advanced life support algorithm. Reproduced with permission from the Resuscitation Council (UK).

Asthma management in adults: British Thoracic Society and SIGN guidelines

Aims
- Minimize symptoms during the day and night.
- Minimize need for reliever medication.
- No exacerbations.
- No limitation on physical activity.
- Achieve best possible pulmonary function.

Treatment
- Initiate treatment at the level most appropriate to the severity of asthma (Table 16.10).
- Step-up treatment, as necessary:
- Before initiating new therapy recheck compliance, inhaler technique and eliminate trigger factors.
  - If trials of add-on therapies are ineffective stop
  - If trials of ↑ steroids are ineffective, return to original dose.
- Step-down treatment levels if control is good:
  - Review regularly while treatment is stepped down.

Table 16.10 Management of chronic asthma in adults

Level	Reliever therapy	Additional therapies	Further advice/therapy considerations
Step 1 Mild Intermittent asthma	Inhaled short-acting B2-agonist PRN		Review patients with high usage of reliever (>10 puffs/day is a marker of poorly controlled asthma)
Step 2 Regular prevented therapy	Inhaled short-acting B2-agonist PRN	Add inhaled steroid (200–800mcg/ daily)	Start at a dose appropriate to the severity and titrate to lowest effective dose. Usual dose is 400mcg/daily Initially, divide dose twice daily; use once daily if a good response is established.

Table 16.10 (Contd.)

Level	Reliever therapy	Additional therapies		Further advice/therapy considerations
Step 3 Add-on therapy	Inhaled short-acting B2-agonist PRN	Add inhaled steroid (200-800m/daily)	Add inhaled long-acting B2-agonist (LABA)	**Good response to LABA**—continue **Improvement with LABA but poor response**—continue and ↑ inhaled steroid to 800mcg/daily —if control is still inadequate, go to step 4 **No response to LABA**—Discontinue LABA and ↑ inhaled steroid dose to 800mcg/daily. If control still inadequate, trial other therapies—eg leukotriene receptor antagonists, theophylline, and slow-release oral B2-agonists If control still inadequate, go to step 4
Step 4 Persistent poor control	Inhaled short-acting B2-agonist PRN	Add inhaled steroid (800mcg/daily)	Inhaled long-acting B2-agonist (unless discontinued because of poor response)	Consider trials of ↑ inhaled steroids, up to 2000mcg/daily. Consider trials of fourth drug—eg leukotriene receptor antagonists, theophylline, and slow-release oral B2 agonists
Step 5 Continuous or frequent use of oral steroids	Inhaled short-acting B2-agonist PRN	High-dose inhaled steroid (2000mcg/daily)	Use oral steroids at the lowest dose for adequate control	Consider other treatments to minimize use of oral steroids. Refer to a specialist

Inhaler techniques

MDIs

The checklist steps for using a pressurized MDI are as follows:

- Sit or stand upright.
- Remove cap and shake the inhaler vigorously.
- Breathe out slowly and completely.
- Hold the inhaler in the upright position.
- Insert mouthpiece into mouth, between closed lips.
- Depress the canister once...
- ...and at this time, begin slow, deep inhalation.
- Remove inhaler, with lips closed.
- Hold breath for 10–15s.
- Wait for 20–30s before starting the second puff.

Emphasize that co-ordination of the commencement of breathing with the release of medicament is very important and can require practice to maximize benefit.

Points for the pharmacist/technician

- Demonstrate the correct method of use with a placebo inhaler, and ask the patient to show you how they use it. Most patients are on long-term therapy and many might have developed bad habits.
- The degree of benefit can be demonstrated to the patient by determining peak expiratory flow rates before dosing and 30mins afterwards.
- Patients with anything other than mild, occasional attacks derive considerable benefit from learning about their disease and how to manage it. They should measure peak-expiratory-flow rates regularly and keep a dairy of the results.

Advice to the patient

- Keep the device clean; replace the mouthpiece cap after use.
- The plastic housing can be cleaned with warm, mild detergent solution; ensure it is dried before use.

Dry-powder inhalers

Several devices are now available to deliver the medicament in a dry-powder inhaler. Because the medicines are dry powder, they must be inhaled fast enough so that the medicine is released.

The basic technique for using a dry-powdered medication is as follows:

- Exhale.
- Put mouthpiece in your mouth.
- Breathe in quickly and deeply.

Diskhaler®

A Diskhaler® is a dry-powder inhaler that holds small pouches (or blisters), each containing a dose of medication, on a disk. The Diskhaler® punctures each blister so that its medication can be inhaled.

The basic technique for using the diskhaler is as follow:

- Remove the cover and check that the device and mouthpiece are clean.

- If a new medication disk is needed, pull the corners of the white cartridge out as far as they will go, then press the ridges on the sides inwards to remove the cartridge.
- Place the medication disk with its numbers facing upwards on the white rotating wheel. Then, slide the cartridge all the way back in.
- Pull the cartridge all the way out, then push it all the way in until the highest number on the medication disk can be seen in the indicator window.
- With the cartridge fully inserted, and the device kept flat, raise the lid as far as it goes, to pierce both sides of the medication blister.
- Move the Diskhaler® away from mouth and breathe out.
- Place the mouthpiece between teeth and lips, making sure that you do not cover the air holes on the mouthpiece. Inhale quickly and deeply. Do not breathe out.
- Move the Diskhaler® away from mouth and continue holding breath for 10s.
- Breathe out slowly.
- If you need another dose, pull the cartridge out all the way and then push it back in all the way. This will move the next blister into place. Repeat the above steps.
- After you have finished using the Diskhaler®, put the mouthpiece cap back on.

Using a turbohaler dry-powder inhaler

The basic technique for using a turbohaler is as follows:
- Remove the cap from the turbohaler by unscrewing it.
- Hold the turbohaler with the mouthpiece up.
- Turn the bottom of the turbohaler all the way to the right and back to the left. You will hear it click.
- Hold the turbohaler away from your mouth and gently breathe out.
- Seal your lips around the mouthpiece.
- Inhale rapidly and deeply. Continue to take a full, deep breath.
- Resume normal breathing.
- Repeat the above steps if more than one puff is prescribed.
- Keep the turbohaler cap on when not in use.

Other points to tell patients include the following.
- When the red dot appears at the top of the window, there are 20 doses left. Plan to get a new turbohaler when you see the red dot.
- When the red dot is at the bottom of the window, the Turbohaler is empty. Start using a new turbohaler.

Accuhaler

- The basic technique for using the Accuhaler is as follows:
- Open the accuhaler by holding the outer case in one hand and putting thumb of the other hand on the thumb grip; push your thumb away as far as it will go, until a click is heard.
- Prime the dose by sliding the lever at the right of the mouthpiece away from you, until a click is heard. Every time the lever is pushed back, a blister is opened and the powder is made available for inhaling. This is shown by the counter.

- Hold the Accuhaler away from the mouth and breathe out as far as comfortable; remember never breathe into the accuhaler.
- Put mouthpiece to lips; suck in quickly and deeply.
- Remove the accuhaler from the mouth; hold your breath for about 10s or for as long as is comfortable.
- Close the Accuhaler by sliding the thumb grip back towards you; it should click shut.

Pain: a definition

The International Association for the Study of Pain defines pain as 'an unpleasant sensory and emotional experience associated with actual or potential tissue damage, or described in terms of such damage.

Pain is always subjective. Each individual learns the application of the word through experiences related to injury in early life. Accordingly, pain is that experience we associate with actual or potential tissue damage. It is unquestionably a sensation in a part or parts of the body, but it is also always unpleasant and, ∴, also an emotional experience.

Many people report pain in the absence of tissue damage or any likely pathophysiological cause; usually this happens for psychological reasons. There is usually no way to distinguish their experience from that caused by tissue damage if we take the subjective report. If they regard their experience as pain and if they report it in the same ways as pain caused by tissue damage, it should be accepted as pain. This definition avoids tying pain to the stimulus.'[1] In view of this, pharmacists should be wary of expressing opinions about whether a particular patient is in pain or not.

Types of pain

Nociceptive pain

'Nociceptive pain' is pain that occurs when nociceptors (pain receptors) are stimulated. This is normal pain in response to injury of the body. The purpose of this type of pain is to discourage the use of injured body parts, thereby potentially extending the injury further. This pain normally responds to conventional analgesics, such as paracetamol, NSAIDs and opioids.

Neuropathic pain

'Neuropathic pain' is pain initiated or caused by a primary lesion or dysfunction in the nervous system. The pain is often triggered by an injury, but this injury might or might not involve actual damage to the nervous system. It seems to have no physiological purpose. The pain frequently has burning, lancinating (stabbing) or electric-shock qualities. Persistent allodynia, pain resulting from a nonpainful stimulus, such as a light touch, is also a common characteristic of neuropathic pain. The pain can persist for months or years beyond the apparent healing of any damaged tissues. These pains might not respond to standard analgesics and might respond to unconventional analgesic treatments, such as antidepressants, anticonvulsants and various other therapies, such as clonidine or capsaicin.

---

1 International Association for the Study of Pain. www.iasp-pain.org

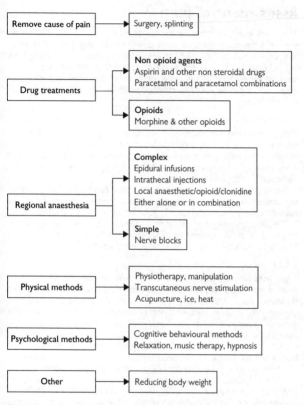

Fig. 16.5 Treating pain—methods available

Assessment of pain

There are good, validated scales for assessing pain. These are usually derived from assessment of both pain intensity and pain relief when analgesics are used. Both visual analogue scales (VASs; a line moving from 'no pain' to 'worst possible pain') or categorical scales (where words such as 'none', 'slight', 'moderate' or 'severe') are employed; often together. They can be useful to monitor progress in patients who are suffering from pain.

Categorical scales

Categorical scales use words to describe the magnitude of the pain. The patient picks the most appropriate word; most research groups use four words (none, mild, moderate and severe). Scales to measure pain relief were developed later. The commonest is the five category scale (none, slight, moderate, good and complete).

For analysis, numbers are given to the verbal categories (for pain intensity, none = 0, mild = 1, moderate = 2 and severe = 3, and for relief, none = 0, slight = 1, moderate = 2, good or lots = 3 and complete = 4).

The main advantages of categorical scales are that they are quick and simple. The small number of descriptors could force the scorer to choose a particular category when none describes the pain satisfactorily.

VASs

VASs, lines with the left end labelled 'no relief of pain' and the right end labelled 'complete relief of pain', seem to overcome this limitation. The standard VAS is 100mm long. Patients mark the line at the point that corresponds to their pain. The scores are obtained by measuring the distance between the 'no relief' end and the patient's mark, usually in millimetres. The main advantages of VASs are that they are simple and quick to score, avoid imprecise descriptive terms and provide many points from which to choose. More concentration and co-ordination are needed, which can be difficult postoperatively or with neurological disorders.

Pain relief scales are perceived as more convenient than pain intensity scales, probably because patients have the same baseline relief (zero), whereas they could start with different baseline intensity (usually moderate or severe). Relief-scale results are then easier to compare. They can also be more sensitive than intensity scales. A theoretical drawback of relief scales is that the patient has to remember what the pain was like to begin with.

Global subjective efficacy ratings, or simply 'global scales', are designed to measure overall treatment performance. Patients are asked questions such as 'How effective do you think the treatment was?' and to answer using a labelled numerical or categorical scale. Although these judgements probably include adverse effects, they can be the most sensitive way to discriminate between treatments.

Judgement of pain by the patient, rather than by a carer, is the ideal. Carers tend to overestimate the pain relief compared with the patient's version (Fig. 16.6).

Instructions

It is important that the use of the scale be explained to each patient. Patients are instructed to place a mark on the line to report the intensity or quality of the sensation experienced. Also, instructions should be written above the scale, eg INSTRUCTION: Put a mark on the line at the point that best describes HOW MUCH PAIN YOU ARE HAVING RIGHT NOW. Notice that what is measured is 'the perception right now', not a comparison such as, what is your pain compared with what you had before.

Fig. 16.7 can be completed to show changes in pain intensity and/or pain relief across time. This can be valuable when introducing changes to analgesia and provides an on going assessment of progress.

A range of pain assessment tools including those in a range of languages and some for children, can be found at the website shown below.[1]

An example of a chart for patients with chronic pain is presented in Fig. 16.7. Patients are asked to assess their pain on a weekly basis and to bring their charts when attending clinics.

(Low end) No pain at all	(High end) Worst possible pain

–> –> –> 100mm <– <– <–

Fig. 16.6 Example of a VAS for pain intensity

1 www.partnersagainstpain.com

OXFORD CHRONIC PAIN RECORD CHART

Patients name

1. Please choose a suitable time and day of the week, and complete the chart on the same day and time every week.
2. Stop when the chart is full, or when the pain returns to the same intensity as it was before the treatment started.
3. If you have more than one pain (e.g. back pain and leg pain) we may ask you to complete a separate chart for each pain.

Type of treatment: ....
Date of treatment: ....

Main Area of Pain:

	Weeks	0	1	2	3	4	5	6	7	8	9	10	11	12	13	14	15	16
How bad has your pain been today?	None																	
	Mild																	
	Moderate																	
	Severe																	
	V Severe																	
How much pain relief have you had today from the injection?	Complete																	
	Good																	
	Moderate																	
	Slight																	
	None																	
Please record the name and number of pain killing tablets taken per week																		
How effective was the treatment this week?	Excellent																	
	Very Good																	
	Good																	
	Fair																	
	Poor																	

Date when full pain returned ....

Fig. 16.7 Oxford chronic pain record chart

Acute pain: incidence

Acute pain is common. A survey of >3000 patients newly discharged from hospital revealed the results shown in Table 16.11.

- Not all of the patients in the survey had undergone surgery, so this is not just a problem for surgical wards.
- Pain can be a problem after operations, dental procedures and wound dressings. Some types of surgery have a less painful recovery than others so analgesia must be tailored.
- The need for pain relief in medical settings such as MI, sickle cell crisis, musculoskeletal disease and renal colic must be considered along with the needs of cancer, trauma, burns and obstetric patients.

Table 16.11 Responses to questions on pain by 3163 inpatients

	Proportion (%) of patients
Pain was present all or most of the time	33%
Pain was severe or moderate	87%
Pain was worse than expected	17%
Had to ask for drugs	42%
Drugs did not arrive immediately	41%
Pain was present all or most of the time	33%

Acute pain

Nonsteroidal anti-inflammatory drugs (NSAIDs) and nonopioids

Effective relief can be achieved with oral nonopioid and NSAIDs. From the NNT chart, it is clear that NSAIDs are superior to paracetamol and paracetamol combined with codeine. Combining paracetamol with an NSAID can enhance pain relief for a number of patients in the acute phase postsurgery. The current vogue of supplying separate paracetamol and codeine is to be discouraged (as a cost-saving exercise) because it leads to confusion in some patients, and there have been cases of codeine (inadvertent), overdosing leading to hospitalization.

There is wisdom in the saying that if patients can swallow, they should receive medicines by mouth. There is no evidence that NSAIDs given rectally or by injection work better or faster than the same oral dose. They do not ↓ the risk of GI damage either. Gastric upset and bleeding are important adverse effects. Ibuprofen is probably the safest in this respect; however, long-term NSAID treatment should be covered with a gastric-protecting agent, such as a proton-pump inhibitor. Beware also of using NSAIDs in patients with pre-existing kidney problems; an NSAID can precipitate acute renal failure, requiring dialysis.

The belief that NSAIDs should not be used after orthopaedic surgery because they inhibit healing is a myth.

Opioids

- These are first-line treatment for acute pain. Intermittent doses might provide effective relief, but patient-controlled analgesia is the preferred method. There are many stories of adequate doses being withheld because of misconceptions, fear and ignorance.
- Dependence is not a problem in acute pain, and respiratory depression is only a problem if the patient is either not in pain or given doses larger than those needed to treat the pain.
- The key principle is to titrate the analgesic until either pain relief is obtained or unacceptable side effects are experienced.
- There is no evidence that one opioid is better than another, although pethidine should be avoided because of its toxic metabolites, which can accumulate, acting as a CNS irritant and eventually inducing convulsions, particularly if underlying renal failure is present. There is no evidence for the view that pethidine is best for renal colic pains.
- The metabolite of morphine (morphine-6-glucuronide) can accumulate in renal disease, with the effect of prolonging the action of morphine. Providing the dose is titrated carefully, this should not be a problem.
- It makes good sense to select one opioid for the treatment of acute pain, so that everyone is familiar with its profile. In most settings, morphine does the job.

Regional anaesthesia

- Regional anaesthesia works by interrupting pain transmission from a localized area. The risk of neurological damage is the main concern.
- Pharmacists should be aware of the compatibility issues surrounding medicines for epidural or intrathecal use, in addition to careful monitoring of the doses used. Preservative-free morphine should be used as a rule (because of the potential neurotoxicity of preservatives), unless patients are in the terminal phase of illness.

Topical agents

- Topical agents can be useful in treating acute injuries, such as strains, sprains and soft tissue trauma. There is limited evidence for the benefits of rubifacients, which work by producing a counter-irritation to relieve musculoskeletal pains. The NNT is ~two, but this is based on three small trials (with 180 participants).
- There is good systematic review evidence to show that topical NSAIDs are effective in acute pain. The NNT for pain relief is two to four based on 37 placebo-controlled trials wing a range of NSAIDs. Ketoprofen, felbinac, ibuprofen and piroxicam are superior to placebo, but indomethacin and benzydamine are no better than placebo. Adverse events for NSAIDs were no different than placebo.

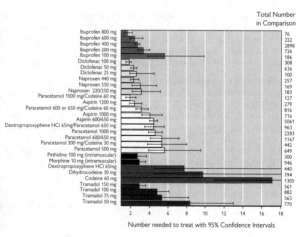

Fig. 16.8 Acute pain treatments: league table of the NNT

Treating cancer pain

Since the introduction of the WHO three-step ladder, potent opioids (usually morphine) have been the analgesics of choice for managing cancer pain (Fig. 16.9).

Morphine is still considered the benchmark by the European Association for Palliative Care mainly because it is available in a number of different dose forms, it has extensive clinical experience and has an ability to provide analgesia. It is not always ideal, however, with wide individual variation in dose needs and active metabolites that can accumulate, particularly in renal failure. There is no maximum dose for morphine, but a systematic review showed that mean daily doses range from 25mg to 300mg and can reach, in unusual cases, 2000mg daily. The adverse effects of morphine are not tolerated in ~4% of patients.

Drugs such as hydromorphone and oxycodone can be substituted, but these offer no real advantages. Transdermal fentanyl has become popular in recent years and can offer less constipation and daytime drowsiness.

Methadone can produce similar analgesia to morphine and has similar side effects, but it has a narrower dose range. It is the safest in renal failure; it also has a long and unpredictable half-life and its potency is often underestimated.

Spinal opioids

A few patients benefit from spinal opioids if they are unable to tolerate oral morphine. Spinal morphine in combination with a local anaesthetic is helpful for incident pain and the addition of clonidine can help neuropathic pain. Spinal opioids are associated with greater risks, especially of epidural abcesses, cerebro spinal fluid leaks and catheter problems.

Dealing with breakthrough pain

Cancer pain often presents as a continuous pain, with intermittent, more serious pains breaking through. This can arise in ≤ 80% of patients with cancer pain. Four episodes daily is about the average, with each pain lasting ~30 mins. There are several dose strategies to manage breakthrough pain, with the usual 4h dose, as needed, every 1–2h (as an instant-release formulation). With transmucosal fentanyl, there seems to be little relationship between the rescue dose and the daily dose.

Use of NSAIDs with opioids

There is good evidence that NSAIDs can ↓ the total dose of opioids and ↓ their adverse effects. Gastric protective agents are needed for chronic long-term dosing.

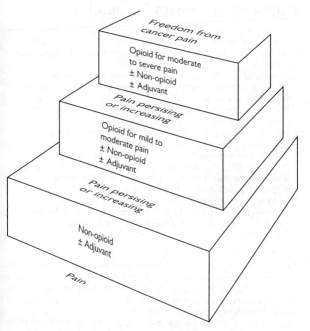

Fig. 16.9 WHO analgesic ladder

Equianalgesic doses for opioids

Calculating equivalent doses is not an exact science, so care is needed. The literature contains much conflicting information, so key points are listed below togther with some external sources for suggested conversion factors.

Key points to consider converting patients from one opioid to another:
- Ratios for acute pain might not be the same as those for chronic pain.
- Ratio tables are for guidance only—they can be useful, but there can be wide variation between individuals. The dose, therefore, needs to be started cautiously and titrated to effect.
- Monitor pain and pain relief—use of pain-assessment tools and adverse-effect monitoring should be considered.
- Tolerance to one opioid might not be carried over to another—this can lead to greater potency than expected. This can be anticipated by ↓ the equianalgesic dose by a further 30–50% and providing further analgesic rescue in the early stages.
- Be careful if treating patients with renal impairment—certain metabolites accumulate in renal impairment, so caution is needed. Fentanyl probably does not produce active metabolites in renal impairment, but caution is still advised.

Further reading

There is an opioid conversion software programme for use on a hand-held computer (and even now a desktop version) at the Johns Hopkins Center for Cancer Pain Research. You can freely download the programme. Free registration required www.hopkinskimmelcancercenter.org/specialtycenters/hop.cfm?facilityid=27;.

Department of anesthesiology and critical care medicine at Johns Hopkins Medical Center has a useful website with additional suggested resources. www.hopkinsmedicine.org/anesthesiology/Team/PDA_Resources.html.

Pereira J, Lawlor P, Vigano A, *et al.* (2001). Equianalgesic dose ratios for opioids. *Journal of Pain and Symptom, Management* **22(2)**: 672–87.

Regnard C (1998). Conversion ratios for transdermal fentanyl. *European Journal of Palliative care* **5(6)**: 204.

Compatibility of drugs in pain and palliative care

There are a number of mixtures in common use, including opioids combined with drugs such as baclofen, midazolam or local anaesthetics.

It is common to differentiate between chemical and physical compatibilities. Ideally, information for the former would be available for all mixtures, but in practice this is often hard to find. Some information is available in the peer-reviewed pharmacy literature and a search of international pharmaceutical abstracts can be helpful.

Time and temperature are two key components affecting chemical reactions, so it is wise to avoid mixtures sitting in syringe drivers for many hours in a warm room. An ↑ number of a drugs mixed together and the greater the concentration will ↑ the risk of incompatibility.

The majority of recommendations are desired from on physical compatibility, ie drugs are mixed and no obvious colour change or precipitation occurs, even when examined microscopically. Additionally, no change in pharmacological effect is seen when the drugs are administered.

Further reading

There are several useful sources for information on common opioid mixtures, as followes:

Trissel L. (2005). *Handbook Of Injectable Drugs.* 13th edition. *Amer. Soc. Health System Pharmacists.*

Dickman A, Schneider J, Varga and J (2005). *The Syringe Driver: Continuous subcutaneous infusions in palliative care.* Oxford University Press, Oxford.

Twycross R, Wilcock A (2002). *Palliative Care Formulary.* Radcliffe Medical Press.

Trissel's Stability of Compounded Formulations 3e (2005). APLA Publications.

Chronic pain

Overview

Chronic pain is a major, undertreated illness. The Pain in Europe study interviewed > 46 000 people and it makes grim reading.

Chronic pain is a widespread problem in Europe, affecting one in five adults. More than one-third of European households have a pain sufferer. Two-thirds of chronic pain sufferers experience moderate pain, wheras one-third of suffers experience severe pain. The most common pain is back pain and the most common cause of this is arthritis.

People with chronic pain have been suffering on average for 7yrs, with one-fifth of suffers reporting a > 20yr history. One-third of suffers have pain all the time. Adequate pain control took >2yrs to achieve, >50% of suffers. Pain has a huge social impact. One in five sufferers have lost their job as a result of their pain. A similar number have been diagnosed with depression as a result of their pain. Generally, patients are satisfied with their care, but only 23% of suffers have seen a pain management specialist and only 1 in 10 have been evaluated using pain scales.

In terms of treatment, two-thirds of suffers report that their pain control is inadequate at times, and one-third of suffers believe that their doctor does not know how to control their pain.

What about the UK?

Almost one in seven people in the UK suffers from chronic pain (~7.8 million people)

One-third of UK households are affected by chronic pain. 50% of chronic pain sufferers report the following:
- Feel tired all the time.
- Feel helpless.
- Feel older than they really are.
- Do not remember what it feels like not to be in pain.

In addition, the following statiztics here been reported:
- One in five sufferers say the pain is sometimes so bad they want to die.
- Two-thirds of sufferers are *always* willing to try new treatments .
- But almost as many sufferers are worried about potential side effects of pain medication.
- Pain sufferers are proactive, with 80% of chronic pain sufferers treating their pain in some way, mainly with prescription medications.
- More than one in five (22%) sufferers have tried, then stopped taking, prescription pain medication.
- Weak opioids are most used class (50%) of pain medication.
- Other commonly prescribed drugs are paracetamol (38%) and NSAIDs (23%).
- The mean number of tablets taken every day is 5.7.

In spite of this much can be done to alleviate the suffering of patients with of chronic pain. The approach to treatment is the same as for acute pain, ie to titrate with analgesics until either pain relief or unacceptable side effects occur. In addition, there are a wide range of medicines other than analgesics that can provide relief.

Analgesics

In treating chronic pain, it is important to start with the simplest and most obvious treatments first, rather than move directly to unconventional analgesics. NSAIDs and/or paracetamol should be tried early. The combination of NSAIDs and paracetamol can be effective and can ↓ the dose of the NSAID needed. The addition of a weak opioid can help in chronic pain. Patients on long-term NSAIDs should be given gastric protection and informed of the reasons for this. Approximately 1 in 120 patients who take an NSAID for >2 months without gastric protection develop a bleeding ulcer, and ~1 in 1200 patients die of a bleeding ulcer.

If simple analgesics are insufficient then there other choices, which include so-called 'unconventional analgesics', such as antidepressants and anticonvulsant drugs. For some patients, a strong opioid can be justified, providing adequate steps are taken to screen patients before initiating treatment.

Nonpharmacological interventions can also help. Weight loss in overweight patients who suffer with arthritis can have a real benefit. Transcutaneous electronic nerve stimulation (TENS) can also be a useful addition. Radiotherapy can be effective in dealing with painful bony metastases. In specialist clinics, nerve blocks and epidural injections can also be helpful. A list of unconventional analgesics that can be effective in chronic neuropathic pain is suggested below. It is usual to start at low doses and titrate the dose upwards until pain relief, unacceptable adverse effects or maximum dose is reached.

- Amitriptyline, 50–150mg at night, or similar tricyclic antidepressants.
- Carbamazepine 100mg three times a day initially, ↑ slowly up to a maximum of 1200mg daily.
- Gabapentin, doses up to 3.6g daily
- Clonazepam, 0.5mg twice daily increasing to 1mg three times a daily.
- Baclofen, 5mg three times daily, increasing to 10mg three times a daily.
- Pyridoxine, 100mg up to five times a daily.
- Capsaicin cream.
- Other anticonvulsants, such as pregabalin, lamotrigine, phenytoin and sodium valproate.
- SSRIs can also be beneficial, but evidence for their use is very limited.

Antidepressant drugs for neuropathic pain

- Neuropathic pain refers to a group of painful disorders characterized by pain caused by dysfunction or disease of the nervous system at a peripheral level or a central level, or both. It is a complex entity, with many symptoms and signs that fluctuate in number and intensity over time. The three common components of neuropathic pain are steady and neuralgic pain paroxysmal spontaneous attacks and hypersensitivity.
- This type of pain can be very disabling, severe and intractable, causing distress and suffering for individuals, including dysaesthesia and paraesthesia. Sensory deficits, such as partial or complex loss of sensation, are also commonly seen.

- The clinical impression is that both antidepressants and anticonvulsants are useful for neuropathic pain, but there are unanswered questions, such as including the following:
  - Which drug class should be the first-line choice?
  - Is one antidepressant drug superior to another?
  - Is there any difference in response to antidepressants in different neuropathic syndromes?
- The mechanisms of action of antidepressant drugs in the treatment of neuropathic pain are uncertain. Analgesia is often achieved at lower dosage and faster (usually within a few days) than the onset of any antidepressant effect, which can take up to 6wks. In addition, there is no correlation between the effect of antidepressants on mood and pain. Furthermore, antidepressants produce analgesia in patients with and without depression.
- Two main groups of antidepressants are in common use. The older tricyclic antidepressants, such as amitriptyline, imipramine and many others, and a newer group of SSRIs. The clinical impression was that tricyclic antidepressants are more effective in treating neuropathic pain. However, SSRIs are gaining acceptance for pain relief.
- Tricyclic antidepressants exhibit more significant adverse effects, which limit clinical use, particularly in the elderly. The most serious adverse effects of tricyclic antidepressants occur within the cardiovascular system
  - Postural hypotension.
  - Heart block.
  - Arrhythmias.
- The most common adverse effects are as follows:
- Sedation.
- Anticholinergic effects (eg dry mouth, constipation and urinary retention).

SSRIs are better tolerated. They are free of cardiovascular side effects, are less sedative and have fewer anticholinergic effects than tricyclic antidepressants.

Basic microbiology

Micro-organisms are classified in many ways. The most important classifications are as follows:

- Category—eg viruses, bacteria and protozoa.
- Genus—ie the 'family' the micro-organism belongs to, such as Staphylococcus.
- Species—ie the specific name, such as aureus.

To correctly name a micro-organism, both the genus and the species name must be used, eg *Staphylococcus aureus* and *Haemophilus influenzae*.

Identifying micro-organisms

To correctly diagnose and treat an infection, the micro-organism must be identified. This is usually done by examining samples of faeces, blood and sputum in various ways.

Microscopy

The sample is examined under the microscope. Sometimes the organism can easily be seen and identified, eg some helminths (worms) and their ova (eggs).

Dyes are used to stain cells so that they can be seen more easily. Differential staining uses the fact that cells with different properties stain differently and can, ∴ be distinguished. Bacteria are divided into two groups according to whether they stain with the Gram stain. The difference between Gram-positive and Gram-negative bacteria is in the permeability of the cell wall when treated with a purple dye followed by a decolourizing agent. Gram-positive cells retain the stain, whereas Gram-negative cells lose the purple stain and appear colourless, until stained with a pink counterstain (Fig. 16.10).

Mycobacteria have waxy cell walls and do not readily take up the Gram stain. A different staining technique is used and then the sample is tested to see if it withstands decolourization with acid and alcohol. Mycobacteria retain the stain and thus are known as acid-fast bacilli (AFB), whereas other bacteria lose the stain.

Examination of stained films allows the shape of the cells to be seen, which can aid identification.

Bacteria are classified as follows:

- Cocci (spherical, rounded)—eg streptococci.
- Bacilli (straight rod)—eg *Pseudomonas* species.
- Spirochaetes (spiral rod)—eg *Treponema* species.
- Vibrios (curved, comma-shaped)—eg *Vibrio cholerae*.

Culture

Bacteria and fungi can be grown on the surface of solid, nutrient media. Colonies of many thousands of the micro-organism can be produced from a single cell. Colonies of different species often have characteristic appearances, which aids identification. For most species, it takes 12–48h for a colony to develop that is visible to the naked eye. Some organisms (eg mycobacteria) multiply much more slowly and can take several weeks to develop.

Samples can be grown in an environment where O_2 has been excluded. Bacteria that grow in the absence of O_2 are known as 'anaerobes' and, bacteria that need O_2 to grow are 'aerobes'. Bacteria are often described as a combination of their Gram staining, shape and anaerobic/aerobic characteristics. This helps to narrow the range of bacteria under consideration before lengthier tests identify the individual organism (Table 16.12).

Other tests that can be used to identify the organism include the following:

- Detection of microbial antigen.
- Detection of microbial products—eg toxin produced by *Clostridium difficile.*
- Using gene probes.
- Polymerase chain reaction.

Discussion of these tests is beyond the scope of this topic. For further information the reader is referred to microbiology texts.

Table 16.12 Examples of pathogens from various types of bacteria

Gram positive cocci	**Gram negative cooci**

Staphylococci:
  coagulase +ve, eg Staphylococcus
    aureus
  coagulase –ve, eg Staph. epidermidis
Streptococci[1]:
  β-haemolytic streptococci
    Streptococus pyogenes (Lancefield
      group A)
    α-haemolytic streptococci
    Strep. mitior
    Strep. pneumoniae (pneumococcus)
    Strep. sanguis
Enterococci (non-haemolytic)[2]:
  Enterococci mutans
  E. faecalis
Anaerobic streptococci

Gram positive bacilli (rods)

Aerobes

  Bacillus anthracis (anthrax)
  Corynebacterium diphtheriae
  Listeria monocytogenes
  Nocardia species

Anaerobes:

  Clostridium
  Cl. botulinum (botulism)
  Cl. perfringens (gas gangrene)
  Cl. tetani (tetanus)
  Cl. difficile (diarrhoea)

Actinomyces:

  Actinomyces israeli, A. naeslundii
  A. odontolyticus, A.viscosus

Obligate intracellular bacteria:

Chlamydia
  Chlamydia trachomatis
  C. psittaci
  C. pneumoniae
Coxiella burnetii
Bartonella
Ehrlichia
Rickettsia (typhus)
Legionella pneumophilia
Mycoplasma pneumoniae

Neisseria:
  Neisseria meningitidis (meningitis,
    septicaemia)
  N. gonorrheae (gonorrhoea)
Moraxella:
  Moraxella catarrhalis (pneumonia)

Gram negative bacilli (rods)

Enterobacteriaceae:
  Escherichia coli
  Shigella species
  Salmonella species
  Citrobacter freundii, C. koseri
  Klebsiella pneumoniae, K. oxytoca
  Enterobacter aerogenes, E.cloacae
  Serratia morascens:
    Proteus mirabilis/vulgaris
  Morganella morganii
  Providencia species
  Yersinia enterocolitica, Y. pestis
  Y. paratuberculosis
  Pseudomonas aeruginosa
  Haemophilus influenzae
  Brucella species
  Bordetella pertussis
  Pasteruella multocida
  Vibrio cholerae
  Camphylobacter jejuni

Anaerobes:

  Bacteroides (wound infections)
  Fusobacterium
  Helicobacter pylori

Mycobacteria:

  Mycobacterium tuberculosis
  M. bovis
  M. leprae (leprosy)

'Atypical' mycobacteria:

  M. avium intracellulare
  M. scrofulaceum, M. kansasii
  M. marinum, M. malmoense
  M. ulcerans, M. xenopi, M. gordonae
  M. fortuitum, M. chelonae, M. flaverscens
  M. smegmatis-phlei

Spirochaetes:

  Treponema (syphilis; yaws; pinta)
  Leptospira (Weil's dis; canicola fever)
  Borrelia (relapsing fever; Lyme dis)

1 Streps are classified according to haemolytic pattern: (α- β or non-haemolytic) or by Lancefield antigen (A–G), or by species (eg Strep. pyogenes). There is crossover among these groups; the above is a generalization for the chief pathogens.
2 Clinically, epidemiologically and in terms of treatment, enterococci behave unlike other streps.

Reproduced with permission from Longmore M, Wilkinson IB, and Rajagopalan S (2004). *Oxford Handbook of Clinical Medicine*, 6th edn. Oxford: University Press.

GRAM +   GRAM –

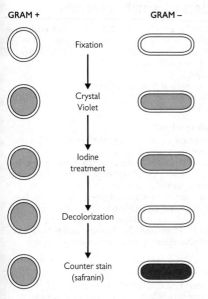

Fixation

Crystal
Violet

Iodine
treatment

Decolorization

Counter stain
(safranin)

Fig. 16.10 The extent of bacterial resistance in the UK

Modes of action of antibacterials

To avoid unwanted toxic effects on human cells, most antibacterials have a mode of action that affects bacterial but not mammalian cells.

There are many possible sites of action of antimicrobial agents. However, the most common mechanisms are as follows:

- Inhibition of cell-wall synthesis.
- Alteration of the cell membrane (usually antifungals).
- Inhibition of protein synthesis.
- Inhibition of nucleic acid synthesis.

Inhibition of cell-wall synthesis

- Mammalian cells do not have a cell wall (only a cell membrane) so this mode of action does not affect mammalian cells.
- Penicillins, cephalosporins and other β-lactam antibacterials interfere with the synthesis of a substance called peptidoglycan. Peptidoglycan is an essential component of bacterial cell walls. If synthesis of peptidoglycan is inhibited, it is unable to support the cell wall and thus the bacteria lose their structure and eventually lyse (disintegrate) and die.
- Isoniazid also acts on the cell wall. It inhibits enzymes that are essential for synthesis of mycolic acids and the mycobacterial cell wall. The mode of action of ethambutol is not clear, but it might be the same as isoniazid.

Inhibition of protein synthesis

- The mechanism of protein synthesis is similar in bacterial and mammalian cells, but there are differences in ribosome structure (involved in protein synthesis) and other target sites, which ↓ the risk of toxicity to mammalian cells.
- Tetracyclines, aminoglycosides, macrolides and chloramphenicol all work by inhibiting synthesis of proteins essential to the growth and reproduction of bacteria.
- Tetracyclines, macrolides and chloramphenicol interfere with the binding of new amino acids onto peptide chains.
- Aminoglycosides prevent initiation of protein synthesis and cause nonfunctional proteins to be created.

Inhibition of nucleic acid synthesis

- Sulphonamides are structural analogues of para-amino benzoic acid (PABA). PABA is an essential precursor in bacterial synthesis of folic acid, which is necessary for the synthesis of nucleic acids. Mammalian cells are not affected as they use exogenous folic acid.
- Trimethoprim is an inhibitor of dihydrofolic acid reductase, an enzyme that reduces dihydrofolic acid to tetrahydrofolic acid. This is one of the stages in bacterial synthesis of purines and thus DNA. Trimethoprim inhibits dihydrofolic acid reductase 50 000 times more efficiently in bacterial cells than mammalian cells.
- Sulphonamides and trimethoprim produce sequential blocking of folate metabolism and, ∴, are synergistic.

- Bacteria use an enzyme called DNA gyrase to make the DNA into a small enough package to fit into the cell. This is called supercoiling. The quinolones inhibit DNA gyrase and supercoiling.
- Rifampicin inhibits bacterial RNA synthesis by binding to RNA polymerase; mammalian RNA polymerase is not affected.
- Nitroimidazoles (eg metronidazole) cause the DNA strand to break (cleavage).
- Pyrazinamide has an unknown mechanism of action.

Selection and use of antimicrobials

To treat or not to treat

The presence of micro-organisms does not necessarily mean that there is infection. The human body hosts a wide range of micro-organisms (mostly bacteria) but these rarely cause infection in an immunocompetent host. These organisms are known as 'commensals' and some have an important role in host defences. For example, *C. difficile* is a pathogen that is normally suppressed by normal bowel flora. Eradication of the bowel flora (eg by broad-spectrum antibacterials) allows overgrowth of *C. difficile*, leading to diarrhoea and, sometimes, pseudomembraneous colitis. Indiscriminate drug therapy can thus ↑ the risk of other infection.

Some organisms might be commensals in one part of the body and pathogens in another, eg *Escherichia coli* is part of the normal bowel flora but if it gets into the bladder it can cause urinary tract infection.

Some pathogenic organisms can reside on the host without causing infection. This is known as 'colonization' and signs and symptoms of infection are absent. A skin or nasal swab positive for methicillin-resistant *S. aureus* (MRSA) does not usually require treatment.

Some infections are self-limiting and resolve without treatment. Many common viral infections resolve without treatment, and in any case, most do not have specific antiviral drugs.

Choice of therapy

If infection is confirmed or is strongly suspected, appropriate therapy must be selected. Ideally, the pathogen is identified before antimicrobial therapy is started. However, identification of an organism by the laboratory usually takes a minimum of 24h and antimicrobial sensitivity tests can take a further 24h. For some slow growing organisms, such as mycobacteria, culture and sensitivity results can take several weeks. Thus, in most cases, therapy will be started using 'best guess' (empiric) antimicrobials and tailored after culture and sensitivity results are known (Table 16.13).

Whenever possible, samples for culture and sensitivity tests should be taken before starting antimicrobial therapy so that growth is not inhibited. However, this delay might not be possible in very sick patients, eg those with suspected bacterial meningitis.

Factors that should be taken into account when selecting an antimicrobial are described below.

Clinical

- Does the patient have an infection that needs treating?
- Diagnosis/likely source of infection.
- Anatomical site of infection.
- Severity or potential severity of infection (and possible consequences, eg loss of prosthetic joint).
- Patient's underlying condition (if any) and vulnerability to infection, eg neutropaenic patients more susceptible to sepsis.
- Patient-specific factors, eg allergies and renal function.

- Does the infection require empiric therapy or can antimicrobials be delayed until culture and sensitivity results are available?
- Foreign material, necrotic tissue and abcesses are relatively impervious to antimicrobials. Abcesses should be drained and necrotic tissue debrided. If possible, foreign material should be removed.

Microbiology

- What are the pathogens?
  - Identified by microscopy or culture.
  - Presumed, according to epidemiology and knowledge of probable infecting organisms for the site of infection.
- Sensitivity of organisms to antimicrobial agents (Table 16.14).
  - National and local resistance patterns.
  - Culture and sensitivity data.

Pharmaceutical

- Evidence of clinical efficacy:
  - Against the organism.
  - At the site of infection.
- Bactericidal versus bacteriostatic agents:
  - Bactericidal drugs generally give more rapid resolution of infection.
  - Bacteriostatic drugs rely on phagocytes to eliminate the organisms and, ∴ are not suitable for infection in which phagocytes are impaired, eg granulocytopenia, or do not penetrate the site of infection, eg infective endocarditis.
- Spectrum of activity:
  - Narrow-spectrum antimicrobials are preferred if the organism has been identified.
  - Broad-spectrum antimicrobials might be required in empiric therapy or mixed infection.
  - Indiscriminate use of broad-spectrum antimicrobials ↑ the risk of development of drug resistance and superinfection, eg *C. difficile*.
- Appropriate route of administration:
  - Topical antimicrobials should be avoided, except where specifically indicated, eg eye or ear infection or metronidazole gel for fungating tumours.
  - Oral therapy is preferred and most antimicrobials have good bioavailability.
  - IV therapy might be necessary in the following circumstances:
    — If the infection is serious.
    — If the drug has poor oral bioavailability.
    — If the patient is unconscious or unable to take oral drugs (eg perioperatively).
- Possible side effects or drug interactions.
- Pharmacokinetics:
  - Tissue penetration—will the antimicrobial get to the site of infection?
  - Clearance in liver/kidney impairment.
- Dose and frequency must be sufficient to give adequate blood levels but avoid unacceptable toxicity. Serum levels four to eight times the minimum inhibitory concentration (MIC) are considered adequate.

- Duration of treatment:
  - Not too long, eg uncomplicated urinary tract infection only requires 3–5days therapy.
  - Not too short, eg bone infection might require therapy for several weeks or months.
- Local policies/restrictions on antimicrobial use.
- Cost.

Combined antimicrobial therapy

Combined antimicrobial therapy might be prescribed for certain indications:

- To give a broad spectrum of activity in empiric therapy—especially in high-risk situations, such as neutropaenic sepsis.
- To treat mixed infection, if one drug does not cover all possible pathogens.
- To achieve a synergistic effect, thus ↑ efficacy but ↓ the dose required of each drug (and thus ↓ the risk of side effects), eg penicillin and gentamicin in the treatment of streptococcal endocarditis. Relatively low doses of gentamicin are used, ↓ the risk of nephrotoxicity.
- To ↓ the probability of the emergence of drug resistance, eg treatment of TB requires a minimum of two drugs and antiretroviral therapy requires a minimum of three drugs.
- To restore or extend the spectrum of activity by including an enzyme inhibitor, eg co-amoxiclav.

Penicillin and cephalosporin hypersensitivity

Up to 10% of people are allergic to penicillins. and ~10% of people who are allergic to penicillin are also allergic to cephalosporins. This can range from mild rash to fever to a serious anaphylactic reaction. Penicillins and cephalosporins should never be used again in a patient who has had a severe hypersensitivity reaction. If a patient has had a severe hypersensitivity reaction to penicillins, it is advisable to avoid cephalosporins, unless there is no alternative. If the penicillin allergy is relatively mild, eg rash, cephalosporins can be prescribed cautiously.

Some patients state that they have had an allergic reaction when they have really only had nausea or a headache. This is not drug allergy and, ∴, it is safe to use penicillins and cephalosporins in these patients.

Ampicillin and amoxicillin can cause rashes in patients who have had glandular fever, leukaemia or are HIV positive. This is not a true allergic reaction and penicillins can be used again in these patients.

Monitoring therapy

It is essential to monitor and review antimicrobial therapy regularly, both to ensure treatment is working and to avoid inappropriate continuation of therapy (Fig. 16.11) The pharmacist should monitor the following parameters:

- Temperature should ↓ to normal (36.8°C). (Note: drug hypersensitivity is a possible cause of persistent pyrexia.)
- Pulse, BP, and respiratory rate revert to normal.
- Raised white cell count decreases.

- raised C-reactive protein decreases (normal, <8).
- Symptoms such as local inflammation, pain, malaise, GI upset, headache and confusion resolve.

Reasons for treatment failure

- Wrong antimicrobial.
- Drug resistance.
- The isolated organism is not the cause of the disease.
- Treatment started too late.
- The wrong dose, duration or route of administration.
- Lack of patient compliance.
- Difficulty getting the drug to the site of infection.
- ↓ immunity of the patient.

Further reading

Wickens H, Wade P (2005). How pharmacists can promote the sensible use of antimicrobials. *Pharmaceutical Journal* **274**: 427–30.

Wickens H, Wade P (2005). The right drug for the right bug. *Pharmaceutical Journal* **274**: 365–8.

Comprehensive recommendations for the management of infection in hospital. www.bsac.org.uk/pyxis/

www.ncht.org.uk/antibiotics

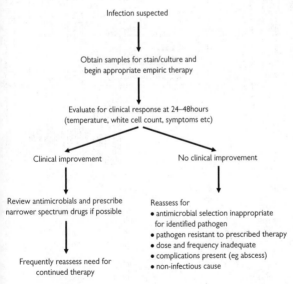

Fig. 16.11 Flowchart of selection and use of antimicrobials

Table 16.13 In vitro activity of antibacterials

✓ = usually sensitive ? = variable sensitivity or inappropriate therapy X = usually resistant or inappropriate therapy

Note: These are generalizations. There are major differences between countries, areas and hospitals. Check local Public Health or Microbiology laboratories for local sensitivity patterns. Antibacterials may not be licensed to treat the bacteria for which they are active.

	Gram positives								Anaerobes			Gram negatives									Atypicals		
	Staphylococcus aureus MSSA	*Staphylococcus aureus* MRSA	*Staphylococcus epidermidis*	Haemolytic streptococci (Strep A, C, G and Strep B)	*Enterococcus faecalis*	*Enterococcus faecium*	*Streptococcus pneumoniae*	*Listeria monocytogenes*	*Clostridium perfringens*	*Clostridium difficile*	*Bacteroides fragilis*	*Neisseria meningitidis*	*Neisseria gonorrhoeae*	*Haemophilus influenzae*	*Escherichia coli*	*Klebsiella* spp	*Proteus mirabilis*	*Proteus vulgaris*	*Pseudomonas aeruginosa*	*Moraxella catarrhalis*	*Legionella* spp	*Mycoplasma pneumoniae*	*Chlamydia* spp
Penicillins																							
Phenoxymethylpenicillin	X	X	X	✓	?	?	✓	?	✓	X	X	✓	?	X	X	X	X	X	X	X	X	X	X
Benzylpenicillin	X	X	X	✓	✓	?	✓	✓	✓	X	X	✓	✓	X	X	X	X	X	X	X	X	X	X
Ampicillin/ Amoxicillin	✓	X	?	✓	✓	?	✓	✓	✓	X	X	✓	?	?	?	X	✓	✓	X	?	X	X	X
Co-amoxiclav	✓	X	?	✓	✓	?	✓	✓	✓	X	✓	✓	✓	✓	✓	✓	✓	✓	X	✓	X	X	X
Flucloxacillin	✓	X	?	✓	X	X	✓	X	X	X	X	X	X	X	X	X	X	X	X	X	X	X	X
Pip+tazobactam (Tazocin®)	✓	X	?	✓	✓	?	✓	✓	✓	X	✓	✓	✓	✓	✓	✓	✓	✓	✓	✓	X	X	X
Cephalosporins																							
Cefradine / Cefalexin	✓	X	?	✓	X	X	✓	X	X	X	X	X	?	X	✓	✓	✓	X	X	✓	X	X	X
Cefotaxime	✓	X	?	✓	X	X	✓	X	X	X	X	✓	✓	✓	✓	✓	✓	✓	X	✓	X	X	X
Cefuroxime	✓	X	?	✓	X	X	✓	X	X	X	X	✓	?	✓	✓	✓	✓	X	X	✓	X	X	X
Ceftriaxone	✓	X	?	✓	X	X	✓	X	X	X	X	✓	✓	✓	✓	✓	✓	✓	?	✓	X	X	X
Ceftazidime	?	X	?	✓	X	X	?	X	X	X	X	✓	?	✓	✓	✓	✓	✓	✓	✓	X	X	X

	Gram positives								Anaerobes			Gram negatives									Atypicals		
	Staphylococcus aureus MSSA	*Staphylococcus aureus* MRSA	*Staphylococcus epidermidis*	Haemolytic streptococc (Strep A, C, G and Strep B)	*Enterococcus faecalis*	*Enterococcus faecium*	*Streptococcus pneumoniae*	*Listeria monocytogenes*	*Clostridium perfringens*	*Clostridium difficile*	*Bacteroides fragilis*	*Neisseria meningitidis*	*Neisseria gonorrhoeae*	*Haemophilus influenzae*	*Escherichia coli*	*Klebsiella* spp	*Proteus mirabilis*	*Proteus vulgaris*	*Pseudomonas aeruginosa*	*Moraxella catarrhalis*	*Legionella* spp	*Mycoplasma pneumoniae*	*Chlamydia* spp
Carbapenems																							
Ertapenem	✓	✗	✓	✓	✗	✗	✓	~	✓	✗	✓	✓	✓	✓	✓	✓	✓	✓	✗	✓		✗	✗
Meropenem / Imipenem	✓	✗	✓	✓	✓	✗	✓	✓	✓	✗	✓	✓	✓	✓	✓	✓	✓	✓	✓	✓		✗	✗
Macrolides/ Lincosamides																							
Azithromycin	✓	✗	✗	✓	✗	✗	✓	✗	✓	✗	✗	✗	✓	✓	✗	✗	✗	✗	✗	✓	✓	✓	✓
Erythromycin	✓	✗	✗	✓	✗	✗	✓	✗	✓	✗	✗	✗	~	~	✗	✗	✗	✗	✗	✓	✓	✓	✓
Clarithromycin	✓	✗	✗	✓	✗	✗	✓	✗	✓	✗	✗	✗	~	~	✗	✗	✗	✗	✗	✓	✓	✓	✓
Clindamycin	✓	~	✓	✓	✗	✗	✓	✗	✓	✗	✓	✗	✗	✗	✗	✗	✗	✗	✗	✗	✗	✗	✗
Aminoglycosides																							
Amikacin	✓	✓	✓	✗	✗	✗	✗	~	✗	✗	✗	✗	✗	✓	✓	✓	✓	✓	✓	✓		✗	✗
Gentamicin	✓	✓	✓	✗	~	~	✗	~	✗	✗	✗	~	~	~	✓	✓	✓	✓	✓	✓		✗	✗
Diaminopyrimidines and sulphonamides																							
Co-trimoxazole	✓	✓	✓	✗	~	~	✓	✓	✗	✗	✗	✗	✓	✓	✓	✓	✓	✓	✗	✓	✓	✗	✗
Trimethoprim	~	~	~	✗	~	~	~	~	✗	✗	✗	✗	~	✓	✓	✓	✓	~	✗	✓	✗	✗	✗
Quinolones																							
Ciprofloxacin	✓	✗	✓	~	~	✗	~	✗	✗	✗	✗	✓	✓	✓	✓	✓	✓	✓	✓	✓	✓	✗	✓
Levofloxacin	✓	~	✓	✓	~	~	✓	✓	✗	✗	~	✓	✓	✓	✓	✓	✓	✓	✓	✓	✓	✓	✓
Moxifloxacin	✓	~	✓	✓	~	~	✓	✓	✗	✗	~	✓	✓	✓	✓	✓	✓	✓	✗	✓	✓	✓	✓
Glycopeptides																							
Vancomycin (IV)	✓	✓	✓	✓	✓	✓	✓	✓	✓	✓	✗	✗	✗	✗	✗	✗	✗	✗	✗	✗	✗	✗	✗
Teicoplanin	✓	✓	✓	✓	✓	✓	✓	~	✓	✓	✗	✗	✗	✗	✗	✗	✗	✗	✗	✗	✗	✗	✗
Nitroimidazoles																							
Metronidazole	✗	✗	✗	✗	✗	✗	✗	✗	✓	✓	✓	✗	✗	✗	✗	✗	✗	✗	✗	✗	✗	✗	✗
Oxazolidinones																							
Linezolid	✓	✓	✓	✓	✓	✓	✓	✓	✓	~	~	✗	✗	✗	✗	✗	✗	✗	✗	✗	✗	✗	✗
Tetracyclines																							
Doxycycline	✓	✓	✓	✓	~	~	✓	~	✓	✗	~	✓	✓	✓	~	~	✗	✗	✗	✓	✓	✓	✓

Miscellaneous	Staphylococcus aureus MSSA	Staphylococcus aureus MRSA	Staphylococcus epidermidis	Haemolytic streptococci (Strep A, C, G and Strep B)	Enterococcus faecalis	Enterococcus faecium	Streptococcus pneumoniae	Listeria monocytogenes	Clostridium perfringens	Clostridium difficile	Bacteroides fragilis	Neisseria meningitidis	Neisseria gonorrhoeae	Haemophilus influenzae	Escherichia coli	Klebsiella spp	Proteus mirabilis	Proteus vulgaris	Pseudomonas aeruginosa	Moraxella catarrhalis	Legionella spp	Mycoplasma pneumoniae	Chlamydia spp
								Gram positives		**Anaerobes**			**Gram negatives**								**Atypicals**		
Chloramphenicol	?	×	×	✓	?	?	✓	×	?	×	✓	✓	✓	✓	✓	?	?	?	×	✓	✓	✓	✓
Quinupristin / dalfopristin (Synercid ®)	✓	✓	✓	✓	×	✓	✓	✓	✓	?	✓	×	✓	?	×	×	×	×	×	✓	✓	✓	✓

¹Sensitive if used synergistically with penicillins/glycopeptides
²IV vancomycin ineffective for *Clostridium difficile*

Table 16.14 Diseases, potential causative bacteria and typical treatment choices[1]

Specific condition	Potential causative bacterial pathogens	Typical empiric treatment
Meningitis	*Streptococcus pneumoniae, Neisseria menigiditis, Haemophilus influenzae.* Group B streptococcus (seen in neonates), *Escherichia coli* and *Listeria monocytogenes*. Other Gram negative bacteria and Staphylococcus spp usually associated with neurosurgery	Cefotaxime and ceftriaxone provide broad cover and good central nervous system penetration. Ampicillin or amoxicillin is required to cover Listeria spp (elderly and neonates). Causative agents can also be mycobacterial, viral or, rarely, fungal and these will require appropriate therapy.
Brain abscess	*S. aureus*, anaerobic streptococci, Bacteroides spp. Gram negatives, such as Escherichia, Proteus, Klebsiella spp	Cefotaxime or ceftriaxone, meropenem if broader cover required (avoid imipenem due to CNS side effects). The condition can occasionally be fungal or parasitic.
Otitis media	Str. pneumoniae, H. influenzae, Moraxella catarrhalis, S. aureus, mixed anaerobes	Antibacterial therapy not always necessary. Amoxicillin or co-amoxiclav. Can also be viral (eg influenza, respiratory syncitial virus, enteroviruses).
Otitis externa	*Pseudomonas aeruginosa* ("swimmer's ear"), S. aureus (pustule)	Topical gentamicin. Less commonly fungal (*Candida albicans*, Aspergillis spp).
Upper respiratory tract infections		
Pharyngitis/tonsillitis	Str. pyogenes (group A)	Phenoymethylpenicillin but note that 50% of sore throats are viral in origin.
Epiglottitis	H. influenzae, Str. pyogenes (group A)	Ceftriaxone or cefotaxime.
Sinusitis	Str. pneumoniae, H. influenzae, mixed anaerobes, S. aureus, M. catarrhalis	Co-amoxiclav. Sinusitis may be viral (eg rhinovirus, influenza) or occasionally, fungal.

Lower respiratory tract infections

Community acquired	Str. pneumoniae, H. influenzae, M. catharrhalis, atypical organisms (Mycoplasma pneumoniae, Chlamydia pneumoniae and, rarely, Legionella pneumophila).	Amoxicillin oral or cefuroxime intravenous (depending on severity) +/- macrolide if atypical organisms are suspected or clarithromycin +/-rifampicin for Legionella.
Hospital acquired	E. coli, Ps. aeruginosa, and other gram negative organisms, methicillin-resistant S. aureus (MRSA)	Broad spectrum antibacterials are required until a definitive diagnosis is made eg meropenem/imipenem/piperacillin+tazobactam (Tazocin), vancomycin + quinolone if MRSA suspected. Infection can be viral. Fungal infection is more likely in immuno-compromised patients.
Endocarditis	Enterococcus spp. Viridans group streptococci, S. aureus, coagulase-negative staphylococci.	Benzylpenicillin and gentamicin (synergistic action) or flucloxacillin and gentamicin if staphylococci are suspected (often seen in injecting drug users).
Gastrointestinal infections	E. coli, Shigella spp. Campylobacter jejuni, Salmonella spp. S aureus, Bacillus cereus (toxin mediated)	Gastrointestinal infections are generally self-limiting and often viral. Fluid replacement may be all that is required. Expert advice should be sought if antibacterials are considered necessary. In severe disease, ciprofloxacin is used for Salmonella spp and erythromycin for Campylobacter.
Urinary tract infections	E. coli, enterococci, Klebsiella spp, Enterobacter spp, Pseudomonas (UTI)/Pyelonephritis spp Proteus spp	For UTI use amoxicillin, cefradine/cefalexin, trimethoprim or nitrofurantoin depending on local resistance patterns. For uncomplicated UTI in a young woman, three days treatment should be sufficient. A longer course may be required in men. Recurrent or complicated UTIs require further investigation, consideration of resistant organisms and use of second-line agents co-amoxiclav, cefuroxime or ceftriaxone (+/- single dose of gentamicin) are often used for pyelonephritis.

Table 16.14 (Contd.)

Specific condition	Potential bacterial pathogens	Typical empiric treatment
Skin and soft tissue infection (cellulitis)	S. aureus, Str. pyogenes (group A)	Penicillin +/– flucloxacillin (oral or intravenously depending on severity). Always check (and treat) for co-existing athlete's foot which can be an entry point for organisms.
Septic arthritis	S. aureus, Str. pneumoniae, occasionally Gram negatives guided by culture results.	Flucloxacillin or cefuroxime empirically, but therapy should be guided by culture results
Osteomyelitis	S. aureus, Str pneumoniae, coagulase negative staphylococci (usually associated with implanted material). Many other organisms infrequently cause disease.	Flucloxacillin or cefuroxime empirically, but therapy should be guided by culture results. Infections involving prostheses will require longer therapy.
Sepsis		
Neutropenic	S aureus (MRSA), Str. viridans, coagulase-negative staphylococci, E. coli, Klebsiella spp, Ps aeruginosa or Pneumocystis jiroveci (carinii) pneumonia (PCP).	Meropenem/imipenem/piperacillin+tazobactam plus gentamicin. Vancomycin if staphylococcus species (including MRSA) suspected. Co-trimoxazole for PCP. If fever persists consider fungal or viral infections
Non-neutropenic	S. aureus (MRSA), Str. spp, E. coli, Pseudomonas spp	Therapy depends on source of infection. Empirically – flucloxacillin/cefuroxime +/– gentamicin. Vancomycin if MRSA suspected. Meropenem/imipenem/piperacillin + tazobactam initially in septic shock

1 Pathogens / therapy may differ in children and neonates – seek specialist advice.
2 See also British Thoracic Society Guidelines for the management of community acquired pneumonia in adults. Thorax (2001) 56 (suppl 4) 1 – 64 www.brit-thoracic.org.uk

Adapted with permission from Wickens H and Wade P (2005) The right drug for the right bug. *The Pharmaceutical Journal*, **274** 365–8.

Antimicrobial prophylaxis

Indiscriminate and prolonged courses of antimicrobials should be avoided, but in some situations, short-term or long-term antimicrobial prophylaxis might be appropriate to prevent infection (and thus further courses of antimicrobials).

Surgical prophylaxis

Antibacterial drugs are given to ↓ the risk of the following:
- Wound infection after potentially contaminated surgery, eg GI or genitourinary surgery and trauma.
- Losing implanted material, eg joint prosthesis.
- Endocarditis in patients with damaged or prosthetic heart valves who are undergoing high-risk procedures, eg dental surgery.

It is important that there are adequate concentrations of antibacterials in the blood at the time of incision ('knife-to-skin time') and throughout surgery. Thus, it is important to administer antibacterials at an appropriate time (usually 30–60mins) before surgery starts and repeat doses of short-acting antibacterials if surgery is delayed or prolonged.

It is rarely necessary to continue antibacterials after wound closure. More prolonged therapy is effectively treatment rather than prophylaxis.

Cefuroxime (with metronidazole, if anaerobic cover is necessary) is the antibacterial most commonly used for surgical prophylaxis. Vancomycin should be used for patients with proven or suspected MRSA colonization[1]. Drugs are usually administered by IV infusion to ensure adequate levels at the critical time.

Medical prophylaxis

Medical prophylaxis is appropriate for specific infections and for high-risk patients, as follows:
- Contacts of sick patients, eg meningitis and TB.
- Immunosuppressed patients, eg organ-transplant recipients, HIV-positive patients and splenectomy patients.
- Malaria.
- Postexposure prophylaxis, following exposure to HIV or hepatitis B.

Further reading

Prophylaxis regimens can be found in the *British National Formulary* and on www.sign.ac.uk

Rahman MH, Anson J (2004). Peri-operative antibacterial prophylaxis. *Pharmaceutical Journal* **272**:743–5.

---

1 Gemmell CG, Edwards DI *et al.* (2006). Guidelines for the prophylaxis and treatment of methicillin-resistant *Staphylococcus aureus* (MRSA) in the UK. *Journal of Antimicrobial chemotherapy* **57** (4): 589–608.

Optimizing antimicrobial use

↓ antimicrobial use might not actually ↓ the rate of resistance, but it might limit the rate at which new resistance emerges. Pharmacists have an important role in optimizing antimicrobial use—often known as 'antimicrobial stewardship'. In the UK, the Department of Health has specifically promoted the role of pharmacists in monitoring and optimizing antimicrobial use. In some hospitals, specialist antimicrobial pharmacists work alongside microbiologists and infectious diseases doctors to promote good antimicrobial stewardship through education, audit and production of prescribing policies. However, all pharmacists, whether in hospitals or the community, have a role in ensuring 'prudent use' of antimicrobials.

Strategies for antimicrobial stewardship

- Use of nonantimicrobial treatment, as appropriate, eg draining abcesses and removing infected invasive devices such as catheters.
- Improved systems for resistance testing and better communication of resistance data in hospital and community setting, to enable better directed therapy:
  - Avoid continued use of ineffective drugs.
  - Enable switching from broad-spectrum to narrower-spectrum antimicrobials.
- Faster diagnosis of infection, to ↓ the amount of unnecessary empiric therapy.
- Ensuring empiric therapy considers the following adjustments, as necessary:
  - Therapy is stopped if infection is ruled out.
  - Therapy is changed, as necessary, when culture results are available.
- Production of antimicrobial prescribing policies and promoting adherence to guidelines.
- Ensuring choice, dose and duration of therapy, including the following:
  - Monitoring serum levels and adjusting doses for antimicrobials that require TDM.
  - Ensuring kinetic factors are taken into account, eg nitrofurantoin is not excreted into the urine in adequate concentrations to be effective in patients with renal impairment.
- Avoiding unnecessary/overlong use of broad-spectrum antimicrobials.
- Appropriate use of antimicrobials for surgical prophylaxis, including avoiding prolonged courses.
- Use of combination therapy if there is a high risk of resistance emerging, eg rifampicin should never be used alone for TB or other infections.
- Avoiding co-prescribing of antimicrobials that have the same or overlapping spectrum of activity, eg co-amoxiclav and metronidazole.
- Considering rotational use of antimicrobials (cycling) in some circumstances.
- Educating patients to take antimicrobials correctly and that some infections do not require antimicrobial therapy.

Points to consider when reviewing a prescription for an antimicrobial

* Is it the right choice for the infection (or appropriate empiric therapy)?
* Does it comply with local policies/restrictive practices?
* Could a narrower-spectrum antimicrobial be used?
* Should it be used in combination with another antimicrobial?
* Is more than one antimicrobial with an overlapping spectrum of activity being used, and if so, why?
* Will the antimicrobial be distributed to the target (infected) organ?
* Is the dose correct taking into account the following?
    * Renal impairment.
    * Severity of infection.
    * Patient weight.
* Is TDM and subsequent dose adjustment required?
* Is the route of administration appropriate?
* Is the duration of therapy appropriate?
* Does the patient understand the dosing instructions and importance of completing the course?

Further reading

Wicken H, Wade P (2005). Understanding antibiotic resistance. *Pharmaceutical Journal* **274**: 501–4.
European Surveillance of Antimicrobials. www.ua.ac.be/esac/
Standing Medical Advisory Committee Sub-Group on Antimicrobial Resistance (SACAR) (1998).
Department of Health. The Path of Least Resistance. London: Department of Health. www.doh.gov.uk/smacful.htm

Patient information sheets on:
* *C. difficile*. www.dh.gov.uk/assetroot/04/11/34/79/04113479.pdf
* MRSA. www.dh.gov.uk/assetroot/04/11/58/84/04115884.pdf
Twelve steps to prevent antimicrobial resistance (advice for clinicians, fact sheets, and posters). www.cdc.gov/drugresistance/healthcare/patients/htm

Antimicrobial prescribing guidelines

Antimicrobials are the second most frequently prescribed class of drugs, after analgesics. In England, about 50 million prescriptions for antimicrobials are dispensed each year. Approximately 80% of antimicrobial prescribing is in the community and though the emergence of 'superbugs' is less of a problem than in hospital, resistance and cost are still an issue. Education of patients and GPs to reduce pressure to prescribe has contributed to a reduction in antimicrobial usage in the community. The remaining 20% of antimicrobial prescribing is in hospital. However, this class represents some of the more expensive drugs used in secondary care and antimicrobial resistance in the hospital setting is an increasing problem, notably with MRSA.

Both WHO and the UK Department of Health have emphasized the need for 'prudent use' of antimicrobials. WHO defines this as:

> 'the cost-effective use of antimicrobials which maximises their clinical therapeutic effect, while minimising both drug-related toxicity and the development of antimicrobial resistance'.

A good antimicrobial prescribing policy or guidelines will contribute to prudent (and thus cost effective) use of antimicrobials.

Type and format of guidance

Antimicrobial prescribing guidelines come in many formats. Before starting to write guidelines both the format and the intent must be decided:

- Advisory or mandatory.
- Policy, guidelines, restricted list.
- Educational.

It has been shown that prescribers prefer an educational approach and this may have the best long term impact. However, it may be necessary to give mandatory advice on the use of certain high cost/sensitive drugs.

The format must be easily accessible to prescribers at the time of prescribing. Computer-based guidelines offer the opportunity to provide additional, educational material and may be linked to a computerized prescribing package. This may be the best approach in the community where most GP practices use electronic prescribing. However, few hospitals in the UK use electronic prescribing and most doctors will not have a computer at the bedside. Thus most hospital guidelines are presented as a booklet, card or filofax insert which can be kept in the pocket. An ideal format is a pocket size ready reference linked to more detailed electronic guidelines.

The amount of detail will be determined by the presentation. As a minimum the recommended drug, (adult) dose, route and duration should be included. More detailed policies might also include side effects, contraindications, use in children, elderly and in pregnancy etc.

Style and layout must be clear and easy to follow. For lengthier guidelines an index or contents list should be provided. Use Plain English throughout and avoid Latin abbreviations (if space permits) such as 'tds'. Note that different countries use different abbreviations which may cause confusion for visiting staff—for example the US abbreviation 'qd' means once a day but may be misinterpreted as the UK 'qds' or four times a day. During the drafting process it is advisable to 'pilot' the guidelines to ensure that potential users interpret them in the way intended.

Hard copy guidelines should be robust, using card (laminated if possible) rather than paper and good quality printing.

Target audience

This should be identified. Are restrictions just applicable to junior doctors or to senior medical staff as well? Write the guidelines as if they are aimed at a doctor who has newly joined the hospital/GP practice and who needs to find quickly and easily what to prescribe in a situation.

Authors

Hospital antimicrobial guidelines are usually produced as a collaboration between microbiology and pharmacy. To ensure local ownership, consultants in the relevant specialities should be invited to contribute or comment eg surgeons for surgical prophylaxis. In the community, guidelines may be produced by a committee of GPs from one or more practice, usually with the assistance of the prescribing adviser. Ideally local primary and secondary care policies should be linked.

Content

Guidelines should:
- Be evidence based and recommendations referenced as appropriate.
- Advise on when **not** to prescribe as this is as valid on advice on when and what antimicrobial to prescribe.
- Discourage unnecessary use of the parenteral route.
- Include contact numbers for microbiology, pharmacy medicines information service.
- Be cross referenced to other relevant hospital/practice guidelines.

Cost may be included but may become outdated before guidelines are due for revision

As a minimum, the following areas should be covered:
- Surgical prophylaxis.
- Meningitis prophylaxis.
- Empirical treatment (first and second choice) for:
  - Meningitis.
  - Urinary tract infection.
  - Lower respiratory tract infection.
  - Sepsis.

Other areas which should be included are:
- Prophylaxis in asplenic patients.
- Empirical treatment for:
  - Gastrointestinal infection.
  - MRSA.
  - Upper respiratory tract infection.
  - Skin infection.

A full list of recommended areas to cover is provided in the SACAR antimicrobial policy template www.advisorybodies.doh.gov.uk/sacar/hospital-antimicrobial-guidelines-template-may05.rtf

Updating

The guidelines should state the issue date and frequency of review. As a minimum guidelines should be reviewed and updated as necessary every two years.

Monitoring and audit

Adherence to the guidelines should be monitored. For example a specific area such as vascular surgery prophylaxis can be audited. If there is significant non-adherence, the reasons should be established and addressed.

Antimicrobial resistance

Resistance is an almost inevitable consequence of antimicrobial use. While bacteria, viruses or other micro-organisms reproduce, mutations can spontaneously occur. These mutations might provide some protection against the action of certain antimicrobials. 'Survival of the fittest' means that when these micro-organisms are exposed to antimicrobials, the fully sensitive ones are suppressed but resistant ones survive, reproduce and become the dominant strain. Most attention has been focused on bacterial resistance, but the principles discussed here apply to all micro-organisms.

Mechanisms of resistance

- Change in cell-wall permeability—thus ↓ drug access to intracellular target sites. The relatively simple cell wall of Gram-positive bacteria makes them inherently more permeable and, ∴ this resistance mechanism is more common in Gram-negative than Gram-positive bacteria.
- Enzyme degradation of the drug—the best known being breakdown of the β-lactam ring of penicillins, cephalosporins and carbapenems by β-lactamases.
- Efflux pumps actively remove the drug from the cell.
- Mutation at the target site:
  - Alteration of penicillin-binding proteins leads to resistance to β-lactam antibiotics.
  - Changes in the structure of the enzyme reverse transcriptase leads to resistance to reverse transcriptase inhibitors.

Some organisms can develop multiple resistance mechanisms—eg *Pseudomonas aeruginosa* manifests resistance to carbapenems through production of β-lactamase, ↑ in efflux pumps and changes to the bacterial cell wall.

Implications of antimicrobial resistance

Antimicrobial resistance leads to ↑ in the following:
- Morbidity:
  - Patients might be sicker for longer.
  - Hospital stays are ↑.
  - Alternative antimicrobials might be more toxic.
  - Residential placements might be difficult.
  - Isolation and institutionalization.
- Mortality.
- Cost:
  - Newer, potentially more expensive antimicrobials might have to be used.
  - Extended hospital stay.
  - More nursing time.
  - ↑ use of disposables eg aprons and gloves.
  - In some cases, equipment might have to be discarded.

New strains of resistant bacteria are appearing at an alarming rate. Within the hospital environment, MRSA has been a problem for many years but the emergence of vancomycin-resistant MRSA (VRSA) and community-acquired MRSA (C-MRSA) is of significant concern. Other increasingly problematic resistant organisms are as follows:

• Vancomycin-resistant enterococci (VRE).
• Extended-spectrum β-lactamases (ESBLs).
• *Acinetobacter baumanii.*

At present, there are agents available to treat these resistant organisms, but they tend to be expensive, with a higher risk of side effects. However, the production of new drugs is not keeping up with development of new resistant bacteria and the possibility of resistant species emerging for which there is no antibacterial therapy available is very real.

Further reading

Standing Medical Advisory Committee, Subgroup on Antimicrobial Resistance (1998). *The Path of Least Resistance.* www.advisorybodies.doh.gov.uk/smacl.htm

Measuring resistance

In-vitro resistance tests generally require the organism to be cultured in the presence of antimicrobials.

Disc diffusion

Disc diffusion involves culturing bacteria on an agar plate that has had samples (impregnated discs) of antibacterial placed on it. If there is no growth around the antibacterial sample, the bacteria are sensitive to the antibacterial, but if the bacteria grow around the sample, this means they are resistant. Partial growth represents intermediate susceptibility.

E-test

The E-test works on similar principles to disk diffusion, but here, an impregnated strip containing a single antibacterial at ↑ concentrations is placed on the agar plate. Bacterial growth is inhibited around the strip after it reaches a certain concentration. This is equivalent to the MIC.

These tests can be problematic for slow-growing bacteria, such as mycobacteria, and for organisms that are difficult to culture such as viruses. Newer tests involve amplifying and examining the genetic material of the organism to look for mutations that are known to be associated with resistance. This technique is used for HIV-resistance testing.

Risk factors for antimicrobial resistance

Excessive and inappropriate antimicrobial use results in selective pressures that facilitate the emergence of resistant micro-organisms. It is estimated that upto 50% of antimicrobial use is inappropriate. Unnecessary antimicrobial use contributes to resistance without any clinical gain. This includes:

- Use of antimicrobials for infection that is trivial or self-limiting.
- Use of antibacterials to treat infection of viral origin, eg the common cold.
- Over long antimicrobial prophylaxis or treatment courses.

Even appropriate antimicrobial therapy is ↑ worldwide, in addition to ↑ use of broad-spectrum antibacterials and prolonged courses. This is owing to the following reasons:

- ↑ numbers of severely ill hospital patients.
- More frequent use of invasive devices and procedures.
- Presence of more severely immunocompromised patients in hospitals and the community.

↑ opportunity for dissemination of infection ↑ the possibility of spread of resistant organisms between patients. This is facilitated by the following:

- Overcrowding in hospital and community healthcare facilities.
- ↑ hospital throughput.
- Poor cleaning and disinfection of rooms, equipment and hands.

Strategies to ↓ or contain antimicrobial resistance

Three main strategies are required to ↓ or contain antimicrobial resistance:

- Prevention of infection through the following mechanisms:
  - Vaccines.
  - Prophylaxis.
  - ↓ use of invasive devices.
  - Good hygiene.
- ↓ dissemination of antimicrobial-resistant organisms (see p.448).
- Limiting or modifying antimicrobial use.

Infection control

Infection control is important in hospital and community residential facilities for the following reasons:
• To prevent cross-transmission of infection.
• To prevent the spread of resistant micro-organisms.
Special attention should be paid to infection control in areas where patients are most vulnerable:
• Intensive care units.
• Neonatal units.
• Burns wards.
• Vascular wards.
• Units treating immunocompromised patients.
Special attention should also be paid to infection control where procedures or devices make patients more vulnerable:
• Urinary catheters.
• Intravascular devices.
• Surgical procedures.
• Respiratory care equipment.
• Enteral or parenteral feeding.
Infection control should be an integral part of the culture of any institution. This requires the following considerations:
• There is an infection control lead clinician or nurse.
• There are written procedures for infection control.
• Staff (including temporary staff and locums) receive education and training on infection-control procedures.
• There are adequate supplies and facilities, eg availability of aprons and, gloves.
• There is documentation of additional infection-control requirements, as necessary, for individual patients.
• Healthcare staff are immunized, as needed, for hepatitis B, TB, chickenpox and influenza.
• There are written procedures for managing occupational exposure to bloodborne viruses and staff are made aware of these procedures.

Universal precautions

Strict attention to hygiene is essential. All body fluids and contaminated equipment, including linen, from all patients should be handled as if infected. This is known as 'universal precautions' and includes taking appropriate measures to ensure the following:
• Prevent contamination, eg wearing apron and gloves and bagging dirty linen.
• Dispose of waste safely eg use of clinical waste bins and sharps boxes.
• Protect staff against occupational exposure to bloodborne viruses (eg hepatitis B and C, and HIV).

Isolation of patients

It might be necessary to nurse patients in isolation in the following circumstances:

- They are a potential source of infection eg MRSA, *C. difficile* diarrhoea and TB.
- They are particularly vulnerable to infection ('reverse barrier nursing'), eg severely neutropaenic patients.

Isolation procedures include the following:
- Nursing patients in a side room or, if more than one patient has the same infection, a cordoned-off area.
- Wearing protective clothing when in contact with the patient. This includes staff who might be in contact with the patient elsewhere in the hospital (eg hospital porters).
- Ensuring equipment is disinfected immediately after use.
- Ensuring aprons, gloves and other disposables are disposed of safely (usually bagged within the room).
- Ensuring visitors take appropriate measures to prevent cross-contamination—eg hand washing and wearing protective clothing for particularly vulnerable patients.

Hand washing or decontamination

Hand hygiene is an essential part of infection control. It is effective for prevention of cross-contamination but unfortunately compliance is often poor—particularly if staff are overworked and stressed.

Education of all staff (clinical and nonclinical) on hand hygiene is essential, in addition to ensuring adequate facilities for washing or decontamination. Hands must be decontaminated at the following times:
- Before any episode of patient contact.
- After any patient contact that could have resulted in hands becoming contaminated.

Visibly soiled or potentially grossly contaminated hands should be washed with soap and water, otherwise alcohol gel can be used. Attention should be paid to ensuring the whole of the hand is decontaminated, including the following para:
- Wrists.
- Thumbs.
- Between the fingers.
- Backs of hands.

Pharmacists and infection control

To avoid contamination of medicines, in addition to presenting a professional appearance, a high standard of cleanliness should be maintained in pharmacy shops and dispensaries. Special attention should be paid to ensuring the following areas are kept clean and tidy:
- Dispensing benches, especially areas where extemporaneous dispensing is carried out.
- Drug refrigerators.
- Toilets.
- Storage areas (often neglected).

Pharmacy staff should have access to handwashing facilities with soap and hot water. Aprons, gloves and (as appropriate) masks should be used when preparing extemporaneous preparations. Tablets and capsules should not be handled—use counting trays and tweezers or a spatula, and disinfect these frequently.

Note that the type of patient contact experienced in a community pharmacy is extremely unlikely to lead to transmission of infection, including MRSA and TB.

Pharmacists do not often have 'hands-on' contact with patient's but they should still observe infection-control procedures. This includes the following:

- Decontaminating hands on entering and leaving clinical areas.
- Wearing gloves and an apron when in close or prolonged contact with high-risk patients, eg those with MRSA.
- Wearing gloves, as appropriate, for 'hands-on' patient contact, eg wound care.
- Checking that new staff, trainees and locums or temporary staff, if necessary, have immunity to chickenpox, TB and hepatitis B.

In the UK, NICE[1] has published guidelines on infection control in primary and community care (including antimicrobial treatment and prophylaxis) in the following areas:

- Standard principles.
- Care of patients with long-term urinary catheters.
- Care during enteral feeding.
- Care of patients with central venous catheters.

1 NICE www.nice.org/page.aspx?0=guidelines.inprogress.infectioncontrolcommunity

Diabetes mellitus

Insulin

Details of the insulins available can be found in the *BNF*, on the Diabetes UK website[1] or on other national websites, such as that hosted by the American Diabetes Association.

There is an ↑ trend towards use of the new insulins such as insulin aspart or insulin lispro. These can be used in an 'inject-and-eat' schedule, ↓ the waiting period between the injection and eating required with older soluble insulins.

Biphasic insulins

Patients need to be counselled about the method needed to adequately resuspend these insulins before injection. Failure to do so leads to a change in the composition of the mix and subsequent hyperglycaemia because of a ↓ dose of the long-acting component.

Insulin pens

These are popular means of delivering insulin, which are generally easy to use, if still somewhat chunky in style. Unfortunately, there is no compatibility between different manufacturer's cartridges.

Although cartridges contain 3mL (300 units) of insulin, the suspension form should not be used beyond 250 units because there is insufficient space to achieve resuspension. Usually, the cartridges have a clear, heavy line. This needs to be considered mind when calculating quantities to be supplied, and patients should be aware of this issue.

1 www.diabetes.org

Monitoring and control

Monitoring

The place of blood glucose monitoring is well recognized in patients with diabetes who require insulin treatment. There are now a wide range of meters available, in addition to finger-pricking devices. It is important to be familiar with a range of machines. The list of those available can be found on the Diabetes UK website[1]. Most companies provide meters at low cost directly to patients and this route is considerably cheaper than purchasing over the counter.

Recent developments have both ↓ the volume of blood required and ↓ the speed of analysis to ~5s. Some can link to computer programmes and estimate average levels according to chosen parameters.

Monitoring of patients with type 2 diabetes tends to be frowned upon by pharmaceutical advisers; however, there are good reasons for regular, if less frequent, monitoring, and it should be encouraged. A sensible pattern might be to monitor twice weekly to ensure no major changes in glucose levels are noted. It is also useful to monitor for lifestyle changes such as ↑ exercise, change of diet, fasting and other influencing factors (eg as mild illness).

Finger-pricking devices are often supplied with meters, which are not prescribable (the lancets are) but can be purchased from community pharmacies. Unfortunately, they all seem to be somewhat painful to use. Laser devices claim to be painless but are very expensive.

Control

Target glucose levels are usually set at 4–7mmol/L for fasting and <9mmol/l for postmeal levels. In the UK, glucose is measured in units of mmol/L. Other countries use mg/100mL. The conversion is 1mmol/L equivalent to 18mg/100mL.

Regular monitoring of HBA_{1c} gives a good pattern of levels in the previous 3 months. Target level for HBA_{1c} should be <7%; however, some authorities set lower levels.

Policy for the administration and handling of cytotoxic drugs

Cytotoxic drugs are used in the treatment of cancers and certain other disorders. They act by killing dividing cells, by preventing their division, but they also act on normal, in addition to malignant, cells. Their use, ∴, poses certain risks to those who handle them. It is important to ensure the safety of staff and patients who come in contact with these drugs.

- Cytotoxic drugs may only be reconstituted in facilities specifically approved for the purpose.
- Staff who prescribe, clinically screen, reconstitute, label, administer and dispose of cytotoxic drugs must be appropriately trained and assessed as competent and must follow the local, approved procedures.
- In areas where cytotoxic drug use is infrequent, a risk assessment must be carried out before a cytotoxic drug is requested. This should assess the availability of appropriate equipment and evidence of training and demonstrate competence in safe administration of the drugs.

Cytotoxic drug procedures

- Any area in the hospital (including the wards, out-patient or daycase areas and pharmacy) using cytotoxic drugs should have available current information on the type of agents used. This information should include relevant health and safety information (control of substances hazardous to health).
- Cytotoxic drugs are occasionally used to treat clinical disorders other than cancer. In such instances, the patient should be referred to a clinical area where cytotoxic drugs are used routinely. Alternatively, a competent practitioner from such an area can administer the drug in the patient's own ward. A trained member of staff must undertake a risk assessment to determine by whom and in what circumstances the drug can be administered.

Prescription, preparation and reconstitution

- All prescriptions must be written legibly and signed in indelible black ink. In some cases, prescriptions might be computer-generated, either on an approved chemotherapy chart or a standard prescription chart.
- Pre-registration house officers can not prescribe cytotoxic drug therapy in some hospitals. Be aware of local policies stipulating who can prescribe chemotherapy.
- The chief pharmacist is responsible for ensuring that cytotoxic drugs reconstitution services are provided in appropriate facilities. In exceptional circumstances, they can designate other areas for reconstitution.

Labelling and transportation

- Syringes, infusion devices and infusion fluids containing cytotoxic drugs must be labelled, to identify the potential cytotoxic hazard, and placed inside a sealed plastic bag.

- Syringes and infusions must be transported in sealed containers identified as containing cytotoxic drugs. The designated cytotoxic drugs reconstitution services must be notified at once if the integrity of a container received is suspect.
- Oral cytotoxic drugs should be transported in the same way as non-cytotoxic medication. In-patient supplies should be labelled as 'cytotoxic' on the normal prescription label.

Administration

- Relevant clinical laboratory results, as defined by chemotherapy protocols, must be reviewed before administration and appropriate action taken.
- The following checks are advised to be made by two qualified staff members, one of whom must be registered as competent in cytotoxic drugs administration, depending on local policy:
  - Visual check of the product (to include signs of leakage, contamination or breakdown products).
  - The drug has been appropriately stored and is within its expiry date.
  - Patients must be identified positively using three patient identifiers, as defined in the trust policy.
  - The following prescription details must be checked:
  - Protocol.
  - Dose.
  - Diluent (if relevant).
  - Route of administration.
  - Frequency.
- Staff should use personal-protective equipment and clothing if handling and administering cytotoxic drugs. This includes gloves, an apron and, in some cases, protection for the face, either goggles or a face shield.

Accidental spillage

- Each clinical area using cytotoxic drugs should have a spill kit available for use at all times. These kits are usually obtained from the pharmacy department. The kit includes instructions on how to proceed safely. Staff should be familiar with the instructions before dealing with a spill.
- A trained healthcare professional should deal with the spill immediately. After use, the spillage kit should be replaced.
- Be familiar with your local policy and location of spillage kits in areas using cytotoxic drugs.

Disposal of product waste

- Cytotoxic waste should be disposed of separately to normal clinical waste, according to local policy. The incorrect disposal of cytotoxic waste can result in prosecution under the Special Waste Regulations, 1996.
- Cytotoxic waste includes vials that have contained cytotoxic drugs, syringes, needles, IV bags and giving sets used to administer cytotoxic drugs, and urinary catheters and drainage bags from patients undergoing cytotoxic therapy.
- Cytotoxic waste should be disposed of according to local policy and clearly marked with cytotoxic residue tape.

- Hospitals have specific policies on the storage and collection of cytotoxic waste, to ensure that cytotoxic waste does not enter the normal clinical waste stream.

Disposal of excreta and blood

- Because cytotoxic drugs have varying half-lives, specific information about them will be found on safety datasheets. If the information is not specified, it is deemed GCP to apply universal precautions for 7 days after administration.
- Patients and relatives (particularly pregnant mothers) who handle body fluids at home should be given appropriate advice.
- Gloves must be worn when handling all body fluids (eg blood, urine, faeces, colostomy and urostomy bags, and nappies) during and after the administration of cytotoxic drugs.
- Linen contaminated with body fluids and cytotoxic drugs must be handled according to the local policy for handling cytotoxic contaminated waste.

Incidents arising from handling and administration of cytotoxic drugs

- Any incident involving prescribing, administration and disposal of cytotoxic drugs must be reported according to the local incident-reporting system.
- The most probable incident for staff is accidental exposure to the drug during the set-up and administration of the drug. This might result from a bag leaking or bursting, or problems with the line *in situ*.
- If there is eye and skin contamination, rinse the affected area with copious amounts of tap water and seek further treatment, if needed. For all cases of staff exposure, the occupational health department should be notified to organize risk assessment and follow-up care plans.
- For patients, the most probable incidents arising are extravasation during treatment.

Handling cytotoxics during pregnancy

Pregnant staff should refer to their local policy with regard to handling cytotoxic drugs, because this group of drugs are potentially mutagenic, teratogenic and carcinogenic. A risk assessment must be undertaken for each local area.

See pp.206–9 for recommendations on handling potentially teratogenic drugs in pregnancy.

Intrathecal chemotherapy

Refer to section on intrathecal administration of chemotheraphy, p.494.

Further reading

Allwood M, Stanley A, Wright P (2002). *The Cytotoxics Handbook*, 4th edn. Abingdon: Radcliffe Medical Press.

Clinical screening of chemotherapy prescriptions

Receipt of prescription for cycle 1

- Check patient's name, date of birth and hospital number against the medical notes.
- Check surface area has been calculated correctly:

$$\text{Surface area} = \sqrt{(\text{Height [cm]} \times \text{weight [kg]})/3600}$$

- Surface area is often capped at $2m^2$ or $2.2m^2$. Check your local policy.
- Check patient's ideal body weight. If the patient is significantly more or less than their ideal body weight, discuss with their doctor.

  $$\text{Ideal body weight} = (\text{height [m]} \times \text{height [m]}) \times 25$$

- Check patient's treatment against the disease protocol.
- Ensure that it is the intended protocol to be prescribed by checking in the medical notes.
- Check patient's age, because some doses/protocols are age-related.
- Check the medical notes for dose modification or variance from the protocol.
- Interpret critical tests to see if a dose modification is required eg impaired renal function, clotting disorders and liver function tests (if appropriate for drug).
- Check the correct drugs have been prescribed.
- Check the frequency of intended cycles and appropriate interval since any previous chemotherapy.
- Check if there are any drug interactions between the chemotherapy and the patient's regular medication.
- Check if there are any drugs contraindicated with the chemotherapy.

Second and subsequent cycles

- Check chemotherapy cycle is correct for protocol.
- Check the correct cycle was ordered.
- Check the drugs were prescribed on the correct days and start dates.
- Check there has been no significant change in the patient's weight that might significantly change the calculated surface area.
- Check response to previous treatment.
  - Blood indices–haematology/biochemical.
  - Tolerability/adverse reactions.
- Check any appropriate modifications have been made in relation to previous response or critical tests (normally in the protocol)

Clinical check

- What type of malignancy does the patient have? Is the chemotherapy appropriate for the malignancy?
- What is the patient's renal and hepatic function? Do any of the doses need adjusting to take this into account?

- Has the patient had any chemotherapy before? Do any of the drugs have a maximum cumulative lifetime dose (eg anthracyclines)?
- Other checks–allergies/reactions to previous chemotherapy and the extent of disease (need for prehydration or allopurinol).
- Critical tests–if white cell count, neutrophils or HB are above a predefined limit, refer to individual protocols.
- Check any appropriate modifications have been made in relation to previous response or critical tests (normally in protocol).
- Check any supportive care has been prescribed–eg antiemetics.

Validating prescription details

- Check doses have been correctly calculated and prescribed.
- Check maximum doses according to the protocol:
  - If it is more than 2 months since a patient has been weighed and no new weight is recorded, ask for the patient to be weighed.
  - Body surface areas are often rounded, do not query a discrepancy unless it is >0.1m^2 for adults.
  - Oncology patients might have their body surface area capped at 2m^2 or 2.2m^2.
  - Eg obese patients—confirm with the prescriber if body surface has not been capped if >2m^2 or 2.2m^2.
  - Haematology patients do not usually have their body surface area capped.
- Check units.
- Check cumulative doses–eg anthracyclines (doxurubicin has a maximum cumulative dose of 550mg/m^2) and bleomycin (a maximum cumulative dose of 300–400 units)
- Rounding doses–be aware that the exact dose might have to be rounded as a result of the manufacturing process.
- Check local policy for variation in the dispensed dose compared with the prescribed dose that has been agreed (often 5% variation is agreed).
- Ensure the doctor has signed and dated the prescription.

Endorsing prescriptions

- Amend any abbreviations.
- Annotate generic names.
- Ensure infusion fluid, volume and rate of administration are stated and appropriate.
- Check that the appropriate route is prescribed.
- For routes other than IV, ensure the route is prescribed in full–eg intrathecal not IT.
- Check oral doses are rounded up or down to account for tablet size.

Annotations

- Sign and date the prescription to confirm the prescription is correct, safe and appropriate.
- The following annotations should be made in the medical notes in black ink:
  - Date.
  - 'Pharmacist' underlined.

- 'Chemo ordered'–'confirmed' or 'awaiting confirmation (TBC)'.
- Cycle number and date the cycle is due.
- Any dose reductions.
- Other relevant notes:
  — With the first cycle, annotate the drugs, doses and frequency in the medical notes, including reasons for alterations—so that it is clear exactly what the patient has received. Include the surface area, height and weight that were used to calculate the doses and relevant biochemistry.
  — On the last cycle, record the cumulative dose of anthracyclines or bleomycin received.
- Clinical pharmacist's signature.
- Bleep number.

Further reading

Allwood M, Stanley A, Wright P (2002). *The Cytotoxics Handbook*, 4th edn. Abingdon: Radcliffe Medical Press.

Royal College of Radiologists' Clinical Oncology Information Network (COIN) (2001). Guidelines for cytotoxic chemotherapy in adults. A document for local expert groups in the United Kingdom preparing chemotherapy policy documents. *Clinical Oncology, (Royal College of Radiology)* **13(1)**; s209–48.

Chemotherapy dosing

Cancer chemotherapy drugs often have a narrow therapeutic window between the dose that is effective and the dose that can be toxic. Inappropriate dose reduction reduces chemotherapy efficacy. However, if doses are not ↓ in patients with organ dysfunction, this can lead to serious or life-threatening toxicity. It is essential that cytotoxic drugs are dosed correctly and adapted to individual patients to enable the maximum probability of a desired therapeutic outcome, with minimum toxicity.

Before administration of chemotherapy, each patient should be assessed for performance status, renal function, liver biochemistry tests, serum albumin level and prognosis. Myelosuppression is the most common and dangerous toxicity of cytotoxics, so all patients must have a blood count before each cycle of chemotherapy. Patients must only be administered chemotherapy if their white blood cell count is $>3.0 \times 10^9$/L (or neutrophil count is $>1.5 \times 10^9$/L) and platelet count is $>150 \times 10^9$/L. There can be exceptions to this in some local policies or for patients with haematological malignancies and those undergoing intensive treatment with specialized support.

Doses of cytotoxics are usually calculated on the basis of body surface area, which is measured in square metres (m^2). The dose is quoted as units (eg milligrammes, grammes or international units) per square metre. The patient's surface area is calculated using a nomogram from patient height and weight measurements or using the following calculation:

$$\sqrt{\frac{\text{Height (cm)} \times \text{weight (kg)}}{3600}}$$

This practice is derived from the relationship between body size and physiological parameters, eg renal function. The performance status of the patient and their renal and liver functions are also taken into account. prior to each cycle of treatment, toxicities must be recorded using common toxicity criteria. Doses are modified if the patient experiences toxicity to treatment. The size of the reduction depends on the nature and severity of the toxicity, taking into account whether the chemotherapy is palliative or curative in intent.

Obese patients have physiological changes that affect drug disposition, including ↑ blood volume, organ size and adipose tissue mass. Body surface area is often 'capped' at 2.0–2.2m^2 in obese patients. The use of ideal body weight can be considered in these settings. However, the possibility of underdosing needs to be considered in curative patients.

Although it is conventional to prescribe chemotherapy according to body surface area, it is acceptable to use preprepared standard doses for commonly used drugs to facilitate bulk preparation and rapid dispensing. This is known as 'dose banding'. The rounded dose must be within agreed limits, eg within 5% of the calculated dose.

There are, however, some exceptions to doses being calculated on the basis of body surface area. Drugs whose doses can be calculated using other parameters include the following:

- Asparaginase—the dosage is IU/kg body weight or IU/body surface area.
- Bleomycin—IU, either per patient surface area or as a fixed dose.
- Carboplatin—The Calvert equation can be used to calculate the dose of carboplatin in patients with or without renal impairment (1):

Dose (mg) = target area under the plasma concentration curve (AUC) X (GFR + 25) (AUC usually 5 to 7)

For example, for a patient with a GFR of 75ml/min, using an AUC of 5, the dose of carboplatin would be as follows:

Dose (mg) = 5(75 + 25) = 500mg carboplatin

- Cytarabine—dosage in mg/kg for certain indications.
- Floxuridine—dosage in mg/kg.
- Mitomycin—dosage in mg/kg for certain indications.

Frequency of chemotherapy administration

Chemotherapy is usually administered at 3wk intervals, up to 8–12 cycles of treatment.

Exceptions to 3wk administration intervals include the following:

- Carboplatin—can be administered every 3wk or 4wk.
- Irinotecan—administered every 2wk
- 5FU—can be administered once weekly on every 2wk, 3wk, or 4wk, depending on dosage schedule.
- Paclitaxel—can be administered once weekly (unlicensed).
- Docetaxel—can be administered once weekly (unlicensed).

Critical tests for chemotherapy to proceed on time

Chemotherapy should only be administered at the full protocol dose if the haematological and biochemical parameters are within the normal range. Biochemical parameters depend on the excreted route of the drug. Creatinine clearance should be monitored for renally cleared drugs and LFTs should be monitored for those drugs metabolized hepatically. Haematological parameters include the white cell count, absolute neutrophil count (>1.5) and platelet count (>100).

If the biochemical or haematological parameters are not within the normal range, dose reduction or delaying subsequent doses must be considered. Doses are usually reduced by 20–25% initially. Chemotherapy is usually delayed by a week at a time.

Further reading

Allwood M, Stanley A, Wright P (2000). *The Cytotoxics Handbook*, 4th edn. Abingdon: Radcliffe Medical Press.

Calvert AH, Newell, DR, Gumbrell, LA, et al. (1989). Carboplatin dosage: prospective evaluation of a simple formula based on renal function. *Jounrnal of Clinical Oncology*; **7**: 1748–56.

Daniels S, Gabriel S (2003). *Dosage adjustment for cytotoxics in hepatic impairment*. UCL Hospitals NHS Trust, www.bopa-web.org/Members/Guidelines.asp

Daniels S, Gabriel, S (2003). *Dosage adjustment for cytotoxics in renal impairment*. UCL Hospitals NHS Trust, 2003. www.bopa-web.org/Members/Guidelines.asp

Myers, P (2002). *Guidelines for the management of cytotoxics in obese adult patients*. The Royal Marsden Hospital, www.bopa-web.org/Members/Guidelines.asp

Royal College of Radiologists' Clinical Oncology Information Network (COIN) (2001). Guidelines for cytotoxic chemotherapy in adults. A document for local expert groups in the United Kingdom preparing chemotherapy policy documents. *Clinical Oncology (R. College Radiololgy)*. **13**(1): s209–48.

Antiemetics for the prophylaxis of chemotherapy–induced nausea and vomiting

- Nausea and vomiting remain two of the most feared side effects of chemotheraphy in cancer patients.
- The goal of antiemetic therapy is to prevent nausea and vomiting completely.
- Antiemetics should be given regularly and prophylactically.
- Combinations of antiemetics are significantly more effective than single agents.
- Clinical practice guidelines ensure appropriate and cost-effective antiemetic use.
- Factors that need to be considered when choosing an antiemetic regimen include the following:
  - The chemotherapy emetic risk (Table 16.15), dose, and schedule.
  - The type of nausea and vomiting being treated (anticipatory, acute or delayed Table 16.16);
  - The patient risk of nausea and vomiting (Table 16.17);
  - Other underlying causes of nausea and vomiting (Table 16.18)
  - The mechanism of action and routes of administration of the antiemetic (Tables 16.19–24);
  - The adverse effects of the drugs.
  - The cost-effectiveness of the drugs.
  - Whether patients can self-administer the antiemetic.

Chemotheraphy drug combinations have an additive emetic effect. If chemotheraphy drugs from the same category are combined, the regimen is classified as a higher emetic risk. If drugs are from different categories, the emetic risk is determined according to the most emetic drug in the combination.

Table 16.15 Emetic risk of chemotherapy

High emetic risk	Moderate-high emetic risk	Low-moderate emetic risk	Low emetic risk
Cisplatin, ≥50mg/m^2	Cisplatin, <50mg/m^2	Procarbazine (oral)	Busulfan (low dose)
Mechloretamine	Cytarabine, >1000mg/m^2	Cyclophosphamide (oral)	Chlorambucil (oral)
Streptozocin	Carboplatin	Mitoxantrone	Fludarabine
Carmustine, >250mg/m^2	Oxaliplatin	Gemcitabine	Hydroxycarbamide
Cyclophosphamide, >1500mg/m^2	Ifosfamide	Docetaxel	Methotrexate, ≤ 50mg/m^2
Dacarbazine	Carmustine ≤ 250mg/m^2	Paclitaxel	Vincristine/ vinblastine/ vinorelbine/vindesine
	Cyclophosphamide ≤ 1500mg/m^2	Etoposide	Bleomycin
	Doxorubicin ≥ 60mg/m^2	Teniposide	Tioguanine
	Epirubicin, ≥ 90mg/m^2	Methotrexate, 50–250mg/m^2	Mercaptopurine
	Actinomycin-D	Mitomycin	Asparaginase
	Lomustine	5-Fluorouracil <1000mg/m^2	Melphalan
	Chlormethine	Doxorubicin, 20–59mg/m^2	Chlorodeoxyadenosine
	Daunorubicin	Treosulphan	
	Idarubicin	Capecitabine	
	Temozolomide		
	Topotecan		
	Irinotecan		
	Doxorubicin (liposomal)		
	Treosulfan		
	Streptozocin		

Table 16.16 Definitions of chemotherapy-induced nausea and vomiting

• Acute nausea and vomiting	Initial 24h after chemotherapy
• Delayed nausea and vomiting	>24h after chemotherapy
• Anticipatory nausea and vomiting	Days to hours before chemotherapy

Table 16.17 Patient risk factors, which predict poor antiemetic control

Patients with more than three or four risk factors should be considered to receive additional antiemetics at the outset.

• ♀ sex
• <30 years old
• History of sickness—in pregnancy/travel sickness/with surgery
• Poor control with prior chemotherapy
• Underlying nausea and vomiting
• Anxiety

Note: high alcohol intake can have a protective effect and ↓ risk of emesis

Table 16.18 Other causes of nausea and vomiting to be considered

• Radiotherapy
• Radiosensitizers
• Infection
• Metabolic disorders
• Electrolyte disturbances
• Constipation
• GI obstruction
• Cachexia syndrome
• Metastases (brain, liver or bone)
• Paraneoplasia
• Emetic medication (eg opioids, antibiotics, antifungals or amifostine)

Table 16.19 Notes on appropriate antiemetic prescribing with chemotherapy

- Antiemetics should be administered regularly, prophylactically, and orally.
- (Serotonin) 5HT-3 receptor antagonists are equally efficacious and should be administered orally, and only for acute nausea and vomiting.
- There is only evidence for the use of 5HT-3 receptor antagonists for an additional day in the delayed phase for cyclophosphamide and carboplatin.
- Neurokinin receptor antagonists (eg aprepitant) can be considered as an adjunct to dexamethasone and a 5HT-3 receptor antagonist to prevent acute and delayed nausea and vomiting with cisplatin-based chemotherapy.
- Optimal emetic control in the acute phase is essential to prevent nausea and vomiting in the delayed phase.
- Dexamethasone is not required when steroids are included in a chemotherapy regimen and for some haematology regimens.
- Consider administering antiemetics by IV infusion, subcutaneously, rectally or sublingually (if available in those formulations), if the patient is unable to take oral antiemetics.
- Metoclopramide can be replaced with domperidone if patient has extrapyramidal side effects.
- If a patient is already taking antiemetics (eg cyclizine or prochlorperazine) for underlying nausea and vomiting before to starting on chemotherapy, these drugs could be continued as a substitute for metoclopramide.

Table 16.20 Combinations of oral antiemetics to prevent Chemotherapy-induced nausea and vomiting

High and moderate/high emetic risk:

Acutely:	Serotonin receptor antagonist, oral 1h before chemotherapy (Table 16.21).
	Dexamethasone, 8mg oral twice daily , starting on the morning of chemotherapy until 24h after highly emetic chemotherapy.
	This is continued for the duration of highly emetic chemotherapy administration.
	Neurokinin receptor antagonist (eg aprepitant, 125mg 1h before chemotherapy) can be added to this combination for cisplatin-based chemotherapy.
Delayed phase:	**For cisplatin only:** dexamethasone, 8mg orally daily (single or divided doses) for 3–4 days, which can be reduced to 4mg daily for 1–2 additional days.
	Neurokinin receptor antagonist (eg aprepitant 80mg daily for 2days) can be given in addition to the dexamethasone.
	For all chemotherapy: metoclopramide 10–20mg orally four times daily for 3–4 days regularly, then if required.

Low–moderate emetic risk:

Acutely:	dexamethasone, 8mg oral twice daily, starting on the morning of chemotherapy, until 24 hours after chemotherapy.
Delayed Phase:	no regular preventative use of antiemetic.
	Metoclopramide 10–20mg oral four times daily for 3–4 days, if required.

Low emetic risk

No routine prophylaxis required.

Metoclopramide, 10–20mg oral four times daily, if required.

Note: for patients <30 years old, consider domperidone instead of metoclopramide if the patient experiences extrapyramidal side effects.

Table 16.21 Recommended oral daily doses of serotonin 5-HT$_3$ receptor antagonists to be administered 1h before to chemotherapy

- Granisetron, 2mg daily
- Ondansetron, 8mg 1h before chemotherapy and another dose 12h later
- Tropisetron, 5mg daily
- Dolasetron, 200mg daily

Table 16.22 Recommended IV doses of 5-HT₃ receptor antagonists to be administered if patients are unable to tolerate medicines by the oral route

- Granisetron,1mg daily
- Ondansetron,8mg daily
- Tropisetron, 5mg daily
- Dolasetron, 100mg daily

Table 16.23 Antiemetics for failure of control

- Dexamethasone is the most useful agent for delayed nausea and vomiting
- To ensure absorption of antiemetics administered, consider subcutaneous, IV, or rectal administration,if available eg prochlorperozine, 25mg rectally twice to four times daily, or domperidone, 30–60mg rectally four times daily.
- Ensure antiemetics cover full period of nausea and vomiting

Table 16.24 Suggested antiemetics for patients refractory to first-line antiemetics

Acutely

1. Use antiemetics recommended for more emetic chemotherapy (for low or moderate emetic risk regimens)
2. If highly emetic chemotherapy, consider **one** of the following options:
   - Add **lorazepam 1mg orally/sublingual/IV every 8h** if anxious (sedative, and amnesic)
   - Consider **levomepromazine, 6.25–12.5mg orally as a single daily dose** instead of metoclopramide
   - Replace lorazepam and metoclopramide **with levomepromazine, 6.25–12.5mg oral or subcutaneous (in the evening) as a single daily dose (Note: 12.5mg oral = 6.25mg subcutaneous)**
   - Prescribe regular lorazepam with prochlorperazine **10mg oral four times daily or 25mg rectal four times daily** instead of metoclopramide
3. For cisplatin–containing regimens, consider adding a neurokinin receptor antagonist to dexamethasone and 5HT-3 receptor antagonist on subsequent cycles of chemotherapy (eg aprepitant, 125mg 1h before chemotherapy, then 80mg daily for 2 days)

Delayed

- **Dexamethasone 4mg twice a day** for up to 1wk after chemotherapy.
- Consider **levomepromazine, 6.25–12.5mg oral as a single daily dose** instead of metoclopramide

Anticipatory

- Consider **lorazepam**, 1mg oral at night (or dose up to 1mg three times daily) orally if anxious or anticipatory nausea and vomiting.

Further reading

Fauser AA, Fellhauer M, Hoffmann M, et al. (1999). Guidelines for antiemetic therapy: acute emesis. *European Journal of Cancer* **35**(3): 361–70.

Gralla RJ, Osoba D, Kris MG, et al. (1999). Recommendations for the use of antiemetics: evidence-based, clinical practice guidelines. *Journal of Clinical Oncology* **17**(9):2971–94.

Stoner NS (2004). Therapy-induced nausea and vomiting: assessment of severity and indications for treatment. In: *The Effective Prevention and Control of Symptoms in Cancer*. Eds: A Hoy, I Finlay, A Miles. Cardiff: The Clyvedon Press Ltd, p. 139–44.

Stoner, NS (2004). Evidence for selection and use of antiemetic agents and regimens: therapy-induced nausea and vomiting. In: *The Effective Prevention and Control of Symptoms in Cancer*. Eds: A Hoy I Finlay, A Miles. Cardiff: The Clyvedon Press Ltd, p. 145–54.

Herrstedt J (2000). European Society for Medical Oncology (ESMO) Recommendations for Prophylaxis of Chemotherapy-Induced Nausea and Vomiting (NV). www.esmo.org/reference/anti_emetics.htm

Principles of extravasation

- Extravasation is the inappropriate or accidental administration of drug into the subcutaneous or subdermal tissues, instead of into the intended IV compartment.
- Extravasation causes pain, erythema, inflammation and discomfort.
- If left undiagnosed or inappropriately treated, extravasation of chemotherapy can cause necrosis and functional loss of the tissue and limb concerned.
- Extravasation can occur with any IV injection. However, it is only considered to be a problem with compounds that are known to be vesicant or irritant.
    - Appropriately treated extravasation, dealt with within 24h should ensure that the patient has no further problems.
    - Risk factors associated with extravasation include the following:
    - Administration technique—↑ risk if staff are inadequately trained.
    - Administration device—use of unsuitable cannulae, eg cannulae 24h old.
    - Location of cannulation site—the forearm is the favoured site.
    - Patient factors:
        - Eg underlying conditions, such as lymphoedema, diabetes and peripheral circulatory diseases.
        - Eg patient age—additional precaution required for paediatrics and elderly patients.
- Concurrent medication—eg steroids and anticoagulants.
- Physical properties of the drugs concerned.
- Prevention of extravasation is best using one or more of the following techniques:
    - Use of central line for slow infusions of high-risk drugs.
    - Administer cytotoxic drugs through a recently sited cannula.
    - Ensure cannula cannot be dislodged during drug administration.
    - Ensure the cannula is patent before administration.
    - Administer vesicants by slow IV push into the side arm of a fast running IV infusion of a compatible solution.
    - Administer the most vesicant drug first.
    - Assess the site continuously for any signs of redness or swelling.
    - Ensure the patient is aware of extravasation risks and reports any burning or pain on administration of the drug.
    - Take time—do not rush.
- Stop the infusion or injection immediately if an extravasation is thought to have occurred and follow the local extravasation policy.
- An extravasation policy and kit must be available in all areas where chemotherapy is administered.
- Check your local extravasation policy, and be aware of the location of extravasation kits.

Further reading

Allwood M, Stanley A, Wright P (2002). *The Cytotoxics Handbook.* 4th edn. Abingdon: Radcliffe Medical Press.

Extravasation of chemotherapy in adult patients

A number of agents used in cancer chemotherapy are extremely damaging if they extravasate or infiltrate into the tissues, rather than remain within the vasculature (Table 16.25). Extravasation might have occurred if there is evidence of the following:

• Any pain on administration, either at the cannulation site or in the surrounding area.
• Swelling around or above the cannulation site.
• Redness or heat at or around the area.

If the patient makes any complaint, stop the administration and check the site. If extravasation is suspected, the nursing/medical staff should follow the directions below:

• The administration of the infusion/injection must be stopped and the cannula left in place.
• The healthcare professional administering the treatment should remain with the patient and ask a colleague to summon a doctor to examine and prescribe the appropriate treatment, according to the local extravasation policy.
• If a vesicant drug (Table 16.25) has been extravasated, the plastic surgical specialist registrar on-call 24h should be contacted according to the local policy. An emergency intervention/antidote might be required, according to the local policy.
• Aspirate 3–5ml of fluid from the extravasation site through the cannula, if possible.
• The area should be marked and the cannula removed.
• Hydrocortisone (100mg) should be administered by IV infusion through a new cannula that is re-sited remotely from the extravasation area.
• Hydrocortisone (100mg; 2mL) can be administered subcutaneously or intradermally in 0.2mL aliquots in a 'pin-cushion' fashion at six to eight points of the compass around and in the extravasated area. Omit this step if the extravasation is around a central line.
• Hydrocortisone 1% cream should be applied topically to the extravasated site three times daily, as long as redness persists.
• The extravasated area should be covered with sterile gauze. Heat can be applied to disperse the extravasated drug or the area can be cooled to localize the extravasation, depending on the drug extravasated and the local policy.
• The site should be elevated while swelling persists.
• Antihistamine cover should be given (eg chlorphenamine, 4mg oral).
• Analgesia should be provided, if required.
• For the management of each individual drug, refer to the management plans in local policy.
• The following documents should be completed within 4h, according to local policy:
  • Standard local documentation for extravasation, and filed in the patients notes.
  • A local incident form.

- The patient's consultant should be informed within 24h (at the discretion of the specialist registrar on-call).

Follow-up care

- If IV chemotherapy is to be continued on the same day as an extravasation incident, avoid, if possible, using the limb where the extravasation has occurred.
- Review the extravasation site (suggested at ~24h and at 7 days). If not ulcerated, advise gradual return to normal use. For subsequent cycles of chemotherapy, consider surgical opinion if persistent pain, swelling or delayed ulceration occurs.
- Inform risk management of the outcome.

Extravasation risk for chemotherapy products

There is no standard test to determine a drug's extravasation risk; the absolute risk is determined by extravasation reports originating from clinical practice and, ∴, controversy will exist for certain drugs.

Definitions of cytotoxic drug classification

- Vesicants—capable of causing pain, inflammation and blistering of the local skin, underlying flesh and structures, leading to tissue death and necrosis.
- Exfoliants—capable of causing inflammation and shedding of skin, but less likely to cause tissue death.
- Irritants—capable of causing inflammation and irritation, rarely proceeding to breakdown of the tissue.

Table 16.25 Classification of cytotoxic drugs according to their potential to cause serious necrosis when extravasated

Vesicants	Exfoliants
• Amsacrine	Aclarubicin
• Carmustine	Cisplatin
• Dacarbazine	Daunorubicin (liposomal)
• Dactinomycin	Docetaxel
• Daunorubicin	Doxorubicin (liposomal)
• Doxorubicin	Floxuridine
• Epirubicin	Mitoxantrone
• Idarubicin	Oxaliplatin
• Mitomycin	Topotecan
• Chlormethine (mustine)	
• Paclitaxel	
• Streptozocin	
• Treosulfan	
• Vinblastine	
• Vincristine	
• Vindesine	
• Vinorelbine	

Irritants
- Carboplatin
- Etoposide
- Irinotecan
- Mesna (undiluted)
- Teniposide

Inflammatory agents
- Aldesleukin
- Etoposide phosphate
- Fluorouracil
- Methotrexate
- Raltitrexed
- Mesna (diluted)

Neutrals
- Asparaginase
- Bleomycin
- Cladribine
- Cyclophosphamide
- Cytarabine
- Fludarabine
- Gemcitabine
- Ifosfamide
- Interleukin 2
- Melphalan
- Pentostatin
- Thiotepa
- α-Interferons

- Inflammatory agents—capable of causing mild-to-moderate inflammation and flare in local tissues.
- Neutral—ostensibly inert or neutral compounds that do not cause inflammation or damage.

Guidelines for the use of an antidote for an extravasated vesicant drug

It is difficult to be certain that the injection of antidotes into the area of extravasation is of benefit, and reports are conflicting. Most small extravasations do not result in serious problems without injection of antidotes; ∴, injection of specific antidotes should probaly be restricted to larger extravasations (>1–2mL).

For large-volume extravasations (10mL or more) of drugs with an acidic pH, the administration of either 1% or 2.1% sodium bicarbonate into the area to neutralize the drug, followed by warm compression to disperse the neutral mixture, has been successful. However, this should only be attempted with extreme care, because if the extravasation has been misdiagnosed or the volume extravasated has been wrongly assessed, the treatment could lead to an alkaline extravasation. Administer the bicarbonate sparingly in 0.2mL aliquots into the 'body' of the injury, not the periphery, and aspirate to remove any excess bicarbonate.

Administering antidotes: (DO NOT USE UNDILUTED):

- To make 10mL of 3% sodium thiosulphate—take 0.6mL of sodium thiosulphate 50% solution and dilute to 10mL with water to make a 3% solution for injection.
- To make 10mL of 1% sodium bicarbonate—take 2.5mL of sodium bicarbonate 4.2% solution and dilute to 10mL with water to make a 1% solution for injection.
- To make 10mL of 2.1% sodium bicarbonate—take 5mL of sodium bicarbonate 4.2% solution and dilute to 10mL with water to make a 2.1% solution for injection.
- To make 1500 units hyluronidase—dissolve one vial of hyaluronidase 1500 units in 1mL of sodium chloride 0.9% solution or water for injection. Note: subcutaneous hyaluronidase administration is very painful for the patient. Therefore, spraying the extravasated area with ethyl chloride before hyaluronidase administration is recommended.
- Dimethylsulfoxide (DMSO)—avoid contact with good skin.

Contents of the extravasation kit:

- Sodium bicarbonate 4.2% solution 10mL injection x 2.
- 1500 units hyaluronidase x 2.
- 100mg hydrocortisone injection x 5.
- 10mL water for injection x 2.
- Diclofenac topical cream x 1.
- DMSO 99% solution 25mL x 1.
- Hydrocortisone 1% cream x 1.
- Cold packs x 2 (one to be stored in the freezer and one to be microwaved for a hot pack).

Further reading

Allwood M, Stanley A, Wright P (2002). *The Cytotoxics Handbook*. 4th ed. Abingdon: Radcliffe Medical Press.

Dorr RT, (1990). Antidotes to vesicant chemotherapy extravasations. *Blood reviews* **4**: 41–60.

Bertelli G, Gozza A, Forno MG *et al.* (1995). Topical dimethylsulfoxide for the prevention of soft tissue injury after extravasation of vesicant cytotoxic drugs: a prospective clinical study. *Journal of Clinical Oncology* **13 (11)**: 2851–5.

Rudolph R, Larson DL, (1987). Etiology and treatment of chemotherapeutic agent extravasation injuries: a review. *Journal of Clinical Oncology* **5:** 116–1122.

Boyle D, Engelking C, (1995). Vesicant extravasation: myths and realities. *Oncology Nursing Forum* **22**: 57–67.

Treatment of chemotherapy drug extravasations in adult patients

Table 16.26

Drug	Suggested antidote
Administer hydrocortisone 100mg subcutaneously or intradermally in a 'pin-cushion' fashion (at points of the compass) around and in the extravasated area.	
Aclarubicin	Apply DMSO 99% solution topically to the extravasated area, every 2h. Once DMSO dries, apply hydrocortisone cream and 30min of **cold compress** every 2h, for the first 24h. Treatment for the next 14days should consist of topical application of DMSO every 6h, alternating with applications of topical hydrocortisone cream every 6h, so that a preparation is applied every 3h on an alternate basis. If blistering occurs, the DMSO should be stopped and further advice sought.
Aldesleukin	If a large volume has been extravasated, aspirate as much fluid as possible. Dispersal of the extravasated drug can be facilitated by the use of subcutaneous hyaluronidase (1500 units in 1mL of water for injection or sodium chloride 0.9% solution) injected around the area of injury. Apply heat and compression to assist natural dispersal of the drug. No further treatment should be required and the patient should be managed symptomatically. Subcutaneous hyaluronidase administration is very painful for the patient, therefore, spraying the extravasated area with ethyl chloride before
Alemtuzumab (MabCampath®)	Not considered to be cytotoxic; therefore, not expected to cause necrosis. No specific treatment is considered necessary. Ask the patient to report any reactions. Symptomatic management only.
Amsacrine	Apply DMSO 99% solution topically to the extravasated area every 2h. Once DMSO dries, apply hydrocortisone cream and 30min of **cold compress** every 2h for the first 24h. Treatment for the next 14 days should consist of topical application of DMSO every 6h, alternating with applications of topical hydrocortisone cream every 6h, so that a preparation is being applied every 3h, on an alternate basis.If blistering occurs, the DMSO should be stopped and further advice sought.

Table 16.26 (Contd.)

Drug	Suggested antidote
Asparaginase Bleomycin	If a large volume has been extravasated, aspirate as much fluid as possible. Dispersal of the extravasated drug can be facilitated by the use of subcutaneous hyaluronidase (1500 units in 1mL water for injections or sodium chloride 0.9% solution) injected around the area of injury. Apply **heat** and compression to assist natural dispersal of the drug. No further treatment should be required and the patient should be managed symptomatically. Subcutaneous hyaluronidase administration is very painful for the patient; therefore, spraying the extravasated area with ethyl chloride before hyaluronidase administration is recommended. If the extravasated area is only small, simply apply a cold compress and elevate. No further treatment should be required.
Carboplatin	Administer hydrocortisone, 100mg IV, then a further 100mg subcutaneous hydrocortisone as 0.2mL injections in a 'pin-cushion' fashion. Apply topical hydrocortisone and cover the area with an **ice pack**. When the initial inflammatory reaction has subsided, the use of a warm compression can aid the dispersal of any residual fluid. There are no specific antidotes for carboplatin, and further management should be symptomatic.
Carmustine*	Infiltrate the area with 1–3mL of sodium bicarbonate 2.1% solution; leave for 2min and aspirate off again. Apply **cold compression**
Cisplatin*	Infiltrate the area with 1–3mL of sodium thiosulphate 3% solution, aspirate back and then give 1500 units of hyaluronidase in 1mL of water for injection or sodium chloride 0.9%, around the area and apply **heat** and compression. Subcutaneous hyaluronidase administration is very painful for the patient; therefore, spraying the extravasated area with ethyl chloride before hyaluronidase administration is recommended.
Cladribine	If a large volume has been extravasated, aspirate as much fluid as possible. Dispersal of the extravasated drug can be facilitated by the use of subcutaneous hyaluronidase (1500 units in 1mL of water for injection or sodium chloride 0.9% solution) injected around the area of injury. Apply **heat** and compression to assist natural dispersal of the drug. No further treatment should be required and the patient should be managed symptomatically. Subcutaneous hyaluronidase administration is very painful for the patient; therefore, spraying the extravasated area with ethyl chloride before hyaluronidase administration is recommended. If the extravasated area is only small, simply apply a cold compress and elevate. No further treatment should be required.

* See Guidelines for the use of an antidote for an extravasated vesicant drug.

Table 16.26 (Contd.)

Drug	Suggested antidote
Cyclophosphamide Cytarabine	If a large volume has been extravasated, aspirate as much fluid as possible. Dispersal of the extravasated drug can be facilitated by the use of subcutaneous hyaluronidase (1500 units in 1mL of water for injections, or sodium chloride 0.9% solution) injected around the area of injury. Apply **heat** and compression to assist natural dispersal of the drug. No further treatment should be required and the patient should be managed symptomatically. Subcutaneous hyaluronidase administration is very painful for the patient; therefore, spraying the extravasated area with ethyl chloride before hyaluronidase administration is recommended. If the extravasated area is only small, simply apply a cold compress and elevate. No further treatment should be required.
Dacarbazine Dactinomycin Daunorubicin Doxorubicin	Apply DMSO 99% solution topically to extravasated area, every 2h. Once DMSO dries, apply hydrocortisone cream and 30min of **cold compress** every 2h for the first 24 hours. Treatment for the next 14days should consist of topical application of DMSO every 6h, alternating with, applications of topical hydrocortisone cream every 6h, so that a preparation is being applied every 3h, on an alternate basis. If blistering occurs, the DMSO should be stopped and further advice sought[1].
Daunorubicin liposomal Doxorubicin liposomal	Aspirate as much fluid as possible, administer hydrocortisone 100mg throughthe venflon and give subcutaneous hydrocortisone as 0.2mL injections in a 'pin-cushion' fashion around the circumference of the affected area. Apply topical hydrocortisone and cover the area with an **ice pack**. Through the liposomes might offer some protection against the cytotoxic drug, if left untreated, the body degrades the liposomes over a period of 2–3 wks, resulting in a full-blown drug extravasation within a further 7–10 days. Therefore, 8–12h after acute treatment, apply DMSO 99% solutionevery 2h for the next 24h and four times daily thereafter for a further 10–14 days. If blistering occurs, the DMSO should be stopped and further advice sought.
Docetaxel	Infiltrate the area with 1–3mL of a mixture of 100mg hydrocortisone and 4mg chlorphenamine (in 10mL water for injection or sodium chloride 0.9% solution), as 0.2mL 'pin-cushion' subcutaneous injections. (Large volume extravasations might need as much as 10mL.) This should be followed by 1500 units of hyaluronidase (in 1mL water for injection or sodium chloride 0.9% solution) and **warm compression**. Warm compression should be alternated with the application of topical hydrocortisone for the next 3 days. In particularly severe cases, oral antihistamines should be given. Subcutaneous hyaluronidase administration is very painful for the patient; therefore, spraying the extravasated area with ethyl chloride before hyaluronidase administration is recommended.

Table 16.26 (Contd.)

Drug	Suggested antidote
Epirubicin	Apply DMSO 99% solution topically to the extravasated area, every 2h. Once DMSO dries, apply hydrocortisone cream and 30mins of **cold compress** every 2h for the first 24h. Treatment for the next 14 days should consist of topical application of DMSO at every 6h, alternating with applications of topical hydrocortisone cream every 6h, so that preparation is being applied every 3h, on an alternate basis. If blistering occurs, the DMSO should be stopped and further advice sought.
Etoposide	Aspirate as much fluid as possible, administer 100mg hydrocortisone through the venflon and give 100mg subcutaneous hydrocortisone as 0.2mL injections in a 'pin-cushion' fashion around the circumference of the affected area. Apply topical hydrocortisone and cover the area with an **ice pack.**
Etoposide phosphate Fluorouracil	Aspirate as much fluid as possible, administer 100mg hydrocortisone through the venflon and give 100mg subcutaneous hydrocortisone as 0.2mL injections in a 'pin-cushion' fashion around the circumference of the affected area. Apply topical hydrocortisone and cover the area with an **ice pack.** When the initial inflammatory reaction has subsided, the use of a warm compression can aid the dispersal of any residual fluid. There are no specific antidotes for these drugs and further management should be symptomatic.
Floxuridine[*]	Administer sodium bicarbonate 1–2.1% solution to the area to neutralize the acidic drug, followed by **warm compression** to disperse the neutral mixture. This requires that the acid-base titration produces a salt and water, where the neutral salt compound is water-soluble. If the salt is nonsoluble in the aqueous-based environment of extracellular fluid, then precipitation of the insoluble salt will causes further problems or damage. However, if the extravasation has been misdiagnosed, or the volume extravasated has been wrongly assessed, the treatment can lead to an alkaline extravasation. Seek specialist advice.

[*] For large volume extravasations (10mL or more) of drugs with an acidic pH, the administration of either 1% or 2.1% sodium bicarbonate into the area to neutralize the drug, followed by warm compression to disperse the neutral mixture, has been successful. However, this should only be attempted with extreme care as if the extravasation has been misdiagnosed, or the volume extravasated has been wrongly assessed, then the treatment could lead to an alkaline extravasation

[*] See Guidelines for the use of an antidote for an extravasated vesicant drug

Table 16.26 (Contd.)

Drug	Suggested antidote
Fludarabine Gemcitabine	If a large volume has extravasated, aspirate as much fluid as possible. Dispersal of the extravasated drug can be facilitated by the use of subcutaneous hyaluronidase (1500 units in 1mL water for injection, or sodium chloride 0.9% solution) injected around the area of injury. Apply **heat compression** to assist natural dispersal of the drug. No further treatment should be required, and the patient should be managed symptomatically. Subcutaneous hyaluronidase administration is very painful for the patient; therefore, spraying the extravasated area with ethyl chloride before to hyaluronidase administration is recommended.
Idarubicin	Apply DMSO 99% solution topically to the extravasated area, every 2h. Once DMSO dries, apply hydrocortisone cream and 30mins of **cold compress** every 2 hours, for the first 24 hours. Treatment for the next 14 days should consist of topical application of DMSO at every 6h alternating with applications of topical hydrocortisone cream every 6h, so that a preparation is being applied every 3h, on an alternate basis. If blistering occurs, the DMSO should be stopped and further advice sought.
Ifosfamide	If a large volume has been extravasated, aspirate as much fluid as possible. Dispersal of the extravasated drug may be facilitated by the use of subcutaneous **hyaluronidase** (1500 units in 1mL water for injection or sodium chloride 0.9% solution) injected around the area of injury. Apply **heat** and compression to assist natural dispersal of the drug. No further treatment should be required, and the patient should be managed symptomatically. Subcutaneous hyaluronidase administration is very painful for the patient; therefore, spraying the extravasated area with ethyl chloride before hyaluronidase administration is recommended. If the extravasated area is only small, simply apply a cold compress and elevate. No further treatment should be required.
Interferon	If a large volume has been extravasated, aspirate as much fluid as possible. Dispersal of the extravasated drug can be facilitated by the use of subcutaneous hyaluronidase (1500 units in 1mL water for injections, or sodium chloride 0.9% solution) injected around the area of injury. Apply **heat** and compression to assist natural dispersal of the drug. No further treatment should be required, and the patient should be managed symptomatically. Subcutaneous hyaluronidase administration is very painful for the patient; therefore, spraying the extravasated area with ethyl chloride before to hyaluronidase administration is recommended. If the extravasated area is only small, simply apply a cold compress and elevate. No further treatment should be required.

Table 16.26 (Contd.)

Drug	Suggested antidote
Irinotecan*	Aspirate as much fluid as possible, administer 100mg hydrocortisone through the venflon and give 100mg subcutaneous hydrocortisone as 0.2mL injections in a 'pin-cushion' fashion around the circumference of the affected area. Apply topical hydrocortisone and cover the area with an **ice pack.** Irinotecan has an acidic pH; therefore large-volume extravasation (>10mL) might require the administration of sodium bicarbonate 1% or 2.1% solution followed by heat.
Iron dextran (Venofer®)	Flush with a small amount of sodium chloride 0.9% solution to dilute and spread the Venofer®. Apply Hydrocortisone cream 1% topically to the extravasated site three times daily, as long as redness persists. Apply a **cold pack** for 30mins every 2h, for 24h.
Melphalan	If a large volume has been extravasated, aspirate as much fluid as possible. Dispersal of the extravasated drug might be facilitated by the use of subcutaneous hyaluronidase (1500 units in 1mL of water for injections, or sodium chloride 0.9%) injected around the area of injury. Apply **heat** and compression to assist natural dispersal of the drug. No further treatment should be required, and the patient should be managed symptomatically. Subcutaneous hyaluronidase administration is very painful for the patient; therefore, spraying the extravasated area with ethyl chloride before hyaluronidase administration is recommended. If the extravasated area is only small, simply apply a cold compress and elevate. No further treatment should be required.
Methotrexate	Aspirate as much fluid as possible, administer 100mg hydrocortisone through the venflon and give 100mg subcutaneous hydrocortisone as 0.2mL injections in a 'pin-cushion' fashion around the circumference of the affected area. Apply topical hydrocortisone and cover the area with an **ice pack**. When the initial inflammatory reaction has subsided, the use of a warm compression can aid the dispersal of any residual fluid. There are no specific antidotes for these drugs, and further management should be symptomatic.
Mitomycin	Apply DMSO 99% solution topically to the extravasated area, every 2h. Once DMSO dries, apply hydrocortisone cream and 30mins of **cold compress** every 2h for the first 24h. Treatment for the next 14 days should consist of topical application of DMSO every 6h alternating with applications of topical hydrocortisone cream every 6h, so that a preparation is being applied every 3h on an alternate basis. If blistering occurs, the DMSO should be stopped and further advice sought.

Table 16.26 (Contd.)

Drug	Suggested antidote
Mitoxantrone	Aspirate as much fluid as possible, administer 100mg hydrocortisone through the venflon and give 100mg subcutaneous hydrocortisone as 0.2mL injections in a 'pin-cushion' fashion around the circumference of the affected area. Apply topical hydrocortisone and cover the area with an **ice pack**. Apply DMSO 99% solution topically to the affected area four times a daily for 5–7 days (this could be alternated with topical hydrocortisone as described previously). If blistering occurs, the DMSO should be stopped and further advice sought.
Chlormethine (Mustine)★	Infiltrate the area with 1–3mL of sodium thiosulphate 3% solution subcutaneously. Introduce a further 100mg hydrocortisone to the infiltrated area, and apply **cold compression** for 30min every 2 hours, for 12 hours.
Oxaliplatin	Infiltrate with 1500 units of hyaluronidase in 1mL water for injections (do not use saline), and a 500mL bag of dextrose 5% solution plus a further 1500 units of hyaluronidase should be administered subcutaneously in the centre of the extravasation area. The area should then be **warmed** to aid dispersion. The fluid should be left for ≤8 hours or until the 500 mL bag has dispersed. Use with caution in diabetic patients. Note: Avoid sodium chloride—chloride ions will exacerbate the situation.
Paclitaxel	Infiltrate the area with 1–3mL of a mixture of 100mg hydrocortisone and 4mg chlorphenamine in a volume of 10mL, as 0.2mL 'pin-cushion' subcutaneous injections. (Large volume extravasations may need as much as 10mL.) This should be followed by 1500 units of hyaluronidase (in 1mL of water for injections, or sodium chloride 0.9%) and **warm compression**. Warm compression should be alternated with the application of topical hydrocortisone for the next 3 days. In particularly severe cases, oral antihistamines should be given. Subcutaneous hyaluronidase administration is very painful for the patient; therefore, spraying the extravasated area with ethyl chloride before to hyaluronidase administration is recommended.
Pentostatin	If a large volume has been extravasated, aspirate as much fluid as possible. Dispersal of the extravasated drug can be facilitated by the use of subcutaneous hyaluronidase (1500 units in 1mL water for injections, or sodium chloride 0.9% solution) injected around the area of injury. Apply **heat** and compression to assist natural dispersal of the drug. No further treatment should be required, and the patient should be managed symptomatically. Subcutaneous hyaluronidase administration is very painful for the patient; therefore, spraying the extravasated area with ethyl chloride beforer to hyaluronidase administration is recommended. If the extravasated area is only small, simply apply a cold compress and elevate. No further treatment should be required.

★ See Guidelines for the use of an antidote for an extravasated vesicant drug

Table 16.26 (Contd.)

Drug	Suggested antidote
Raltitrexed	Aspirate as much fluid as possible, administer 100mg hydrocortisone through the venflon, and give 100mg subcutaneous hydrocortisone as 0.2mL injections in a 'pin-cushion' fashion around the circumference of the affected area. Apply topical hydrocortisone and cover the area with an **ice** pack. When the initial inflammatory reaction has subsided, the use of a warm compression can aid the dispersal of any residual fluid. There are no specific antidotes for these drugs, and further management should be symptomatic.
Rituximab (MabThera®)	Not considered to be cytotoxic; therefore, not expected to cause necrosis. No specific treatment is considered necessary. Ask the patient to **report** any reactions. Symptomatic management only.
Streptozocin	Apply DMSO 99% solution topically to the extravasated area, every 2h. Once DMSO dries, apply hydrocortisone cream and 30min of **cold compress** every 2 hours, for the first 24h. Treatment for the next 14days should consist of topical application of DMSO every 6h, alternating with applications of topical hydrocortisone cream every6h, so that preparation is being applied every 3h, on an alternate basis. If blistering occurs, the DMSO should be stopped and further advice sought.
Teniposide	Aspirate as much fluid as possible, administer 100mg hydrocortisone through the venflon, and give 100mg subcutaneous hydrocortisone as 0.2mL injections in a 'pin-cushion' fashion around the circumference of the affected area. Apply topical hydrocortisone and cover the area with an **ice pack**.

Thiotepa	If a large volume has been extravasated, aspirate as much fluid as possible. Dispersal of the extravasated drug may be facilitated by the use of subcutaneous hyaluronidase (1500 units in 1mL water for injections, or sodium chloride 0.9%) injected around the area of injury. Apply **heat** and compression to assist natural dispersal of the drug. No further treatment should be required and the patient should be managed symptomatically.
	
	    Subcutaneous hyaluronidase administration is very painful for the patient; therefore, spraying the extravasated area with ethyl chloride before to hyaluronidase administration is recommended.
	
	    If the extravasated area is only small, simply apply a cold compress and elevate. No further treatment should be required.

Table 16.26 (Contd.)

Drug	Suggested antidote
Topotecan[*] Treosulfan[*]	Administer 1–3mL of sodium bicarbonate 1%–2.1% solution to the area in order to neutralize the acidic drug, leave for 2min and then aspirate off again. Followed this with **warm compression** to disperse the neutral mixture. This requires that the acid–base titration produces a salt and water, where the neutral salt compound is water-soluble. If the salt is nonsoluble in the aqueous-based environment of extracellular fluid, then precipitation of the insoluble salt will causes further problems or damage. However, if the extravasation has been misdiagnosed, or the volume extravasated has been wrongly assessed, the treatment can lead to an alkaline extravasation. Seek specialist advice.
Venofer® (Iron dextran)	Flush with a small amount of sodium chloride 0.9% solution to dilute and spread the Venofer®. Apply hydrocortisone 1% cream topically to the extravasated site three times a day, as long as redness persists. Apply **cold pack** for 30min every 2 hours, for 24h.
Vinblastine Vincristine Vindesine Vinorelbine	Infiltrate the area with 1500 units hyaluronidase (in 1mL water for injections or sodium chloride 0.9% solution), as 0.2mL injections subcutaneously (with a 25g needle), over and around the circumference of the affected area. Anaesthetize the skin surface with ethyl chloride spray if the patient cannot tolerate the subcutaneous injections. Apply **heat** and compression for the first 24 hours. For the next 7 days apply a topical NASID cream to the affected area four times a day.

References

Allwood M, Stanley A, Wright P (2002). *The Cytotoxics Handbook*, 4th edn. Abingdon: Radcliffe Medical Press.

Dorr RT (1990). Antidotes to vesicant chemotherapy extravasations. *Blood Reviews*. **4**: 41–60.

Further reading

Bertelli G, Gozza A, Forno MG et al. (1995). Topical dimethylsulfoxide for the prevention of soft tissue injury after extravasation of vesicant cytotoxic drugs: a prospective clinical study. *Journal of Clinical Oncology*, **13**(11): 2851–5.

Rudolph R, Larson DL (1987). Etiology and treatment of chemotherapeutic agent extravasation injuries: a review. *Journal of Clinical Oncology*, **5**: 116–1122.

Boyle D, Engelking C (1995). Vesicant extravasation: myths and realities. *Oncology Nursing Forum* **22**: 57–67.

[*] For large volume extravasations (10mL or more) of drugs with an acidic pH, the administration of either 1% or 2.1% sodium bicarbonate into the area to neutralize the drug, followed by warm compression to disperse the neutral mixture, has been successful. However, this should only be attempted with extreme care as if the extravasation has been misdiagnosed, or the volume extravasated has been wrongly assessed, then the treatment could lead to an alkaline extravasation.

Extravasation of chemotherapy in paediatric patients

Central venous catheters

- The majority of chemotherapy administered to children is given through indwelling central venous catheters.
- It is very unusual for administration of chemotherapy through indwelling central venous catheters to result in any problems with extravasation.
- The very occasional problems that occur with leakage or rupture of indwelling lines must be dealt with on their individual merits, taking account of such factors as the site of the leak, type of drug being administered and volume of drug thought to have been extravasated.

Peripheral catheters

- The same principles and treatment of extravasation apply to paediatric patients as for adult patients.
- During the administration of bolus chemotherapy, very careful attention must be paid to ensure that there is no evidence of extravasation at the time of the injection.
- Administration must be stopped immediately if there is swelling around the site of the cannula. Some patients can experience discomfort during IV injection and, ∴, pain is a less reliable sign of extravasation. Some drugs can induce marked amounts of flare, even when being delivered safely into the vein and, ∴, the presence of flare is not an indication that extravasation is occurring.
- Infusion chemotherapy should be administered using a pressure-monitoring pump, with the pressure limit set as low as possible.
- Antidotes are usually avoided in paediatric extravasations, because some antidotes can cause more damage than the extravasation itself.
- Problems of extravasation are most likely to occur with the administration of vincristine or vinblastine. Extravasations with vincristine or vinblastine should be regarded as an emergency. Should there be an extravasation of either of these two drugs, it is appropriate to call the plastic surgeons so that the site of the extravasation can be extensively irrigated. Arrangements should be made quickly for the patient to be taken to theatre and anaesthetized and the area irrigated.

Further reading

Allwood M, Stanley A, Wright P (2002). *The Cytotoxics Handbook*, 4th edn. Abingdon: Radcliffe Medical Press.

Common toxicity criteria (CTC)

The CTC are a grading scale used for the side effects of chemotherapy drugs. The adverse events are graded from 0 (none) to 4 (severe) for all possible side effects. The CTC are used in cancer clinical trials to ensure uniform capture of toxicity data. The full table of Common Toxicity Criteria is available from the website[1]:

Intrathecal administration of chemotherapy

Background

- Intrathecal chemotherapy is mainly used to treat CNS complications of haematological malignancy.
- The only chemotherapy drugs that can be given intrathecally are cytarabine and methotrexate.
- However, other noncytotoxic drugs can be administered by this route and include bupivicaine, opioids, baclofen, clonidine, gentamicin, hydrocortisone, and vancomycin.

Neurotoxicity of vincristine

Vincristine and the other vinca alkaloids don't pass through the blood–brain barrier; they are always used intravenously. Peripheral neurotoxicity is one of the main side effects, which ↑ in a cumulative fashion with the total dose of treatment. Hence, when vinca alkaloids are inadvertently injected into the cerebrospinal fluid the outcome is normally fatal. Since 1975, 14 people have died in the UK because vincristine was mistakenly given intrathecally—ie as a spinal injection.

Safe practice

- Within the UK, there is a national policy that encompasses a range of standards that hospitals must comply with to enable staff to administer intrathecal chemotherapy[1].
- To prevent inadvertent mix-up with other drugs, intrathecal chemotherapy is segregated from IV chemotherapy. The separate delivery and locations for these drugs help assure that IV drugs are never present in the same location as intrathecal medications.
- To facilitate this, intrathecal medications should only be administered in a designated location, such as an anaesthetic room, at a standard time by competent registered staff. In this way, the pharmacy can release intrathecal medications to the doctor immediately before they are needed.
- Also, at least two health professionals should independently verify the accuracy of all intrathecal doses before administration.

Frequently asked questions

Which drugs are contraindicated for use through the intrathecal route?
Vinca alkaloids, eg vincristine, vinblastine, vinorelbine and vindesine, must never be given by this route. Vincristine is the most commonly used drug of this group.

1 www.dh.gov.uk

Explain the intrathecal route of administration?

Chemotherapy is injected into the area of the lower spine into cerebrospinal fluid. This injection is also termed 'spinal' or subarachnoid. It is mainly indicated when patients show clinical signs that their disease has spread into the CNS. Drugs can also be administered through an Ommaya reservoir, which is discussed below.

Why have people been given the wrong drug intrathecally?

The main problem occurs as a result of inexperienced health profession-als becoming involved in the process. With the result that the drug vincristine (intended solely for the IV route) is administered in error using the intrathecal route. This results in immediate neural damage that normally results in death.

How are intrathecal products to be labelled?

The label on the product states that the drug is intended for intrathecal use only. The product is packaged and transported in a separate container from other IV chemotherapy products and collected by the person who is going to give the drug.

How should vincristine to be labelled?

The label will state 'for IV use only—fatal if given by other routes'. The dose is be diluted to a fixed volume of 20mL for all adults and to a fixed concentration of 0.1mL/mL for paediatric patients. The other vinca alkaloids are also diluted to 20mL for adult patients, but the national policy only specifies the dilution for vincristine when used for paediatric patients.

What range of volumes is administered intrathecally?

Generally, the volume administered varies with the dose, but the typical volume tends to be ~5mL.

Who is allowed to administer intrathecal products?

Only doctors at registrar or consultant level who are registered are allowed to administer chemotherapy products intrathecally. Obviously, anaethetists also administer intrathecal products, but are not allowed to administer cytotoxic chemotherapy unless there are deemed competent and are authorized on the trust's register. Senior hospital officers can only be involved in administration if a risk assessment has been undertaken and a waiver signed by the chief executive that endorses their involvement.

What is an Ommaya reservoir?

It is a small plastic dome-like device with a small tube. The reservoir is placed under the scalp and the tube is placed into the ventricles so that it connects with cerebrospinal fluid. The Ommaya reservoir is permanent, unless there are complications. This device allows certain drugs to be administered into the cerebrospinal fluid and allows cerebrospinal fluid sampling without repeated need of lumbar puncture.

How are intrathecal products administered?

A spinal needle is inserted past the epidural space until the dura is pierced and enters the cerebrospinal fluid, which should flow from the needle. When cerebrospinal fluid appears, care is needed not to alter the position of the spinal needle while the syringe of chemotherapy is being attached. The syringe is attached firmly to the hub of the needle and then injected slowly. When the injection is complete, the needle is removed.

Pertinent points for tasks involving medical staff

Prescribing

Prescription, collection and administration of intrathecal chemotherapy can only be performed by registrars and consultants who are registered after competency assessment. Prescribing should be performed on an approved intrathecal prescription chart.

Collecting

The doctor who is to administer the intrathecal chemotherapy should collect the drug in person by presenting the intrathecal prescription and any other chemotherapy prescriptions for that patient. The doctor must check the drug against the prescription before accepting drug. It must be released only by a pharmacist authorized to do so. The drug should be carried to the patient from pharmacy in a dedicated container.

Administering

Frequently asked questions about administering include the following:

Where can intrathecal chemotherapy be administered?

This must be done only in designated areas.

When can intrathecal chemotherapy be administered?

This can only be done at designated times that have been approved locally, and must be undertaken within normal working hours.

Who checks the intrathecal chemotherapy at the bedside?

This should be done by a staff nurse authorized to perform this task. A final check must always be done by the administering doctor just before injection.

How should intrathecal chemotherapy be administered?

Access to cerebrospinal fluid should be obtained by a standard lumbar puncture procedure to obtain free flow of cerebrospinal fluid. Injection of the chemotherapy must only be performed when the physician is confident that the spinal needle is in the intrathecal space. If assistance from an anaesthetist is required to perform the lumbar puncture, the chemotherapy must only be injected intrathecally by an authorized doctor, as above.

Pertinent points for nursing staff

For nurses to be able to check intrathecal drugs, they have to have taken specific training related to these drugs and must be registered locally after competency assessment.

Pertinent points for pharmacists

Clinically screening prescriptions

Pharmacists must have been assessed as competent and registered to screen chemotherapy. Follow the chemotherapy screening protocol.

Releasing the product to medical staff

Only pharmacists who have been authorized and registered are involved in this process. The doctor who is due to administer the intrathecal product presents the correct prescriptions to an authorized pharmacist who releases the product providing there is documented evidence that any IV chemotherapy intended on the same day has already been administered.

Administration sets

A standard administration set, which does not have a filter chamber is suitable for most IV infusions, except the following:

- Blood and blood products—a blood administration set has an integral filter chamber.
- Platelets—special administration set is usually supplied with platelets.
- Neonates and paediatrics—a burette should be used.

These sets deliver different number of drops/mL.

Rates

- Standard administration set—20 drops/mL.
- Blood administration set—15 drops/mL.
- Burette—60 drops/mL.
- Note: an amiodarone infusion alters the surface tension of the infusion, resulting in a different number of drops/mL.

Changing administration sets

Administration sets should normally be changed every 24h as a precaution on microbiological grounds, although a number of studies have shown that during administration of crystalloid infusions, there isn't an ↑ in infection rates if administration sets are left unchanged for up to 72h. Contamination of infusion fluid during manufacture is extremely rare; however, if drugs are added to infusion fluids at ward level, the risk of microbial contamination is high and sets must be changed every 24h.

However, administration sets should be changed every 24h for the following:

- Parenteral nutrition.
- Blood and blood products.
- Infusions to which drugs have been added.

Calculating flow rates

If an infusion depends on gravity for its flow, there will be a limitation to its rate and accuracy of delivery.

The rate of administration also needs to be calculated, using the following formula:

$$\text{Number of drops/min} = \frac{\text{Quantity to be infused (mL)} \times \text{number. of drops/mL}}{\text{Number of h over which the infusion is to be delivered} \times 60\text{min}}$$

Table 16.27 Cannula sizes

Size (gauge)	Colour	Use	Flow rate mL/min
22Ga	Blue	For small fragile veins	35
20Ga	Pink	For IV drug and fluid administration in patients who have fragile veins	60
18Ga/17Ga	Green/ Yellow	Standard size for IV drug and fluid administration	100
16Ga	Grey	For patients requiring rapid IV fluid replacement	200
14Ga	Brown	Used in theatres for rapid transfusion	350

The number of drops/ml is dependent on the administration set and viscosity of the fluid. If greater safety is required, a burette administration set can be used, particularly if large bolus volumes could be harmful, eg in children or in patients with cardiac failure.

The burette set has a discreet 150–200mL chamber that can be filled from the infusion bag, as necessary, depending on the flow rate. This enables the nurse to ensure that the patient receives no more than the prescribed hourly rate.

Intravenous (IV) administration pumps and other devices

Classification

The Medical Devices Agency (MDA) developed a classification for pumps according to the perceived risk and suitability of a device for a specific clinical purpose, as follows:
• Neonatal—the highest risk category.
• High-risk infusions—infusion of fluids in children, where fluid balance is critical, or the infusion of drugs (eg cardiac inotropes) or cytotoxic drugs, where consistency of flow and accuracy are important.
• Lower-risk infusions—delivery of simple electrolytes, parenteral nutrition and infusional antibiotics.

Neonatal

The required characteristics of neonatal devices are as follows:
• High accuracy.
• Consistency of flow delivery, with very low flow rates.
• Flow rate increments in mL/h.
• Very short occlusion and low-pressure alarm times.
• Very low bolus volume on release of occlusion.

High-risk infusion pumps

The required characteristics of high-risk infusion pumps are as follows:
• High accuracy.
• Consistency of flow delivery.
• Short occlusion and low pressure alarm times.
• Low bolus volume on release of occlusion.

Lower-risk infusion pumps

The required characteristics of lower-risk infusion pumps are as follows:
• Lower accuracy over the long and short terms.
• Less consistent flow.
• Rudimentary alarm and safety features.
• Higher occlusion alarm pressure.
• Poorer overall occlusion alarm response.

IV pumps and syringe drivers are increasingly being used to control infusions in general wards, in addition to specialist clinical areas. Operators have a responsibility to ensure they are fully conversant with any device being used. Training is provided initially by company representatives, although long-term local on-the-job competency training is the usual method employed.

There is a continuously expanding range of infusion devices, which vary slightly in design; however, there are normally a number of common features that operators need to be familiar with and understand the appropriate clinical use of each device.

Most devices require a specific administration set, cassette or syringe. The use of the incorrect type can have a detrimental effect on patient care. If a pump is designed to use a variety of sets or syringes, it normally must be programmed with information regarding the type and size being used.

Devices can be grouped into four main types as follow:

- Infusion devices using a syringe:
  - Syringe infusion pumps.
  - Syringe drivers.
  - Anaesthetic pumps.
  - Patient-controlled analgesia pumps.
- Infusion devices using gravity controllers:
  - Drip-rate controllers.
  - Volumetric controllers.
- Infusion pumps:
  - Drip-rate pumps.
  - Volumetric pumps.
  - Patient-controlled analgesia pumps.
- Ambulatory pumps:
  - Continuous infusion.
  - Multimodality pumps.
  - Patient-controlled analgesia pumps.

Syringe infusion pumps:

These are devices in which a syringe containing fluid or a drug in solution is fitted into the pump and the plunger of the syringe is driven forwards at a predetermined rate. These pumps are usually set to run at mL/h.

Application

Designed for the accurate delivery of fluids at low flow rates. Syringe pumps are ∴, ideally selected for the safe infusion of fluids and drugs to neonates or children and drugs to adults. Often used in anaesthesia and critical care areas; commonly used for the administration of patient-controlled analgesia.

Gravity controllers

Electronic devices that achieve the desired infusion rate on the principle of restricting flow through the administration set by an infusion force that is dependant on gravity (drip-rate control) or by way of a dedicated rate-controlling administration set.

Application

Suitable for most low-risk infusions such as IV fluids (eg sodium chloride or dextrose 5% solutions). Not recommended for TPN.

Volumetric pumps

Application

Preferred for larger flow rates. They usually weigh between 3kg and 5kg, and are designed to be 'stationary'. Volumetric pumps have the facility to work off mains power or a battery. The infusion rate is set using mL/h and most devices can be programmed to between 1mL/h and 1000mL/h, although if used at rates <5mL/h, accuracy might ↓. Most pumps use a linear peristaltic pumping action.

Can often programme the pump to stop infusing after a set volume, useful if have to give a proportion of an infusion bottle or bag.

Ambulatory pumps

Small portable devices

They can use a small syringe but most use a reservoir bag of 100–250mL. Pumps are preprogrammable.

Implanted pumps

Implanted pumps have been developed for those ambulatory patients who need long-term low-volume therapy. These pumps are small and are implanted subcutaneously. The drug is then infused through an internal catheter into a vein, an artery or an area of dedicated tissue.

Disposable pumps

Nonelectronic devices; generally, very lightweight and small. Usually very 'user-friendly', requiring the minimum of input from the patient. They do not require a battery.

Disposable pumps work on a variety of principles:

- An elastomeric balloon, which is situated inside a plastic cylinder. When the balloon is filled with the infusion fluid, the resulting hydrostatic pressure inside the balloon is enough to power the infusion. The drug is infused through a small-bore administration set, which usually has a rate restrictor at the patient end.
- Sidekick that exerts mechanical pressure from a spring-loaded device.
- Smartdose works by generation of CO_3 in the space between rigid plastic outer and infusion bag.

Management of flow control devices

Any technical equipment will only function optimally if maintained appropriately, and standardized because devices are often moved with patients through various wards and departments. Care should be taken to comply with the manufacturer's instructions regarding storage of their product.

Guidelines for the treatment of hypomagnesaemia

The normal range of magnesium is 0.7–1.0mmol/L.

Preparations for replacement

- Magnesium glycerophosphate tabs (4mmol)
- Magnesium hydroxide mixture (14mmol/10mL)
- Magnesium sulphate 50% solution 5g in 10mL (20mmol/10mL).

Mild hypomagnesaemia (0.5–0.7mmol/L) or asymptomatic patients

- Magnesium glycerophosphate tablets (4mmol), one or two tablets three to four times daily. Unlicensed, but shows greatest absorption and least side effects (diarrhoea).
- Magnesium hydroxide mixture (14mmol/10mL), 5–10mL three to four times daily.
- Dosing can be increased up to 50mmol orally, but can be limited by side effects.

Moderate–severe hypomagnesaemia (<0.5mmol/L) or symptomatic patients

Magnesium sulphate injection of 10–20mmol (2.5–5g) in 1L normal saline over 12h daily until serum magnesium is within normal range.
The volume of fluid is not critical but consider the following:

- The maximum peripheral concentration is 20% (20mmol in 25mL) because the injection has a very high osmolality.
- The maximum rate is 150mg/min (20mmol over a period of 40mins).

Magnesium sulphate is compatible with sodium chloride 0.9% solution, dextrose 5% solution and sodium chloride/dextrose solution.

Monitoring

Magnesium levels for symptomatic patients should be checked daily until corrected; note that plasma levels might be artificially high while magnesium equilibrates with the intracellular compartment. However, if toxicity is suspected treatment should be discontinued.

Treatment guidelines for hypophosphataemia

The normal range of phosphate is 0.8–1.45mmol/L.

Preparations for IV replacement;

Because of current acquisition costs and the need to restrict IV K^+ additions to bags at ward level, the following are ranked in preference order:

- First choice: disodium hydrogen phosphate (Na_2HPO_4) 21.49% solution.
  - 6mmol phosphate in 10mL (9mmol phosphate in 15mL).
  - 12mmol sodium in 10mL.
- Second choice: potassium phosphate 17.42% solution.
  - 5mmol phosphate in 5mL (9mmol phosphate in 9mL).
  - 10mmol K^+ in 5mL.
- Third choice: Addiphos®
  - 40mmol phosphate in 20mL.
  - 30mmol K^+ in 20mL.
  - 30mmol sodium in 20mL.

Doses (expressed as phosphate ions)

Standard dose–phosphate level 0.3–0.79mmol/L

- A peripheral infusion of 12mmol of phosphate in 250–500mL sodium chloride 0.9% solution over 12h. Ensure the bag is shaken well. Repeat, as necessary, after checking plasma phosphate level.
- If the patient has a central line, 12mmol of phosphate can be given in 50mL of sodium chloride 0.9% solution and administered over 4h.

High dose–phosphate level <0.3mmol/L (Ideally for use in critical areas only)

- An infusion of 24mmol phosphate diluted to 50mL with sodium chloride 0.9% solution administered through a central line using a syringe driver over 4h.
- Potassium phosphate 17.42% solution–use only if the patient is hypernatraemic (>150mmol/L) or hypokalaemic (<3.5mmol/L)
- An infusion of 20mmol phosphate diluted to 50mL with sodium chloride 0.9% solution through a central line using a syringe driver over 4h.
- If the patient has only peripheral access, dilute in 500mL sodium chloride 0.9% solution and administer over 12h.

Re-feeding syndrome–phosphate level <0.3mmol/L

- Re-feeding syndrome manifests on introduction of nutrition in malnourished patients, which results in abnormal distribution shifts intracellularly of phosphate and magnesium as a consequence of the action of endogenous insulin.
- One vial of Addiphos®, (20mL), containing 40mmol phosphate in 500mL dextrose 5% solution, administered over 6h. Ensure the bag is shaken well. (Note that vial also contains 30mmol of K^+, so ensure serum K^+ level is checked and within range before treatment.)

Monitor

The frequency of serum phosphate monitoring depends on the severity of the hypophosphataemia but should probably be determined at the end of the infusion.

Monitor sodium/K^+ concurrently if administering repeated infusions (depending on the salt used) to avoid hypernatremia/hyperkalaemia.

Side effects

- Hyperphosphataemia, hypotension with rapid infusion, hypocalcaemia with large doses or run accidentally at accelerated rate.
- Hypernatremia/hyperkalaemia, depending on the salt used.

Preparations for oral supplementation

Phosphate Sandoz tablets contain 16.1mmol phosphate per tablet in addition to 20mmol sodium and 3mmol K^+.

The usual dose is two tablets twice or three times daily.

Side effects

Oral supplementation (Phosphate tablets) can cause diarrhoea, so ensure adequate fluid intake at the time of administration.

Renal impairment

Hypophosphataemia is unlikely in patients with chronic renal failure; doses of IV and oral phosphate might need to be reduced in renal impairment. Patients receiving haemofiltration are likely to have hyper-phosphataemia and ∴, phosphate therapy should be avoided.

Parenteral potassium

- In July 2002, the National Patient Safety Agency (NPSA) in the UK issued a patient safety alert to prevent further fatalities following accidental overdose with IV potassium chloride concentrate that had been misidentified for sodium chloride 0.9% solution and water for injections.
- The risks associated with IV potassium chloride are well known. Potassium chloride, if injected too rapidly or in too high a dose, can cause cardiac arrest within minutes. The effect of hyperkalaemia on the heart is complex—virtually any arrhythmia could be observed.
- The true incidence of K^+ related fatalities and incidents is unknown.
- The alert identified safe-medication-ractice recommendations concerning the prescribing, distribution, storage and preparation of potassium chloride solutions in hospitals.
- The NPSA recommended withdrawal of concentrated potassium solutions from ward stock to be replaced by ready-to-use infusion products.
- The NPSA recommended that new control arrangements be introduced in critical-care areas continuing to use potassium chloride concentrate ampoules.
- Although ↓ the risk to patients, it did result in a number of initial consequences, as follows
  - Treatment delay as a result of new control arrangements and uncertainty about the correct process.
  - Range of ready-to-use K^+ infusions not sufficiently comprehensive for the number of clinical indications required.
  - ↑ cost.
  - Requirement of training and competency assessment for safe use of IV K^+.
- Although recommendations have ↓ the risk to patients, staff still need to be vigilant to minimize and prevent harm to patients from incompetent/dangerous practice.

Minimizing risk: points pharmacists should encourage

K^+ containing fluids (see Table 16.28)

- Labelling: the labelling format used differs between different manufacturers; the font size of K^+ details should be ↑ to improve identification. Historically, there has been a reliance on specifying the K^+ concentration as a percentage on products as the primary focus rather than mmol/volume, which should become main emphasis in the future.
- Storage: decanting from boxes should be discouraged, although most ward areas have limited storage space it is GCP to segregate K^+-containing bags from other infusion fluids.
- Range of infusions.

Table 16.28 K^+ containing IV fluids

Approved name	Manufacturer	Bag price	Notes
Potassium chloride 0.15%, glucose 2.5%, sodium chloride 0.45% (500mL)	Baxter	£5.30	Discontinued recently
Potassium chloride 0.15%, glucose 10% (500ml)	Baxter	£4.58	10mmol in 500mL
Potassium chloride 0.15%, glucose 10% sodium chloride 0.18% (500mL)	IVEX	£3.55	10mmol in 500mL
Potassium chloride 0.15%, glucose 2.5%, sodium chloride 0.45% (1000mL)	Fresenius Kabi		20mmol in 1L
Potassium chloride 0.15%, glucose 4% sodium chloride 0.18% (1000mL)	Fresenius Kabi	£0.82	20mmol in 1L
Potassium chloride 0.15%, glucose 4%, sodium chloride 0.18% (500mL)	Fresenius Kabi	£0.77	10mmol in 500mL
Potassium chloride 0.15%, glucose 4%, sodium chloride 0.45% (500mL)	IVEX	£2.47	10mmol in 500mL
Potassium chloride 0.15%, glucose 5% (1000mL)	Fresenius Kabi	£0.79	20mmol in 1L
Potassium chloride 0.15%, sodium chloride 0.9% (1000mL)	Fresenius Kabi	£0.81	20mmol in 1L
Potassium chloride 0.15%, sodium chloride 0.9% (500mL)	Fresenius Kabi	£0.68	10mmol in 500mL
Potassium chloride 0.3%, glucose 4%, sodium chloride 0.18% (1000mL)	Fresenius Kabi	£0.79	40mmol in 1L
Potassium chloride 0.3%, glucose 4%, sodium chloride 0.18% (500mL)	Fresenius Kabi	£0.68	20mmol in 500mL

Table 16.28 (*Contd.*)

Approved name	Manufacturer	Bag price	Notes
Potassium chloride 0.3%, glucose 5%, sodium chloride 0.45% (500mL)	Fresenius Kabi	£2.95	20mmol in 500mL
Potassium chloride 0.3%, glucose 5% (1000mL)	Fresenius Kabi	£0.82	40mmol in 1L
Potassium chloride 0.3%, sodium chloride 0.9% (1000mL)	Fresenius Kabi	£0.82	40mmol in 1L
Potassium chloride 0.3%, sodium chloride 0.9% (500mL)	Fresenius Kabi	£0.68	20mmol in 500mL
Potassium chloride 0.45%, sodium chloride 0.9% (1000mL)	Baxter	£3.65	60mmol in 1L
Potassium chloride 0.6%, sodium chloride 0.9% (500mL)	Baxter	£2.94	40mmol in 500mL
Potassium chloride 0.6%, sodium chloride 0.9% (1000mL)	Baxter	£3.70	80mmol in 1L
Potassium chloride 3%, sodium chloride 0.9% (100mL)	Baxter	£1.76	40mmol in 100mL

* Prices listed as guide only. Cost will vary locally

The NPSA recommended the manufacture of five new products to ↓ reliance on ampoules. Pharmacy departments should provide a formulary of all K^+ containing solutions held locally to promote better information to doctors and nurses.
• Staff competency needs to be established for IV fluid administration.

Concentrated K^+ containing products
Critical areas, high-dependency areas and, cardiac theatres that are allowed to locally store ampoules of potassium chloride should have a risk assessment performed periodically to overview the prescribing, ordering, storage and administration processes. However, other areas, such as general theatres, should not have access to concentrated ampoules of K^+.
Training development—the process from prescribing through to administration needs to be mapped and used as a backbone to develop multi-disciplinary training.

Developing policies to support prescribing and administration
For example, policy on the use of IV K^+ within theatres.
- All prescribing of K^+ must be expressed in terms of millimoles of K^+ and must include the rate of infusion and whether it is to be administered peripherally or centrally.
- Ampoules of K^+-containing solutions will not be stocked within theatres.
  - A local range of K^+ containing fluids available should be displayed within the department.
- All K^+ containing infusions must be administered through a suitable infusion pump, to control the infusion rate and volume.
- All patients treated with IV K^+ are to have had a recent measurement of serum K^+ level undertaken before administration commences (Table 16.29).

Table 16.29 Treatment of hypokaleamia

Serum potassium level (mmol/L)	Degree of hypokalaemia	Treatment
3.5–5.0 (normal)	Prophylaxis against hypokalaemia	20mmol in 1L of sodium chloride 0.9% solution or dextrose 5% solution administered peripherally (or centrally) over at least 8h, as part of a normal fluids regimen.
3.0–3.4	Mild or nonurgent hypokalaemia	40mmol in 1L of sodium chloride 0.9% solution or dextrose 5% solution administered peripherally (or centrally) over at least 6h
<3.0	Severe or very urgent hypokalaemia	40mmol in 500mL sodium chloride 0.9% solution or dextrose 5% solution administered peripherally (or centrally) over at least 4h or over at least 2h through a central line with continuous ECG monitoring of heart rate and rhythm

Guidelines for the treatment of hypocalcaemia

- The normal range of total calcium 2.15–2.60mmol/L.
- The normal range of ionized calcium 1.1–1.4mmol/L.
- The most common cause of low total serum calcium is hypoalbuminaemia; ∴, it is important to measure ionized calcium or correct the total serum calcium.

Preparations for replacement

- Calcium gluconate 10% (0.1g/mL). Injection contains 0.22mmol/mL of calcium.
- Calcium chloride 14.7% (0.147g/mL). Injection contains 1mmol/mL of calcium.

Calcium solutions (especially calcium chloride) are irritants and care should be taken to prevent extravasation.

Dilution

A calcium gluconate 10% injection can be given neat or diluted in glucose 5% solution or sodium chloride 0.9% solution.

A calcium chloride 14.7% solution should ideally be diluted in at least twice its volume of glucose 5% solution or sodium chloride 0.9% solution for peripheral administration. Calcium chloride can be given neat by central line administration only.

Emergency elevation of serum calcium in symptomatic patients

- Give 2.25mmol IV stat over 10min
- Equate either of to the following:
  - 10mL of calcium gluconate 10% solution.
  - 2.25mL of calcium chloride 14.7% solution.

Hyperkalaemia and disturbance of ECG function

- 2.25–4.5mmol of calcium over 10–20min, depending on dose (up to a maximum rate of 0.2mmol/min).
- Equate to either of the following:
- 2–4mL of calcium chloride 14.7% injection.
- 10–20mls of calcium gluconate 10% injection.
- Titrate dose according to ECG.

Monitoring

For symptomatic patients calcium and albumin levels should be checked daily until corrected; serum phosphate and magnesium levels should be monitored periodically.

Suggested dosing in asymptomatic hypocalcaemic patients

IV infusion to give 9mmol/daily, which might need to be repeated at intervals of 1–3 days, as follows:

- 40mL of calcium gluconate 10% injection over 4h can be given neat or diluted in glucose 5% solution or sodium chloride 0.9% solution.
- 9mL of calcium chloride 14.7% injection over 4h diluted in 100mls of glucose 5% solution or sodium chloride 0.9% solution.

If the patient is absorbing oral medication, consider the use of soluble calcium tablets in divided doses.

Prescribing IV fluids

The aim of fluid therapy is to facilitate the patient's recovery by maintaining the following.
- Blood volume.
- Fluid and electrolyte balance.
- Renal function.

Three phases that need to be considered when planning a suitable fluid regimen are as follows.
- Maintenance.
- Correction of pre existing dehydration.
- Abnormal losses—eg fluid management of the surgical patient.

Fluids for maintenance
- A patient who is unable to take fluid by mouth needs a basic IV regimen. In temperate climates, this is $1.5L/m^2$ surface area of fluid or 30–40mL/kg body in 24h.
- Basic electrolyte requirements are sodium, 1mmol/kg body weight/day, potassium, 1mmol/kg body weight/day.
- The patient can manage with lower sodium intakes because of efficient conservation processes; however, if there are obligatory losses of K^+ and insufficient replacement, patients become K^+ depleted.
- Remember that febrile patients will have ↑ insensible losses.

Correction of existing dehydration
- Need to identify the compartment(s) from which the fluid has been lost and the extent of the losses.
- Check fluid charts, and any note loss from drains or catheters.
- Most body fluids contain salt, but in lower levels than plasma, and thus replacement requires a mixture of sodium chloride and glucose.

Table 16.30 Composition of gastrointestinal body fluid

	Volume (L/24h)	Na^+ (mmol/L)	K^+ (mmol/L)	Cl^- (mmol/L)	HCO_3^- (mmol/L)	pH
Saliva	0.5–1.5	20–80	10–20	20–40	20–60	7–8
Gastric juice	1.0–2.0	20–100	5–10	120–160	0	1–7
Bile	0.5–1.0	150–250	5–10	40–120	20–40	7–8
Pancreatic juice	1.0–2.0	120–250	5–10	10–60	80–120	7–8

- Clinical history and examination are vital but can be assisted by the measurement of changes in electrolytes, PCV and plasma proteins.
- Patients with heart failure are at greater risk of pulmonary oedema if overhydrated. They also are unable to tolerate ↑ salt load because sodium retention accompanies heart failure.

- Patients with liver failure, despite being oedematous and often hyponatraemic, have ↑ total body sodium; ∴ sodium chloride is best avoided in fluid regimens.

Abnormal losses: fluid management of the surgical patient

Planning an IV fluid therapy regimen:
- Ensure adequate preoperative hydration.
- Minimize insensible losses during surgery.
  - Humidify inspired gases, minimise sweating by ensuring adequate anaesthesia and, cover the patient where possible to ensure adequate ambient temperature.
- Replace losses, such as blood loss.

Preoperative considerations

For routine elective surgery, the patient is kept NBM for 6–12h and takes little oral fluid for 6h postoperatively. A fluid deficit of 1000–1500mL arises but this will be quickly corrected when the patient is drinking normally. IV fluid therapy is not required for many routine operations in adults, providing the patient isn't dehydrated. IV therapy is indicated preoperatively if the patient is likely to be NBM for >8h. Anaesthetists might set up an IV infusion of Hartmann's solution just before induction. On return to the surgical ward, this should be switched to sodium chloride or dextrose as required, because as there no evidence that further treatment with Hartmann's solution has a clinical benefit compared other crystalloids.

Perioperative considerations and blood loss

Operative blood loss of up to 500mL can be replaced with crystalloid solution (remembering that four times as much crystalloid solution will be needed).
Using the following replacement fluids for blood loss:
- <500mL: use crystalloid solution.
- 500–1000mL: use colloid solution.
- >1000mL or haemegiobin<10gdL: use whole blood.

Other replacement fluid is more appropriate if there is excess fluid loss from a specific compartment.

Hartmann's solution causes the least disturbance to plasma electrolyte concentrations and avoids postoperative fluid depletion. An allowance of 1mL/kg body weight /h should be begin at the start of anaesthesia intraoperatively to replace essential losses intraoperatively.

Postoperative considerations

- Normal fluid requirement is 2–3L/24h.
- Electrolyte requirements: sodium 2mmol/kg body weight K⁺ 1mmol/kg body weight.
- Low urine output (night after surgery) is almost always results from inadequate fluid replacement, but might be consequence of the anaesthetic technique. (K⁺ is not normally administered during the first 24h in such patients.) Check JVP/CVP for signs of cardiac failure and consider fluid challenge, if appropriate.
- Check operation notes for extent of bleeding in theatre.

- Losses from gut–replace NGT aspirate volume with sodium chloride 0.9% solution.
- Losses from surgical drains–replace significant losses.

However, calculate (24h) total fluid loss as follows:
- Estimate skin and lung loss = (10 × body weight) mL.
- Estimation of stool losses = 50mL.
- Estimation of urine losses, normally measured directly.
- Drain loss/NGT loss.

Design a fluid regimen
- Calculate fluid losses and replace them (as above).
- Calculate sodium and K^+ requirements.
  - Measure plasma U&Es if patient is ill.
- Start oral fluids as soon as possible.

For example, a fluid regimen for 60kg patient would be as follow:
- Fluid losses:
  - Patient urine output 1500mL.
  - Fluid losses = (10 × 60)+1500 + 50mL = 2150mL.
  - NGT loss = 1000mL.
- Sodium requirement = 2 × 60 = 120mmol.
- K^+ requirement = 1 × 60 = 60mmol.
- Volume of sodium chloride 0.9% solution that will provide sodium requirement = 1000mL (154mmol sodium).
- Amount of K^+ required = 60mmoL
- Remember that dextrose 5% solution can be considered as isotonic water and will be used to make up the difference for the patient's fluid requirement.
- NGT replacement = 1000mL sodium chloride 0.9% solution.
- Hence, a suitable 24h regimen for a 60kg patient with 1.5L urinary output and 1L NGT losses would be as follow:
  - 2 × 1000mL sodium chloride 0.9% solution + 20mmol potassium chloride.
  - 1000mL dextrose 5% solution + 20mmoL potassium chloride.
  - Each bag runs for a period of 8h.
- Start oral fluids as soon as reasonable, depending on the patient's condition/indication for surgery.

Special conditions that need more specialist fluid knowledge
- Haemorrhagic/hypovolaemic shock.
- Septic shock.
- Heart or liver impairment.
- Excessive vomiting.

Fluid balance

During a lifetime, the water content and fluid compartments within the body alter. In infants fluid content represents 70–80% of their body weight; this progressively ↓, reaching 60% of body weight at 2yrs. In adults, the content accounts for 60% of the body weight in ♂ and 55% in ♀, and the ratio of extracellular fluid (ECF) to intracellular fluid (ICF) is 1:3.

For example, the fluid content of a 70kg is as follows:
- Total fluid = 42L.
- Intracellular fluid (ICF)–67% of body water = 28L.
- Extravascular space (ECF)–33% of body water = 14L. (25% intravascular space = 3.5L 75% interstitium = 10.5L).

Compartment barriers

- The fluid compartments are separated from one another by semi-permeable membranes through which water and solutes can pass. The composition of each fluid compartment is maintained by selectivity of its membrane.
- The barrier between plasma and the interstitium is the capillary endothelium, which allows free passage of water and electrolytes but not large molecules, such as proteins.
- The barrier between the ECF and the ICF is the cell membrane.

Transport mechanisms

- Simple diffusion: movement of solutes down concentration gradients.
- Facilitated diffusion: again depends on concentration gradient differences, but also relies on the availability of carrier substances.
- Osmosis: movement of solvent through semipermeable membranes.
- Active transport: eg sodium/k$^+$ exchange pump.

Osmolality

- Osmotic pressure is generated by colloids impermeable to the membrane.
- Water distributes across in either direction if there is a difference in osmolality across the membrane.
- Osmolarity is the number of osmoles/L of solution.
- Osmolality is the number of osmoles/kg of solvent or solution.
- Osmolality of blood is 285–295mOsm/L.

Tonicity

Molecules that affect the movement of water eg sodium and glucose, are called 'effective osmoles', which contribute to compartments osmolality (sometimes referred to or termed 'tonicity'). The normal range of serum osmolality is 285–295mOsm/L. The measured osmolality should not exceed the predicted value by >10mOsm/L. A difference of > 10mOsm/L is considered an osmolal gap. Causes for a serum osmolal gap include mannitol, ethanol, methanol, ethylene glycol and other toxins in very high concentration, usually small molecules. (The propylene glycol in lorazepam can cause hyperosmolarity and hyperosmolar coma in some patients, particularly when the lorazepam is used as a continuous infusion.)

Serum osmolality is calculated as follows: 2 x (sodium + K$^+$) + glucose/18 + BUN/2.8

Units for equation
- Sodium and K$^+$–mmol/L.
- Glucose and BUN–mg/dL. For glucose conversion from mmol, divide by a factor of 0.05551 For BUN conversion from mmol, divide by a factor of 0.3569.

Knowledge of fluid distribution
- Dextrose 5% solution distributes through the ECF with a resultant fall in ECF osmolality, 'water distributes into the cells and as such dextrose 5% solution distributes throughout the body water.
- Conversely, a person marooned on a life raft with no water loses water from all compartments.
- Sodium chloride 0.9% solution contains 154mmol/L of sodium with an osmolality of 300mOmol/L. When infused, most of the solution stay in the ECF, which is of a similar osmolality.
- Conversely, losing water and electrolytes together (eg severe diarrhoea) loses fluid mainly from the ECF.
- With ECF losses, sodium and water are lost together, so the sodium concentration in the remaining ECF does not change.
- However, protein and red cells are not lost so their concentration rises.
- If plasma alone is lost, only PCV rises.
- Extra fluid for continuing losses should, of course, resemble as closely as possible the fluid that has been lost.

Table 16.31 Fluid balance–average daily water balance

Input (mL of water)	Output (mL of water)
Drink: 1500	Urine: 1500
In food: 800	Insensible losses (lungs and skin): 800
Metabolism of food: 200	Stool: 200
Total: 2500	Total: 2500

The body is normally in positive water balance, with the kidney adjusting for varying intakes and losses by altering water clearance. The kidney requires 500mL of water to excrete the average daily load of osmotically active waste products at maximal urinary concentration.

Table 16.32 Composition of replacement fluids

Fluid type	Osmolality mosmol/kg	Na⁺ (mmol/L)	K⁺ (mmol/L)	Ca²⁺ (mmol/L)	HCO₃⁻ (mmol/L)	Glucose (mmol/L)	pH
Sodium lactate solution (Hartmann's)	280	130	5	2	29	0	6.5
0.18% sodium chloride	61	30	0	0	0	0	5.9
0.45% sodium chloride	154	77	0	0	0	0	5.2
0.9% sodium chloride	308	150	0	0	0	0	5.5
1.8% sodium chloride	616	308	0	0	0	0	5.9
0.18% sodium chloride + 4% dextrose	300	30	0	0	0	40	4.5
0.45% sodium chloride + 5% dextrose	406	77	20	0	0	50	4.8
5% dextrose	278	0	0	0	0	50	5.6
10% dextrose	505	0	0	0	0	100	5.6
20% dextrose	1250	0	0	0	0	200	5.6

Practical issues concerning parenteral nutrition

The identification and selection of patients who require parenteral nutrition, and the subsequent provision and monitoring of this treatment, consists of a number of overlapping phases.

If there is concern with regard to a patient's nutrition they should have been referred to the ward dietician for a full assessment.

Initiation of parenteral nutrition

Once referred to the nutrition support team, the patient will be formally assessed, and if it is felt appropriate, line access will be planned. For short term parenteral nutrition (7–10 days), this will usually be a peripherally inserted venous catheter (PICC), and a tunnelled central line will be used if the anticipated duration of parenteral nutrition is longer or peripheral access is limited.

Before to initiating parenteral nutrition , baseline biochemistry should be checked (Table 16.33) and fluid and electrolyte abnormalities corrected. In those at risk of developing re-feeding syndrome, additional IV vitamins might be required.

Early monitoring phase

During the first week of parenteral nutrition (and subsequently if the patient is 'unstable' with respect to fluid and electrolyte or metabolic issues) the patient is monitored intensively. This consists of a minimum set of mandatory ward observations, and appropriate blood and other laboratory tests. The aim is to optimize nutritional support, while remaining aware of the other therapeutic strategies in the patient's overall care plan.

It might be necessary to modify either nutritional support or the overall patient care plan to obtain the best patient outcomes.

Stable patient phase

After the patient is stabilized on parenteral nutrition a less intensive monitoring process is required.

Reintroduction of diet

At a certain point, diet or enteral feed is usually introduced in a transitional manner. Liaison with the ward dietician is essential and, if appropriate, reduction or cessation of parenteral nutrition is recommended.

Cessation of parenteral nutrition

Parenteral nutrition is usually stopped when oral nutritional intake is deemed adequate for the individual patient. As a general rule of thumb, cessation of parenteral nutrition is determined on a variety of factors and is a multidisciplinary decision.

IV access

Peripheral cannulae (Venflons) should not routinely be used for the administration of parenteral nutrition and should only be used in the short term for the administration of 'peripheral formulated' parenteral nutrition.

PICC lines are usually used for medium then to long-term venous access (2–6 months).

Tunnelled, cuffed central venous catheters (CVs) are inserted via the subclavian (or jugular) vein for long term feeding.

A dedicated single-lumen line is the safest route for parenteral nutrition administration. There is a greater risk of infection the more times a line is manipulated. Obviously, aseptic technique should be used. Nothing else should be given through this lumen, nor should blood be sampled from the line under normal circumstances (it might be appropriate for blood sampling in patients receiving parenteral nutrition at home).

If a multilumen line must be used for clinical reasons; one lumen should be dedicated for parenteral nutrition use only. Again, ideally, nothing else should be given through this lumen, nor should blood be sampled from it.

Prescribing parenteral nutrition

Patients' nutritional requirements are based on standard dietetic equations. A regimen close to a patient's requirements should be provided in a formulation prepared to minimize risk.

Nitrogen

Protein in parenteral nutrition is provided in the form of amino acids. Individual nitrogen requirements are calculated.

Carbohydrate and lipid

The energy in parenteral nutrition is generally described as nonprotein calories (ie the figure excludes the energy provided from amino acids).

Total energy intake is best given as a mixture of glucose and lipid, usually in a ratio of 60:40. This might be varied if clinically important glucose intolerance develops or if there is a requirement for a lipid-free parenteral nutrition bag.

Volume

The overall aim is to provide all fluid volume requirements through parenteral nutrition, including losses from wounds, drains, stomas and fistulae etc. However, if these losses are large or highly variable, they should be replaced and managed separately.

Electrolytes

These are modified according to clinical requirements, and with particular regard to extrarenal losses.

Electrolytes should be reviewed daily and modified as necessary. Monitoring of urinary electrolyte losses is useful.

Vitamins, minerals and trace elements

These are added routinely on a daily basis. Extra zinc or selenium might be required in patients with large GI losses. Patients on long-term parenteral nutrition will have routine micronutrient screening undertaken (Table 16.33).

Other medications

No drug additions should be made to the parenteral nutrition on grounds of stability, unless stability work is undertaken; certain drug additions are known to lead to incompatibility, eg heparin.

Recommended monitoring/care

- Daily weight (before starting parenteral nutrition and daily thereafter).
- Take temperature and BP reading every 4–6h. (Also observe for clinical evidence of infection, and general well-being.)
- Accurate fluid-balance chart and summary (to maintain accurate fluid balance and homeostasis). Bag change should be undertaken at same time of day.
- Capillary glucose monitoring (BMs) 6h during the first 24h, then twice or once daily stable (generally, the glucose target should be 4–10mmols/L). Return to BMs every 6h on when parenteral nutrition being weaned off.
- Daily assessment for CVC/PICC site infection or leakage.
  change dressing for CVs at least every 72h and more frequent if loose, soiled or wet. Change PICC dressings weekly.
- 24h urine collections for nitrogen balance and electrolytes should be undertaken according to local practice.

Storage of parenteral nutrition on ward

Bags not yet connected to the patient must be stored in a refrigerator (at between 2°C and 8°C). Bags stored in a drug refrigerator must be kept away from any freezer compartment to prevent ice crystal formation in the parenteral nutrition.

Bags that have been refrigerated should be removed at least 1–2h before being hung and infused, to enable the solution to reach room temperature. Bags connected to the patient should be protected from light using protective covers.

Table 16.33 Suggested monitoring guide (please refer to local guidelines)

	Baseline	New patient or unstabe	Stable patient
Blood biochemistry			
Urea and creatinine	Yes	Daily	Three times weekly
sodium	Yes	Daily	Three times weekly
K$^+$	Yes	Daily	Three times weekly
Bicarbonate	Yes	Daily	Three times weekly
Chloride	Yes	Daily	Three times weekly
LFTs: bilirubin	Yes	Daily	Three times weekly
Alk phos	Yes	Daily	Three times weekly
AST or ALT	Yes	Daily	Three times weekly
Albumin	Yes	Daily	Three times weekly
Calcium	Yes	Daily	Three times weekly
Magnesium	Yes	Daily	Three times weekly
Phosphate	Yes	Daily	Three times weekly
Zinc	Yes	Weekly	Every 2 weeks
Copper	Yes	Monthly	Every 3 months
CRP	Yes	Three times weekly	Three times weekly
Full blood count	Yes	Three times weekly	Weekly
Coagulation			
APTT	Yes	Weekly	Weekly
INR	Yes	Weekly	Weekly
Lipids			
Cholesterol	Yes	Weekly	Weekly
Triglycerides	Yes	Weekly	Weekly

Nutritional support in adults

Parenteral support

Poor nutritional status is a major determinant of a patient's morbidity (as a consequence of depressed cell-mediated immunity and wound healing) and mortality.

The decision to provide nutritional support must be as a result of a thorough clinical assessment of the patient's condition. Parenteral nutritional support should be for patients who are malnourished or likely to become so, and in whom the gastrointestinal tract is not sufficiently functional to meet nutritional needs or is inaccessible.

Appropriate indications for parenteral nutrition

- Short bowel syndrome.
- GI fistulae.
- Prolonged paralytic ileus.
- Acute pancreatitis if jejunal feeding is contraindicated.
- Multiple injuries involving the viscera.
- Major sepsis.
- Severe burns.
- Inflammatory bowel disease.
- Malnourished patients in whom the use of the intestine is not anticipated for >7 days after major abdominal surgery.
- Conditions severely affecting the GI tract, such as severe mucositis following systemic chemotherapy.

Guide to calculating parenteral nutritional requirements in adults

Nutritional assessment

Assessment is essential for the correct provision of nutritional support. A variety of techniques are available to assess nutritional status.

Some of the common criteria used to define malnutrition are recent weight loss and body mass index (BMI) changes.

Identifying high risk-patients

- Unintentional weight loss – 5–10% is clinically significant.
- ↓ oral intake – can result from vomiting, anorexia or NBM.
- Weight loss – take oedema, ascites or dehydration into consideration.

$$BMI = \frac{Weight\ (Kg)}{Height^2 (m)}$$

Normal

♀ 20–25

♂ 22–27

BMI is useful for identifying malnourished underweight patients, but a normal BMI does not rule out malnutrition, especially in an increasingly obese population.

Normal nutritional requirements

The Schofield equation is used typically in the UK; the Harris–Benedict and Ireton–Jones equations are commonly referred to in US texts.

It is always best to be cautious and start low and titrate up, depending on tolerance and clinical response. Use actual bodyweight if BMI >30kg/m^2: the methods used to calculate requirements in the obese are complex and poorly defined. A useful starting point in obese patients is to use 75% of body weight or alternatively feed-to-basal metabolic rate (BMR), without stress or activity factors added.

Macronutrients
- Calories
- Schofield equation
- Calculate BMR (W = weight in kg).

Table 16.34

♀ (kcal/day)		♂ (kcal/day)	
18–29yrs	(14.8W) + 692	18–29yrs	(15.1W) + 692
30–59yrs	(8.3W) + 846	30–59yrs	(11.5W) + 873
60–74yrs	(9.2W) + 687	60–74yrs	(11.9W) + 700
>75yrs	(9.8W) + 624	>75yrs	(8.3W) + 820

Add activity factor and stress factor as follows:
- Activity:
  - Bedbound/immobile: +10%.
  - Bedbound mobile/sitting: +15–20%.
  - Mobile: +25% upwards.
- Stress: % added for stress varies widely depending on the clinical condition, but it is typically in the range 0–30%.

Harris–Benedict equation

BW = body weight in kilograms, HT = height in cm, age in years

♂: BMR = 66.473 + 13.751*BW + 5.0033*HT - 6.755*age

♀: BMR = 655.0955 + 9.463*BW + 1.8496*HT - 4.6756*age

(Total caloric requirements = the BMR × by the sum of the stress and activity factors. Stress conditions and activity factors then need to be factored to calculate specific requirements)

Composition of parenteral nutrition regimens
- If possible, a balance of glucose and lipids should be used to provide total amount calories calculated.
- Glucose provision should be within glucose oxidation rate (GOR) if possible.
- Normal GOR is 4–7mg/kg body weight/min.

Nitrogen

- Normal nitrogen requirements are 0.14–0.2g/kg body weight.
- Requirements in catabolic patients can be in the range of 0.2–0.3g/kg body weight.
- Nonrenal nitrogen losses should be taken into consideration, eg wound, fistula and burn losses.

Electrolytes

- Sodium (normal range 0.5–1.5mmol/kg body weight).
  - Sensitive to haemodilutional effects; actual low sodium level is usually only as a result of excessive losses, and a moderately low levels is unlikely to be clinically significant.
  - Renal excretion can be a useful indicator. Aim to keep urine sodium >20mmol/L.
- K^+ (normal range 0.3–1.0mmol/kg body weight).
  - Affected by renal function, drugs or excessive losses.
- Calcium (normal range 0.1–0.15mmol/kg body weight).
  - Sensitive to haemoconcentration and heamodilution. Minimal supplementation generally adequate in short term parenteral nutrition.
- Magnesium (normal range 0.1–0.2mmol/kg body weight)
  - Renally conserved, minimal amounts generally suffice, unless patient has excessive losses.
- Phosphate (normal range 0.5–1.0mmol/kg body weight)
  - Influenced by renal function, re-feeding syndrome and onset of sepsis.

Trace elements and vitamins

Commercial multivitamin and mineral preparations eg Solivito® N, Decan®, Additrace®, and Cernevit® are suitable for most patients in the short to medium term, For long-term patients, requirements are dictated by monitoring.

How specific clinical conditions can affect parenteral nutrition requirements and provision

Re-feeding syndrome

- Start with low calories/day (max 20kcal/kg **body weight**/day).
- Monitor and supplement K^+, megnesium and phosphate as required.
- Ensure adequate vitamin supply, especially thiamine.

Acute renal failure

- Consider fluid, K^+ and phosphate restriction.
- Sodium restriction can also help to ↓ fluid retention.

Chronic renal failure

- Influenced by dialysis status.
- Consider need for nitrogen, K^+ and phosphate restriction.

Acute liver failure
- Use dry body weight (especially. if ascites are present) to calculate requirements.
- Patients might require sodium and fluid restriction. Protein restriction is not necessary.
- Provision of nutrition usually outweighs risks of abnormal LFTs.

Congestive cardiac failure
- Consider need for sodium and fluid restriction.

Children's parenteral nutrition regimens

Parenteral nutrition in children

Infants and children are particularly susceptible to the effects of starvation. The small (1kg) pre-term infant contains only 1% fat and 8% protein and has a nonprotein caloric reserve of only 110kcal/kg. body weight With growth, the fat and protein content rises, so a 1yr-old child of 10kg will has a nonprotein calorie reserve of 221kcal/kg. body weight All nonprotein content and one-third of the protein content of the body is available for calorific needs at a rate of 50kcal/kg body weight/day in infants and children.

A small preterm baby <1.5kg has sufficient reserve to survive only 4 days of starvation and a large preterm baby >3kg has enough for approximately 10–12 days. With ↑ calorific requirements associated with disease this might be reduced dramatically to <2 days for small preterm infants and perhaps 1 week for a large preterm baby.

Indications for parenteral nutrition

Some patients only require short-term parenteral nutrition in the following clinical situation:
- Major intestinal surgery.
- Chemotherapy.
- Severe acute pancreatitis.
- Multiorgan failure in extensive trauma, burns or prematurity.

Others will need long-term parenteral nutrition if there are prolonged episodes of intestinal failure eg in the following clinical situations:
- Protracted diarrhoea of infancy.
- Short bowel syndrome.
- Gastroschisis.
- Chronic intestinal pseudo-obstruction.

Nutritional requirements (see Table 16.35)

Fluid requirements also depend on the patient's size, abnormal losses (eg diarrhoea, fever), surgical procedures and disease state. The requirements for fluid to body weight are much greater in very small children than in older children and adults. Infants have a much larger body surface area relative to weight than older patients. Infants lose more fluid through evaporation and dissipate much more heat/kg. The use of radiant heaters and phototherapy further ↑ a neonate's fluid loss, resulting in a ↑ fluid requirement. Patients with high urinary outputs, ↑ ileostomy or gastrostomy tube outputs, diarrhoea and vomiting should have replacement fluids for these excessive losses, in addition to their maintenance fluid requirements.

The patient's weight and assessment of intake and output can be used to estimate hydration status. It is important that patients receiving parenteral nutrition are weighed regularly (initially daily, then twice to three times weekly with growth plotted when their condition stabilizes) and fluid balance monitored when parenteral nutrition is prescribed.

Energy sources

The body of a child requires energy for physical growth and neurological development.

Carbohydrate

Glucose is the carbohydrate source of choice in parenteral nutrition. To prevent hyperosmolality and hyperinsulinaemia, glucose infusions are introduced in a stepwise manner. In infants, glucose is introduced at 5–7.5% glucose and ↑ by 2.5% each day, to an upper limit of 4–7mg/kg body weight/min glucose infusion rate. In older children parenteral nutrition is started at 10–15% and ↑ daily to 20%, as tolerated.

The amount of glucose depends on the type of feeding line inserted. The dextrose concentration in parenteral nutrition infused peripherally is limited to 12.5%. If central access is available up to 20% glucose can be infused. Infusion of parenteral nutrition with glucose concentrations >20% has been associated with cardiac arrhythmias.

The very low birth weight infant has low glycogen reserves in the liver and a diminished capacity for gluconeogenesis. Hepatic glycogen is depleted within hours of birth, depriving the brain of metabolic fuel. Providing exogenous glucose through parenteral nutrition is thus a priority. Preterm infants, especially those with birth weights <1000g, are relatively glucose intolerant because of insulin resistance. Infusion of glucose >6 mg/kg body weight/min may can lead to hyperglycaemia and serum hyperosmolality, resulting in osmotic diuresis. Tolerance to glucose improves on subsequent days. It is generally recommended that the glucose infusion rate does not exceed 9mg/kg body weight/min for premature infants after the first day of life and that ↑ be implemented gradually as the infant develops.

Lipids

- Regimens require fat as a source of essential fatty acids. Fat is an important parenteral substrate because it is a concentrated source of calories in an isotonic medium, which makes it useful for peripheral administration.
- It is a useful substitute for carbohydrate if dextrose calories are limited because of glucose intolerance. Fat is available as emulsions of soybean, soybean–safflower oil mixtures or olive oil. The major differences are their fatty acid contents.
- Essential fatty acid deficiency can develop in the premature newborn during the first week of life on lipid-free regimens. A maximum lipid utilization rate of 3.3–3.6g/kg body weight/day. Above these values, ↑ risk of fat deposition 2° to the incomplete metabolic utilization of the infused lipid.
- IV fat should be commenced at a dose not exceeding 1g/kg body weight/day and ↑ gradually to a maximum of 3g/kg body weight/day, depending on age. Tolerance should be assessed by measuring serum triglyceride and free fatty acid concentrations.

Nitrogen

Nitrogen is needed for growth, the formation of new tissues (eg wound healing) and the synthesis of plasma proteins, enzymes and blood cells.

Requirements vary according to age, nutritional status and disease state. Infants and children experiencing periods of growth have higher nitrogen requirements than adults. Low birth weight infants have relatively high total amino acid requirements to support maintenance, growth and developmental needs.

Amino acid intakes of 2.0–2.5g/kg body weight/day result in nitrogen retention comparable with to the healthy enteral-fed infant. Rates of up to 4g/kg body weight/day might be required. because the amino acid profile varies between commercial brands, their nitrogen contents are not equivalent and protein requirements are calculated as grammes of amino acids rather than grammes of nitrogen in children.

Choice of amino acid solution

The proteins of the human body are manufactured from 20 different amino acids. There are eight essential amino acids. Premature infants and children are unable to synthesize/metabolize some of the amino acids that are 'nonessential' for adults. The use of amino acid solutions designed for adults have resulted in abnormal plasma amino acid profiles in infants. Infants fed with adult amino acid solutions have been shown to develop high concentrations of phenylalanine and tyrosine and low levels of taurine.

Paediatric amino acid solutions (see Table 16.36)

Amino-acid solutions specifically designed for neonates have been developed, as follow:

- Higher concentration of branch-chain amino acids (leucine, isoleucine and valine) and lower content of glycine, methionine and phenylalanine.
- Higher percentage of amino acids essential for preterm infants, with wider distribution of nonessential amino acids.
- Contain taurine.

The amino acid preparations available are based on either the amino acid profile of human milk (Vaminolact®) or placental cord blood (Primene®).

Table 16.35 Estimated average requirements for fluid, energy, protein, and nitrogen

Age (yrs)	Fluid (mL/kg body weight/day)	Energy (Kcal/kg body weight/day)	Protein (g/kg body weight/day)	Nitrogen (g/kg body weight/day)
Preterm	150–200	130–150	3.0–4.0	0.5–0.65
0–1	110–150	110–130	2.0–3.0	0.34–0.46
1–6	80–100	70–100	1.5–2.5	0.22–0.38
6–12	75–80	50–70	1.5–2.0	0.2–0.33
12–18	50–75	40–50	1.0–1.3	0.16–0.2

Table 16.36 Normal baseline electrolyte requirements

Electrolytes	Requirements according to age mmol/kg body weight/day	
	Infants	Children
Sodium	2.0–3.5	1.0–2.0
K^+	2.0–3.0	1.0–2.0
Calcium	1.0–1.5	0.5–1.0
Magnesium	0.15–0.3	0.1–0.15
Phosphate	0.5–1.5	0.12–0.4
Chloride	1.8–1.5	1.2–2

Trace elements (see Table 16.37)

Table 16.37 Requirements for trace elements

Element (mcg/kg body weight/day)	Preterm	Infant	Children
Zinc	100–500	50–100	50–80
Copper	30–60	20–50	20
Selenium	n/a	2–5	2
Manganese	n/a	1	1
Iron	100–200	20–100	100

Vitamins
Water-soluble vitamins

Table 16.38 Requirements for water-soluble vitamins

Vitamin	Preterm	Infant	Children
B1 (mg)	0.1–0.5	0.4–1.5	1.0–3.0
B2 (mg)	0.1–0.3	0.4–1.5	1.0–3.0
B6 (mg)	0.08–0.4	0.1–1.0	1.0–2.0
B12 (mcg)	0.3–0.6	0.3–30	20–40
C (mg)	20–40	20–40	20–40
Biotin (mcg)	5–30	35–50	150–300
Folate (mcg)	50–200	100–200	100–200
Niacin (mg)	2–5	5–10	5–20

Fat soluble vitamins

Table 16.39 Requirements for water soluble vitamins

Vitamin	Preterm	Infant	Children
A (mcg)	75–300	300–600	500–800
D (mcg)	5–10	10–20	10–20
E mg	3–8	3–10	10–15
K (mcg)	5–80	100–200	N/a

Administration of nutrition

- The aqueous phase runs over a period of 24h and the solution is filtered using a 0.2 micron filter.
- Lipid normally runs over a period of 20h–24h and is filtered using a 1.2 micron filter, although some centres prefer not to use filters.
- The weight used for calculation is usually the actual weight of the child.

Complications

Catheter-related

Complications could be due to catheter insertion (eg malposition, haemorrhage, pneumothorax, air embolism, or nerve injury) or might occur subsequently (eg infection, occlusion, or thromboembolism).

Metabolic- related

In stable patients with no abnormal fluid losses or major organ failure, severe biochemical disturbances are unusual.

Parenteral nutrition-associated cholestasis

Aetiology seems to be multifactorial, including absence of enteral feeding, overfeeding, prematurity, surgery and sepsis. It might progress to cirrhosis. Excessive calories, particularly glucose overload, can lower serum glucagon concentrations, which ↓ bile flow. Early initiation of oral calorie intake is the single most important factor in preventing or reversing cholestasis. Small intestinal bacterial overgrowth, which often occurs in the presence of intestinal stasis, can impair bile flow, leading to cholestasis.

Monitoring of children receiving parenteral nutrition in hospital

Requires clinical and laboratory monitoring, observations and assessment of growth. Growth is conveniently assessed by accurate measurement of weight and height, and development assessment is plotted over time. Fluid balance, temperature and DAILY BM's need to be assessed daily.

Laboratory monitoring

- Initial assessment—daily for first 3–4 days, then twice weekly)
- Full blood count.
- Blood test: sodium, K^+, urea, glucose
- Calcium, magnesium, phosphate, bilirubin, ALP, AST, ALT, blood glucose albumin, triglycerides and cholesterol.
- Cu, Zn, Se, vitamin A & E: baseline measurement
- Urine: sodium and K^+ (baseline).

Continued monitoring depends on the child's clinical condition.

Enteral feeding

Types of tube feeding

Intragastric feeding

- Nasogastric.
- Percutaneous endoscopic gastroscopy (PEG).

Post-pyloric feeding

- Nasojejunal.
- Percutaneous endoscopic gastrojejunostomy.
- Percutaneous endoscopic jejunostomy.
- Surgically placed jejunostomy.

Enteral feeding should be considered in patients with a functioning GI tract who are unable to meet requirements with ordinary diet, food fortification and/or oral nutritional supplements

Postpyloric feeding is indicated if there is gastric outflow obstruction or severe pancreatitis or if patient is at risk from aspiration with intragastric feeding.

Feeding-tube-specific issues

Site of delivery

- Gastric tube ends in the stomach, whereas jejunal tube ends in the jejunum.
- Sterile water must be used for jejunal tubes because of gastric-acid barrier bypass.

Number of differences between tubes apart from site of feed delivery

- Bore size—fine-bore tube is designed for administration of feeds and, wide-bore tube is designed for aspiration.
- Number of lumens.
- Rate of flow.
- Length.

Complications of tubes

- Removal by patient.
- Oesophageal ulceration or strictures.
- Incorrect positioning of tube.
- Blockage.

Categories of feeds

Polymeric feeds

Contain whole protein, carbohydrate and fat and can be used as a sole source of nutrition for those patients without any special nutrient requirements. Standard concentration is 1kcal/mL but they can vary in energy density (0.8–2kcal/mL) and can be supplemented with fibre, which can help improve bowel function, if problematic.

Elemental feeds

Contain amino acid and glucose or maltodextrins; fat content is very low. Used in situations of malabsorption or pancreatic insufficiency. Because of their high osmolality, they should not be used in patients with short bowel syndrome.

Disease-specific feeds and modular supplements

Certain clinical conditions require adjustment in diets; for example, high-energy low-electrolyte feeds for patients requiring dialysis and low-carbohydrate and high-fat diets for patients with CO_2 retention (for certain patients on ventilators) as carbohydrate leads to more CO_2 production compared with calorific equivalent amounts of protein or fat.

Modular supplements are used for a variety of conditions eg malabsorption and hypoprotein states. They are not nutritionally complete and hence not suitable as a sole source of food.

These feeds contain extra substrates that are claimed to alter the immune and inflammatory responses. Include substrates glutamine, arginine, RNA, omega-3 fatty acids and antioxidants.

Administration of tube feeds

For intragastric feeds, diet can be delivered either by continuous rate delivering over a period of 16–18h daily.

Alternatively administration of intermittent boluses of 50–250mL by syringe over a period of 10–30min can be suggested, although complications such as aspiration and delayed gastric transit times have been reported more frequently with this approach.

Postpyloric feeding is generally performed by continuous infusion because it is deemed more physiological.

Complications from feeds

Diarrhoea

This is the commonest complication; management is to exclude other explanations (eg colitis, laxative use, antibiotics and malabsorption).

Concomitant medications need to be rationalized, antidiarrhoeal medication codeine phosphate and/or loperamide are often useful and fibre can help in some cases.

If diarrhoea persists after treatment, consider switching to the postpyloric route.

Constipation

Usually a result of a combination of inadequate fluid, dehydration, immobility and drugs. If functional pathology is excluded, management is by laxatives, suppositories and fibre feeds.

Vomiting, aspiration or reflux

Both nasogastric and postpyloric feeding can ↑ the risk of aspiration, both can interfere with oesophageal sphincter function and wide bore tubes cause more problems than fine-bore tubes. Standard antiemetics and prokinetics are usually effective.

Metabolic complications

Re-feeding syndrome

Excess carbohydrate stimulates insulin release, which leads to intracellular shifts of phosphate, magnesium and K^+ that can lead to cardiac arrhythmias or neurological events. Emaciated patients must have their feed introduced gradually at a rate of 20kcal/kg body weight and electrolytes replaced in accordance to daily blood levels.

Vitamin/trace element deficiencies

Incidence is rare as commercially available feeds are nutritionally complete. Patients being fed over extended periods should have appropriate monitoring undertaken.

Hyperglycaemia

Important in the critically ill, it is imperative that blood glucose is monitored and controlled because good control glycaonic improves mortality rates in the critically ill.

Drug administration in patients with feeding tubes

The administration of medication to patients with feeding tubes can be challenging and a number of issues need to be considered in parallel with the patient's medical problems.

These issues include the following:
- The continued need for the patient's regular medicines and, the consequences of medication withdrawal or administration delay, both medically and legally.
- The intention to tube feed and subsequent compliance of the patient to retain the tube.
- Institutional ability to site percutaneous tubes
- Availability and appropriateness of different formulations of medication

Formulation difficulties

Pharmacists will be involved in influencing the choice of medication formulation on the basis of their training and experience.

Is there a formulation available for use by a licensed route, eg rectal, buccal or parenteral, that is appropriate for your patient?

Pharmacists should also be able to calculate the cost implications of the different formulations, and importantly, should facilitate long-term choice, particularly if the parenteral route cannot be used in the long term.

Does a commercial oral solution, suspension or soluble solid dose form exist?
- Soluble tablets dissolved in 10mL of water are often best option for tube-fed patients.
- Refer to specific manufacturer's advice for feed-tube administration.
- Remember to shake liquid preparations before administration.
- Viscous liquids might have to be diluted with water to ↓ tube blockage.
- Liquids with high osmolality or sorbitol content can lead to diarrhoea.
- Does the crushed tablet or capsule contents disperse fully or form a workable suspension that will not clog or block the feeding tube?

Is the parenteral formulation of the product suitable for enteral use?
- Osmolality concerns for parenteral product.
- However, additives in injections might make administration through a tubes unsuitable.

Is there therapeutic substitution that can be administered through a tube?

Administration of medication through a tube
- Do not add medication directly to the feed.
- Only administer one medication at a time.
- Use an oral syringe if possible.
- Flush the tube with 50mL water. immediately after stopping the feed
- Add the volume of water used to fluid-balance charts.
- Draw identified formulation into appropriate 50mL syringe.
- Attach the tube and apply gentle pressure.
- Flush with a minimum 15mL of water between different medicines.

- Flush with 50mL of water after the last medication.
- If drug is to be taken on an empty stomach, for gastric tubes, stop feed for 30min before the dose and resume feeding 30min after words. These measures are obviously not relevant for jejunal tubes.
- Add the total volume of flushes and medicine to the fluid-balance chart.

Specific drug/tube feeding problems

Drug-specific issues
- Absorption could be unpredictable because the tube might be beyond the main site of absorption for the specific drug.
- Formulation issues of medication being administered through feeding tubes.
- Crushing destroys the formulation properties of tablets, altering peak-and-trough levels.
- Detrimental clinical effect for certain slow-release products eg nifedipine LA, causing severe hypotension, if inadvertently given crushed.

Adsorption onto feeding tubes
For example phenytion, diazepam and carbamazepine. Dilute with at least 50mL of water and flush the tube well.

Interactions causing blockage
Antacids and acidic formulations could cause precipitation because of an acid–base reaction.

Feed ↓ drug absorption
For example carbamazepine, theophylline, warfarin and ciprofloxacin absorption is ↓, feeds should be stopped 2h before and after the drug is given Remember to flush the tube well.

Drug–feed interactions
If vitamin K^+ is in present feed it means that doses of warfarin might need to be amended.

Bioequivalence
Different formulations might necessitate adjustment of dose, eg phenytoin tablets and liquid.

IV therapy at home

Patients who are medically stable but require prolonged courses of IV drugs (usually antimicrobials) can benefit from IV therapy at home. Suitable indications or therapies are as follows:

- Bone infections.
- Endocarditis.
- Cystic fibrosis.
- Cytomegalovirus infection.
- Total parenteral nutrition.
- Immunoglobulins.

The advantages of treating these patients at home are as follows:

- Releases hospital beds for other patients.
- Avoids patient exposure to hospital-acquired infection.
- ↑ patient autonomy.
- Improved patient comfort and convenience.
- Some patients could to return to work or study while therapy continues

Despite the potential benefits, IV therapy at home should not be undertaken lightly. All IV therapy is potentially hazardous and complications, such as line sepsis or blockage, are potentially more probable and risky in the community.

It is recommended that a multidisciplinary home IV team is set up to oversee the process and that guidelines are drawn up to ensure home IV therapy is done safely and effectively[1].

Home IV therapy team

The following people should be included in the team; they might not have hands on involvement in every patient but should be available for advice and support:

- Clinician with an interest in home IV therapy (eg microbiologist, infectious diseases physician)
- Home IV therapy specialist nurse(s)/community liaison nurse(s).
- Pharmacist.
- Community representative (GP or community nurse).

24h access to key member(s) of the team (usually the specialist nurse and/or a clinician) is essential.

For individual patients, the medical and nursing team responsible for the patient's care should liaise with the home IV team and be involved in assessment, discharge planning and follow-up.

IV access

Venous access through short peripheral lines ('Venflons') is unsuitable for home delivery because it is designed for short term use and should be replaced every 48–72h. Peripheral access is also unsuitable for irritant or hyperosmolar infusions, eg TPN. Central venous access is preferred for the following reasons:

- Can remain in place for prolonged periods.
- Can be used for irritant or hyperosmolar infusions.

1 Nathwani D and Conlon C (1998). Outpatient and home parenteral antibiotic therapy (OHPAT) in the UK: a consensus statement by a working party. *Clinical Microbiology and infection* **4**: 537–51.

- Easier for patients to self-administer through a central line.

Three types of central IV access are used for home IV therapy, as follow:

- **Central line (eg Hickman or Groshong)**—the line is inserted, usually through the subclavian vein and is threaded through a subcutaneous tunnel to exit on the chest wall. The tip lies in the superior vena cava or just inside the right atrium. Central lines are inserted under general or local anaesthetic. In some hospitals specialist nurses insert central lines. Central lines might have one or more lumens, but for IV therapy at home, a single lumen line is recommended to ↓ complications. These lines can remain in place for many months.

- **Port-A-Cath**—a central venous access device, consisting of a small reservoir (the port) attached to a catheter. The port is implanted into the chest wall, with the catheter inserted into the subclavian or internal jugular vein. The reservoir is covered with a thick rubber septum, which is accessed through the skin using a special needle known as a 'Huber needle'. Port-A-Caths are inserted under general anaesthetic. They can remain in place for years. Due to the cost and complexity of insertion, Port-A-Caths are only suitable for patients who require prolonged or repeated IV therapy eg cystic fibrosis patients.

- **Peripherally inserted central catheters (PICC)**—these are fine, flexible catheters inserted into the basilic or cephalic vein at the antecubital fossa, in a similar manner to peripheral venous access. Using a guidewire, the catheter is threaded up the axilliary vein and into a central vein. PICC lines are inserted under local anaesthetic and are the least complex of the three types to insert. They can remain in place for several weeks or months. PICC lines are the least costly and complex and, ∴ are usually the preferred type of access.

To preserve the patency of central lines and avoid septic complications, guidelines should give advice on handling the line, including the following:

- Aseptic technique for drug administration.
- Flushing the line between doses.
- Use of heparinized saline to avoid clot formation within the line.
- Dressing and cleaning the insertion site.
- Care of the line when not in use.
- Procedure if the line is blocked or damaged.
- Procedure if there are signs of infection/cellulitis around the insertion site or signs/symptoms of sepsis.

Assessment and discharge planning

The home IV team should take responsibility for assessing whether the patient is suitable for IV therapy at home and for planning the discharge jointly with other nursing/medical staff caring for the patient. It is important that sufficient time is allowed to ensure that assessment, training and general organization of the discharge is carried out adequately. Guidelines should advise a minimum of 48h notice and ideally longer.

Patients should be as follows:

- Medically stable.
- Not likely to misuse the line.
- Psychologically able to cope with IV therapy at home.
- Willing to have IV therapy at home.

- Able to recognize problems and act accordingly.

The patient's home circumstances must also be taken into account:

- Is there another responsible adult who can support the patient and, if necessary, contact medical services themselves?
- Does the patient have a telephone?
- Are there reliable water and electricity supplies?
- Is there somewhere cool, dry and safe to store drugs (out of reach of children)?
- Does the patient have a fridge, if needed, for drug storage (and do children have unsupervised access to this fridge)?
- Are there children or other people in the house who might be distressed by seeing drugs being administered IV?
- Does the patient have some means of transport to outpatient appointments?

Procedures for children receiving IV therapy at home are much the same as for adults but special attention must be paid to ensuring home circumstances are suitable and that parents do not feel too pressured, especially if they are responsible for administering the drugs.

The discharge plan should be written in the patients medical records (Table 16.40). A copy should be supplied to the GP, and patients should be supplied with written information on the drugs, administration, side effects, and given monitoring and emergency contact details.

Drug selection and administration

Drug selection primarily depends on the condition being treated. Ideally drugs that are administered once daily should be used. In most UK schemes, IV infusions are avoided and wherever possible drugs are administered by slow IV push because this is a less complex and time consuming method of drug administration. Where IV infusion cannot be avoided (eg vancomycin) the drug should be administered through a volumetric pump, rather than a gravity drip. In some situations, it can be more appropriate to use an ambulatory infusion device such as an elastomeric pump (eg Homepump) or other system (eg Sidekick), rather than a volumetric pump. Discussion of these devices is beyond the scope of this topic.

Guidelines should give advice on drug administration. Issues that must be considered are:

- Who will administer the drug, eg patient, carer, community nurse?
- What training will they require?
- Who will do the training?

Many patients or their carers are capable of administering IV therapy provided they receive suitable training and support. However, if therapy is only to continue for a week or less it is probably not worth the time taken to train a patient or carer. In some areas community nurses can administer the drugs, but they might also need additional training. Training is usually provided by a specialist nurse

Training should include recognition of adverse effects and what action to take. This includes possible allergic or anaphylactic reactions. Protocols for administration of drugs by patients/carers or community nurses to treat anaphylaxis should be in place and an 'anaphylaxis kit' kept in the patients home. These protocols should follow UK Resuscitation Council guidelines[1].

It is recommended that the first one or two doses of the drug should be administered in hospital so that the patient can be monitored for acute side effects.

Guidelines should include procedures for disposal of clinical waste (eg used dressings), sharps and empty vials. These should follow local practice, eg some areas might accept sharps boxes for disposal in the community, whereas others might require them to be returned to the hospital.

Community support

The patient's GP should be willing for the patient to go home with IV therapy. Even if they are not administering the drug, community nurses might be involved in other aspects of patient care and so should be kept informed. Good communication between the home IV therapy team and community healthcare workers is essential. Contact details for the hospital clinician and specialist home IV therapy nurse should be provided—including out of hours contact details

Follow-up

Before discharge, follow-up arrangements should be planned. This should include the following:

- What to do if the patient has a significant ADR—who is responsible for managing this?
- Blood tests for monitoring ADR and TDM:
  - Who will take blood?
  - What tests are required?
  - Frequency.
  - How will the results be communicated and to whom?
  - Who will act on the results?
- The specialist home IV therapy nurse will usually be the main point of contact.
- The referring team should follow-up the patient with respect to presenting indication, in addition to follow-up from the home IV therapy team.
- Duration of IV therapy is usually decided before discharge. It should be agreed which team is responsible for review of this and for provision of oral follow-on therapy.
- The home IV therapy team is usually responsible for line removal (as appropriate) at the end of the IV course.

---

1 UK resuscitation council guidelines. www.resus.org.uk/pages/reaction.htm

The role of the pharmacist

The pharmacist is an important member of the home IV team. Their role includes the following responsibilties:

- Advice on drug stability and compatibility.
- Advice on drug administration including infusion rates and, ambulatory infusion devices.
- Ensuring the supply of IV and ancillary drugs on discharge.
- Ensuring follow-on oral therapy is prescribed.
- Provision of anaphylaxis kits.
- Liaison with home delivery companies
- Supporting the training of patients, and community nurses.

The American Society of Health System Pharmacists has published guidelines on the pharmacist's role in home care which includes home IV therapy at home[1]. It should be borne in mind that these guidelines reflect the US system of healthcare and so some aspects might not be relevant to non-US pharmacists.

Drugs for home IV therapy at home fall into the 'hospital-at-home' category and, as such, all supplies should come from the hospital. Thus community pharmacists are rarely involved in IV therapy at home. However, it is important that hospital pharmacists liaise with their community colleagues, as appropriate, eg where oral follow on therapy might be prescribed by the GP.

---

1 American Society of Health System Pharmacists (2000). ASHP guidelines on the pharmacist's role in home care. *Amercan Journal Health Systems Pharmacy* **57**:1252–7.

Table 16.40 Checklist of information to be included in the discharge plan

Patient	Vascular access device	Treatment
• Relevant past medical history	• Type of device	• Pathology and infecting organism
• Problems/side effects experienced	• When inserted or placed, and by whom	• Details of antibiotic regimen—drug and dose regimen
• Frequency and timing of clinic visits during treatment	• If centrally placed, where is the tip?	• Administration details
• Blood monitoring and frequency	• Possible complications—signs, symptoms, prevention and management	• Side effects
• Length of time on treatment	• Day-to-day care of the line	• Monitoring requirements and action required if results are abnormal
• Finish/review date for the treatment	• Who to contact if there are any difficulties with the device	
• How to access help	• Who will remove the device and how	

Sodium content of parenteral drugs

A number of parenteral formulations contain a significant amount of sodium ions (Table 16.41). This sodium load is unlikely to be important in most patients but could be clinically significant for some patient groups, eg neonates and patients with significant liver impairment. Table 16.41 is not exhaustive but lists the sodium content of more frequently used drugs or drugs in which the sodium level is especially high. The absence of a drug from the table does not necessarily mean that it has a low sodium content—check additional sources. If a drug is reconstituted or infused with sodium chloride 0.9% solution this further ↑ the sodium load (by 15mmol sodium for each 100mL of sodium chloride 0.9% solution).

Note that some oral preparations, especially soluble tablets, might have high sodium levels.

Other sources that quote the sodium content of parenteral formulations

Royal College of Paediatrics and Child Health and the Neonatal Paediatric Pharmacists Group (2003). *Medicines for Children*. London: RCPCH Publications Ltd.

Barber N and Willson (1999). *A Clinical Pharmacy Survival Guide*. Churchill Livingstone.

Shulman R *et al* (ed) (1998). *Injectable Drug Administration Guide*. Blackwell Science Ltd.

Table 16.41 Summary of product characteristics

Name	Vial/ampoule size	Sodium content per vial (mmol)
Acetylcysteine	2g	12.78
Aciclovir	250mg	1
Addiphos®	20ml	30
Amoxicillin	250mg	0.7
Ampicillin	250mg	0.7
Amphotericin lipid complex (Abelcet®)	100mg	3.13
Amphotericin liposomal (Ambisome®)	50mg	<0.5
Atenolol	5mg	1.3–1.8
Benzylpenicillin	600mg	1.68
Cefotaxime	500mg	1.1
Ceftazidime	500mg	1.2
Ceftriaxone	1g	3.6

Table 16.41 (Contd)

Name	Vial/ampoule size	Sodium content per vial (mmol)
Cefuroxime	750mg	1.8
Chloramphenicol sodium succinate	1g	3.14
Chlormetiazole	500mL	15–16
Ciprofloxacin	200mg	15.4
Co-amoxiclav	600mg	1.6
Co-trimoxazole	480mg	1.7
Desmopressin	4mcg	0.15
Diazoxide	300mg	15
Disodium hydrogen phosphate	10mL	12
Ertapenem	1g	6
Flucloxacillin	250mg	0.5
Fluconazole	200mg	15
Flucytosine	2.5g	34.44
Folinic acid	15mg	0.2
Foscarnet	1g	15.6
Furosemide	250mg	1
Ganciclovir	500mg	2
Granisetron	3mg	1.17
Heparin	25000IU/mL	0.625–0.8
Human albumin solution (all concentrations)	100ml	100–160 (check label for exact amount)
Hydrocortisone:		
sodium phosphate	100mg	0.66
sodium succinate	100mg	0.37
Imipenem	500mg	1.72
Levofloxacin	500mg	15.4
Meropenem	1g	3.9
Metoclopramide	10mg	0.27
Metronidazole	500mg	13–14.55
Ofloxacin	200mg	15.4

Table 16.41 (Contd)

Name	Vial/ampoule size	Sodium content per vial (mmol)
Pamidronate:		
dry powder	15mg	0.1
	30mg	0.2
	90mg	0.3
solution	15mg	1.1
	30mg	1.1
Phenytoin	250mg	1.1
Piperacillin + tazobactam	4.5g	9.4
Rifampicin	300mg	<0.5
	600mg	< 0.5
Sodium bicarbonate	1.26%	150/litre
	4.2%	500/litre
	8.4%	1000/litre
Sodium chloride	0.9%	150/litre
Sodium nitroprusside	50mg	0.34
Sodium valproate	400mg	2.41
Sotalol	40mg	0.5
Teicoplanin	200mg	<0.5
	400mg	<0.5
Terbutaline	500mcg	0.15
Thiopental sodium	500mg	23.26
Ticarcillin + clavulanic acid	3.2g	16
Verapamil	5mg	0.3
Vitamins B and C		
Pabrinex high-potency IV	1+2 ampoules	2.95
Pabrinex high-potency IM	1+2 ampoules	2.92

Wound care

The skin is the largest organ of the body and has the primary function of protecting underlying tissues and organs. Breaching this barrier exposes the underlying tissues and organs to the following:
- Mechanical damage.
- Dehydration.
- Microbial invasion.
- Temperature variations.

The ideal wound dressing replicates the skin's protective qualities, in addition to promoting wound healing.

Factors affecting the healing process

For a wound to heal the following factors are required:
- Moist, but not excessively wet.
- Warmth.
- O_2.
- Nutrition.
- (Relatively) free of contamination with microbes or foreign bodies—including slough and necrotic tissue.

A wound dressing should provide all these factors.

Some patients experience delayed wound healing and can develop chronic wounds, eg leg ulcers, despite good wound care. This might be caused by patient-related factors, which inhibit wound healing, and these must be addressed as far as possible (Table 16.42).

Classification of wounds

Various classifications for wounds exist. For the purposes of wound care, the following descriptions are most useful because they correspond to dressing choice. Note that some wounds may show more than one of the following features:
- Epithelializing or granulating—a clean, red or pink wound, usually shallow with minimal exudates.
- Sloughy—yellow slough covers part or all of the wound. This might be a dry or wet wound. Note that visible bone or tendon appears yellow.
- Necrotic—dead tissue creates a black, dry, leathery eschar.
- Infected—yellow or greenish in colour, with possible surrounding cellulitis of unbroken skin. The wound might have an offensive smell.
- Exuding—all the above (except necrotic) might produce exudates to varying degrees. High levels of exudates can lead to maceration of surrounding skin.
- Cavity—the wound might form a deep or shallow cavity. Sinuses are narrow cavities, which can extend to some depth, including tracking to bone or between two wounds.
- Malodorous—fungating tumours and infected and necrotic wounds can all have an offensive smell.

These classifications broadly represent the stages of wound healing. Thus, as the wound heals, the type of dressing appropriate to the wound can change. Slough and necrotic tissue are effectively foreign bodies that inhibit wound healing. After these have been removed, the underlying tissue should be granulating. Patients should be warned that as debridement occurs the wound might appear to get bigger before it starts to heal. Occasionally pain associated with the wound can ↑ as the wound heals because damaged nerve endings also heal.

It is important to review wound care on a regular basis. Frequency of reviews (and dressing changes) depend on the severity and nature of the wound. An infected or highly exuding wound might require daily dressing changes, but a granulating wound might only require re-dressing every few days. It is important to avoid renewing a dressing unnecessarily becuase this can expose the wound to cooling, dehydration or mechanical damage. It is good clinical practice to prepare a wound-care chart (Table 16.43). This ensures that all staff are informed about the nature of the wound, which dressings are being used and the frequency of dressing changes/review. Including photographs of the wound enables progress (or deterioration) to be monitored.

Selection of wound dressing

There is no universal wound dressing and different types of dressing, suit different wounds. The ideal dressing fulfils all the requirements described, in Table 16.44 according to the environment in which it is being used. Dressings are divided into the following two categories:

- Primary dressings–applied directly to the wound surface.
- Secondary dressings–which are placed over the primary dressings to hold them in place and/or provide additional padding or protection.

It is less important for secondary dressings to fulfil the ideal requirements.

Each time a dressing is changed, it exposes the wound to contamination, dehydration and cooling. Thus, ideally, the frequency of primary dressing changes should be kept to a minimum. Secondary dressings can be changed more frequently, without disturbing the primary dressing.

Wound care has advanced greatly since the introduction of 'interactive' dressings. These dressings provide active wound management, usually by interacting with the wound surface (eg alginates form a gel on contact with exudates) rather than simply acting as a barrier. Selection of the correct dressing is important both to ensure that the wound is healed as efficiently as possible and to ensure cost-effective use because interactive dressings are usually more expensive than noninteractive dressings (Table 16.45).

Use of topical antimicrobials

These agents are usually not recommended because of the risk of development of resistance and high incidence of local sensitivity reactions (which could ultimately lead to systemic allergic reactions). There is little evidence that topical antimicrobials work and infection should be treated systemically.

The following preparations are recommended in particular situations:

- Povidone iodine preparations, either as impregnated dressings (Inadine) or as solutions (Betadine aqueous), can be used on wounds infected with bacteria, fungi or protozoa. These should be stopped as soon as the infection is under control as povidone iodine has been shown to inhibit wound healing.

- Silver, either as silver sulfadiazine cream (Flamazine®) or as silver-impregnated dressings (AquacelAg®), is active against Gram-negative infection, eg Pseudomonas infection in burns, and MRSA. These preparations are often used inappropriately for any 'infected' wound. Use should be restricted because they are expensive and excessive use of the cream can cause irreversible black skin staining (argyria) because of deposition of silver into the skin.
- Metronidazole gel is used to inhibit anaerobic bacteria, which cause the malodour associated with fungating tumours or necrotic wounds. Liberal application of metronidazole suppresses bacterial growth and thus ↓ odour. The surrounding skin should be protected from the gel to avoid maceration. Excessive use could (theoretically) lead to the emergence of metronidazole resistance. Where metronidazole gel is unavailable—eg in developing countries—the tablets can be crushed to a fine powder and sprinkled over the wound or mixed with an aqueous gel (eg KY jelly) before application.

Chlorinated desloughing agents, such as Eusol® and Chlorasol®, are no longer recommended. Although effective for debriding sloughy wounds, they are potential irritants and can delay healing because of cell toxicity and ↓ capillary blood flow. With more modern desloughing dressings available, the disadvantages of these agents outweigh the benefits.

Sugar paste and honey dressings can be used on sloughy, infected and/or malodorous wounds. The antibacterial effect of the sugar or honey ↓ odour. Bacterial growth is inhibited because of the ↑ osmotic pressure in the wound, and honey (especially Manuka honey) has some inherent antimicrobial effect. These dressings debride sloughy wounds and can promote angiogenesis.

Sugar pastes are made from preservative-free icing or caster sugar. Thin pastes can be used in wounds with small openings—using a syringe to dribble the paste into the wound—and thick pastes are used for larger, cavity wounds. The disadvantage of these dressings is that they might require frequent changes—twice daily or more.

Vacuum assisted closure (VAC) therapy is a form of wound care where negative pressure is applied to a special porous dressing, which is placed in the wound cavity or over a flap or graft. VAC helps to remove excess exudates and mechanically draws the edges of the wound inwards, promoting healing. It is suitable for any chronic open wound or acute and traumatic surgical wounds and is used in plastic surgery to promote healing of grafts and flaps. VAC therapy should not be used on infected wounds (including those involving osteomyelitis) unless these are being treated with systemic antimicrobials. VAC is unsuitable for fistulae, which connect with body cavities or organs, and malignant or necrotic wounds and should be used with caution on bleeding wounds.

Larval (maggot) therapy—larvae of the common greenbottle are used in the management of necrotic or sloughy wounds. To feed, the larvae produce proteolytic substances that degrade dead tissue but have no adverse effect on living tissue.

Table 16.42 Patient factors that inhibit wound healing

- Poor perfusion, eg peripheral vascular disease
- Older age (usually linked to poor nutrition or other disease)
- Concurrent disease, eg diabetes, cancer or anaemia
- Drugs, eg steroids, cytotoxics or NSAIDs
- Smoking
- Immobility

Table 16.43 Wound care plan

Patient's name: _____   Date: _____

Photograph/diagram   **Description of wound(s)**
(number each wound and use
numbering scheme when describing wounds):

Dressings (number, as above):   **Frequency of dressing changes:**

Other information (eg analgesia required with dressing changes):

Review date: _____
Signature: _____

Table 16.44 Characteristics of the ideal wound dressing

- Maintain moist environment
- Manage excessive exudates
- Allow oxygenation
- Provide a barrier to micro-organisms
- Maintain a warm environment (approx 37 °C)
- Not shed particles or fibres
- ↓ or eliminate odour
- Cost-effective
- Acceptable to the patient

Larvae are supplied either in a gauze bag—various sizes contain different numbers of larvae—or loose. The former presentation is often more acceptable to patients (and nurses) and can be used on cavity wounds, where it might be difficult to locate and retrieve free larvae.

Larvae should be used within 48h of receipt, otherwise they will die because of lack of nutrients, and will generally survive 3–5days feeding on the wound. During this time, they ↑ in size, and as long as they are still active and increasing in size, they are still effective.

The gauze bag or individual larvae are applied directly to the wound and covered with a nonadherent dressing, which is soaked in saline to ensure larvae are kept moist (but not drowning!). A nonocclusive secondary dressing should be used to cover them to prevent drying out and to ensure they have sufficient O_2 to survive. Most interactive dressings are unsuitable (and unnecessary) for use on a wound being treated with larvae because they might kill them due to ↑ osmotic pressure or ↓ O_2 supply. During treatment, the amount of exudate can ↑ and appear greenish in colour, but this is normal. It might be necessary to protect surrounding healthy skin from maceration caused by ↑ exudates by applying a barrier film, such as Cavilon®.

Further reading

A peer-reviewed online wound care journal, sponsored by industry but with a code of practice to limit bias. www.worldwidewounds.com

Table 16.45 Matching the dressing to the wound

Dressing type	Examples	Suitable for	Comment
Alginate	Sorbsan®, Sorbsan® plus Kaltostat®	Exuding, sloughy. Ribbon or rope—cavity or sinus	'Plus' versions have a highly absorbent backing, suitable for highly exuding wounds
Foams	Lyofoam®, Allevyn®	Exuding or highly exuding wounds	Avoid adhesive versions on fragile skin
Films and Membranes	Opsite®, Tegapore®	Shallow, granulating	
Hydrocolloid	Granuflex®, Comfeel® Tegasorb®	Sloughy, light-to-medium exudates	Not suitable for infected wounds or if frequent dressing changes required Avoid on fragile skin
Hydrofibres	Aquacel®	Sloughy, medium-to high-exudates. Ribbon—cavity or sinus	
Hydrogels	Intrasite®, Granugel®	Dry, sloughy	Always requires a secondary dressing
Low adherent	Melolin®, N–A®	Dry, lightly exuding, granulating	Even 'nonadherent' versions can stick to wound, causing trauma on removal
Odour absorbing	Actisorb®, Carbonet®	Malodorous	Apply over primary dressings
Padding	Gamgee®	Highly exuding	Secondary dressing only
Paraffin gauze	Jelonet®	Granulating	
Polysaccharide beads	Debrisan®, Iodosorb®	Deep cavities	Not suitable for deep or tortuous sinuses

Introduction to critical care

For the purposes of critical care in the UK, patients are grouped into one of four levels of care, an allocation that changes according to severity of illness and degree of actual or potential organ support required by the patient:

- Level 0: patients have needs that can be met by normal ward care.
- Level 1: patients have needs that can be met on an acute ward, with additional advice and support from the critical care team. They are at risk of their condition deteriorating or have recently been relocated from higher levels of care.
- Level 2: patients require more detailed observation or intervention, including support for a single failing organ system or postoperative care and patients stepping down from higher levels of care (formally known as high-dependency unit (HDU) patients).
- Level 3: patients require advanced respiratory support alone or basic respiratory support together with support of at least two organ systems. This level includes all complex patients requiring support for multiorgan failure (formally known as intensive care unit (ICU) patients).

This classification has meant that critical care has come to define a type of therapy, rather than a specific place where such therapy is administered. Critical care teams work in ICUs, HDUs, specialist surgical units, recovery areas, perioperative care and on general wards, with outreach teams. Critical care, ∴, encompasses a diverse area for pharmacists who work within, and pharmacists working on general wards are increasingly coming into contact with critically ill patients. For the pharmacist who commits to a career in critical care, a competency framework describing various levels of specialist pharmacist practice has been drawn up and is published on the Department of Health's website[1].

Tips, hints and things you should bear in mind

Critical care can be a daunting area within which to work at first. Patients are on the extremes of the physiological spectra, often accompanied by a frightening array of equipment that bristles with buttons, gaudy displays and issuing all manner of warning squeaks, pips and beeps. The patient is cared for by experienced, efficient nurses and calm, intelligent doctors and can be surrounded by teams of personnel attending to various functions of care. An enormous variety and quantity of data are generated, with the patient's notes quickly expanding in size. All of this activity is watched by tense, tired and often tearful relatives or carers, who are constantly looking for the slightest sign that their loved ones condition is either improving or deteriorating.

---

1 http://www.dh.gov.uk/PolicyAndGuidance/OrganisationPolicy/EmergencyCare/KeyEmergency CareDocuments/fs/en

Put the patient first

In all your endeavours and work, you must put the patient first. If there are limited resources and you have several patient care responsibilities, you must do the best you can for the patients who need you the most.

Not all patients are model citizens. They might have led very colourful lives and this can complicate their medical management and dealings with relatives or affect your own personal feelings for them. You must put these aspects aside to do your best for them.

You will have to come to terms with the fact that a significant proportion of patients will die despite your best efforts. This of course reflects the severity of their illness, not your performance, and you will need to remind yourself of this from time to time.

Remember the relatives, carers and friends

The patient is not always alone. Loved ones visit and stay by the bedside without restrictions on visiting hours. As a member of the team, you will be asked about various aspects of the patient's care. As a junior pharmacist, you should defer giving information about progress or planning to a member of the medical team. This ensures that visitors receive consistent information. You might still need to talk to relatives, to obtain information about medications or possibly because you are asked to discuss a specific aspect of care with them by the medical team. When you do so, employ great sensitivity. Loved ones have a lot of time to think and dwell on the consequences of the illness that brings the patient to critical care and as such, can be extremely fragile. Remember that certain aspects of the patient might not be known to them, and should not be divulged to them, sometimes at the specific request of the patient. This can give rise to some extraordinary circumstances, yet you must still employ strict patient confidentiality. Because of the situation they find themselves in, visitors might not take in everything you are saying. They might also make their own interpretation of any information you are giving them or asking of them. Be as clear and concise as you can. Note the key points of conversation in the patient's notes, and if possible, ensure that the patient's nurse is party to the conversation. In addition to acting as a witness, they can dig you out of a hole.

Do not worry

You might not know the nuances and subtleties of various standard critical care interventions, such as vasopressors or sedation and analgesia. You are, in fact, unlikely to, unless you have committed to a career in critical care pharmacy. Fortunately, intensivists tend to know a fair bit about these agents, and so you should be assured that at more junior levels of practice, such in depth knowledge is not necessary to contribute meaningfully to the team.

Nor are you be expected to know the function of every piece of kit available at the bedside, and no one expects you to be able to interpret pressure waveforms or scan results. Your role is not the same as everyone else's. In time, you might understand the intricacies of the available monitoring and supporting equipment, but for now, concentrate on the area you know best: basic clinical pharmacy.

Develop a methodical approach

Every critical care patient requires a high degree of pharmaceutical care/medicines management. You must know the patients medical history, drug history, allergy history, admitting complaint, progress, pharmacokinetic reserve and prescription as a minimum dataset from which to work. Making professional notes is important to record all pertinent information and aid in planning the patient's care (including follow-up).

Do not get overloaded with the huge amount of information available. Always summarize trends if possible. It is usual to think in terms of individual body systems to avoid missing anything out, but these are of course inter-related and so you must always step back and consider the patient as a whole. Remember that medicines are only one of the tools that can be used in the care of a patient. Try to think beyond just drugs (eg there are mechanical methods for venous thrombus prophylaxis, in addition to anticoagulants).

Draw on what you know …

Your broad generalist knowledge of medicine is a bonus. Critical care teams are highly specialist, and despite the broad case mix, many of the patients present to intensive care for the same sorts of reasons and require the same sorts of treatments. It is very useful to the team that you know a bit about other medications found outside critical care.

Despite the fact that the majority of critically ill patients have disturbances of organ function that necessitate adjustments of dose, route or choice of agent, this area is often not consistently tackled by medical staff, and is one area where you can make a major contribution. Examples include dose adjustment in renal dysfunction and changes in the route of administration because of surgery.

Keeping a look out for, or avoiding ADRs/interactions is very important. This can sometimes be more about refuting that such a reaction has taken place rather than the more usual situation of trying to avoid problems before they arise.

…and say when you don't know

Knowing your limitations is something to be respected. Do not blag your way through an issue, it is obvious when you do and nobody likes it. It can result in inappropriate interventions in the short term and appropriate advice or interventions being ignored or treated as suspect in the future.

Recognize others' expertise

Everyone has expertise, medics, surgeons, nurses, physiotherapists, dietitians, relatives and loved ones. There are overlaps, in addition to gaps in knowledge and differences in opinion. Learn to live with it and collaborate. Do not create conflict; this will not help the patient.

Be aware and use other resources

Liaise with pharmacists from the service that the patient came from. Critical care is a support service, treating the sickest patients from many other services. Obtaining valuable advice from pharmacists who routinely work in those services greatly aids in the provision of appropriate care for the patient.

Critical care units do not work in isolation from each other. Each unit is part of a larger network or group of units that covers a distinct geographical location. This means that within each network or group, there are other critical care pharmacists with whom you can talk to or draw support from. Find out who they are and introduce yourself to them (face to face, by telephone or e-mail), before you need their advice in a crisis. Each network or group has standards of practice and therapeutic protocols (often called 'care bundles'). Obtain copies and be familiar with them.

Mechanical ventilation

Mechanical respiratory support might be required in patients with a certain degree of respiratory failure. Typically, such failure can be described in terms of a failure to oxygenate blood, such as during an acute asthma attack (type 1 respiratory failure), or a failure to ventilate the lungs resulting in CO_2 retention, such as in exacerbations of COPD (type 2 respiratory failure). Patients who do not protect their airway (eg through the consequences of traumatic head injury) might also require respiratory support.

Non-invasive ventilation

Selected patients might initially be managed using a form of tight-fitting face mask, which acts as the interface between patient and ventilator. These come in a variety of shapes and sizes. A nasogastric tube is usually *in situ* to decompress the stomach, which frequently can become inflated through air swallowing.

Invasive ventilation

The more typical method for connecting a ventilator to a patient is through the insertion of a plastic pipe into the patient's trachea, placed either through the upper airways (nasal passages or mouth) or through a stoma in the patients neck under the larynx. An inflatable cuff at the end of the tube secures it in the trachea. The ventilator is attached to the other end of the tube. The act of tube placement is known as 'intubation'.

Drugs used to facilitate intubation

Feeding a large-diameter tube through the mouth or nose into the trachea generates all manner of physiological responses, none of which are described as 'pleasant'. Various agents are used to manage or attenuate such a noxious stimulus.

Rapid sequence induction (RSI)

This technique is used to rapidly secure a patients airway while minimizing the risk of soiling the airways with stomach contents. A sedative agent, such as thiopentone (3–4mg/kg body weight), is used in combination with a muscle relaxant, such as suxamethonium (1–1.5mg/kg body weight), to facilitate the technique. Other sedative agents used include propofol (2mg/kg body weight), etomidate (0.1–0.4mg/kg body weight) or, occasionally, ketamine (1–2mg/kg body weight). Alternative muscle relaxants include rocuronium (1mg/kg body weight) or succinylcholine (2mg/kg body weight).

Awake intubation

Used to secure an airway if a difficult intubation is anticipated (eg because of previous history or airway obstruction), unstable cervical spine fracture or if anaesthetic induction is dangerous for the patient. Comfort for the patient is provided using topical anaesthetics, such as lidocaine 4% solution, possibly with light sedation with an agent such as midazolam (1–2mg). Atropine (400–600mcg) or glycopyrolate (200–400mcg) is given to dry secretions.

Ventilation modes

There is a bewildering array of ventilation modes in use; the following is intended to be a brief overview of those most commonly used.

Continuous mandatory ventilation (CMV)

The ventilator controls movement of gas through the patient's lungs according to the parameters set and takes no account of any residual breathing effort the patient might make. Set parameters can be volume-based or pressure-based, or a mixture of both.

Assist control ventilation (ACV)

The ventilator controls movement of gas through the patient's lungs according to the parameters set, either when the patient triggers a breath (assisted breaths) or at the set respiratory rate if the patient fails to trigger a breath (controlled breaths).

Intermittent mandatory ventilation (IMV)

The ventilator controls movement of gas through the patient's lungs according to the parameters set at a mandatory respiratory rate, but allows spontaneous breathing to occur between mandatory breaths.

Synchronous intermittent mandatory ventilation (SIMV)

The ventilator controls movement of gas through the patient's lungs according to the parameters set at a mandatory respiratory rate, but allows spontaneous breathing to occur between mandatory breaths. Assisted breaths are synchronized with spontaneous breaths when their timing is sufficiently close.

Pressure support ventilation (PSV)

The ventilator augments the flow of gas moving into the patient's lungs to maintain a preset pressure in the ventilator circuit during inspiration. When the flow rate falls below a set value, the expiration cycle begins. PSV can be combined with other modes of ventilation to support spontaneous breaths.

Continuous positive airway pressure (CPAP)

The ventilator maintains the ventilator circuit pressure at a constant value above the ambient pressure during spontaneous breaths.

Positive end-expiratory pressure (PEEP)

The ventilator maintains the ventilator circuit pressure at a constant value above the ambient pressure during ventilator generated breaths.

Bilevel positive airway pressure (BiPAP)

The ventilator maintains the ventilator circuit pressure at one value above the ambient pressure during inspiration and a lower value (still above ambient pressure) during expiration.

Motility stimulants

The provision of early enteral feed is an important goal in critically ill patients and has several advantages over parenteral feeding. Haemodynamic disturbance, pre-existing disease states and drug use in the critically ill patient frequently result in the failure of the patient to absorb enteral feed.

It is usual to use markers, such as bowel sounds and gastric residue volume on aspiration, to assess gut motility, although neither method is particularly reliable.

Metoclopramide

Metoclopramide is widely used to promote gut motility; however, the evidence base in the critically ill is very poor. This dopamine antagonist possibly works through blockade of dopaminergic neurons in the stomach and small bowel that would normally inhibit GI motility. It also ↑ lower oesophageal sphincter tone. A typical dose is 10mg three times daily.

Erythromycin

The evidence base for erythromycin is stronger than that for metoclopramide and comes from several small-scale studies, but it is often reserved for second-line therapy, after metoclopramide, because of concerns about promoting antimicrobial resistance. Erythromycin acts as a motilin receptor agonist. The addition of erythromycin to a metoclopramide regimen is not evidence-based, although simultaneously targeting different motility pathways could prove beneficial.

Typical doses range from 250mg IV twice daily to 200mg IV three times daily. Doses as small as 70mg have been shown to have an effect in adults. It is believed that smaller doses are more effective than larger doses and this is consistent with the well known upper GI effects of erythromycin.

Neostigmine

Neostigmine infusions have been used to promote normal bowel function in the critically ill. Neostigmine directly stimulates acetylcholine release from nerve plexi within the gut wall. A continuous infusion of 0.4–0.8mg/h is an effective prokinetic on the basis of the frequency of stool production.

Domperidone

There is no evidence to either support or refute the usefulness of domperidone for gut motility. Activation of dopaminergic fibres found in the smooth muscle of the GI tract inhibit smooth-muscle contraction and, ∴, blockade of these fibres by dopamine antagonists might encourage smooth-muscle contraction. It is ∴, possible that a role for domperidone and other dopamine antagonists might be found in the future.

Renal-replacement therapy

Acute renal failure is a common feature of critical illness. Renal function recovers completely in the majority of patients, although a proportion go on to require chronic renal support. During the period of time it takes for the kidneys to recover, renal-replacement therapy is required to undertake some of the functions that the healthy kidneys would perform.

Terminology

Confusion often arises over the various techniques used for renal-replacement therapy. Abbreviations add to the confusion, but there are basically two main renal replacement modes, with a hybrid of the two also being commonly employed. The process is usually continuous, but can be intermittent. Blood follows a pressure gradient that is either generated by taking blood from an artery and returning it to a vein (arteriovenous; AV) or taking blood from a vein and using the machine to generate the pressure gradient required before returning the blood to a vein (venovenous; VV). Putting the various abbreviations together with the form of renal replacement gives the appropriate abbreviation for the technique (eg continuous venovenous haemodiafiltration [CVVHDF])

Haemodialysis (HD)

Not normally used in critical care, but may be used where a patient already has chronic renal failure. Blood is pushed through thousands of small tubes made of a semi-permeable membrane (Fig. 16.13). Clearance of small, water-soluble molecules occurs by diffusion through a semipermeable membrane into dialysis fluid that bathes the tubes. Water can also be drawn off by altering the concentration of glucose in the dialysis fluid.

Clean fluid can be infused back into the patient if required, although this is unusual for this form of renal replacement.

Haemofiltration (HF)

Blood passes through thousands of small tubes made of a membrane full of small holes (typically 20 000Da, in diameter). A pressure gradient pushes the patients plasma through the holes (filtration) and this eluent is discarded (Fig. 16.14).

Clean fluid is infused back into the patient.

Haemodiafiltration (HDF)

A hybrid form that adds a dialysis element to haemofiltration by allowing dialysis fluid to be added to the eluent generated from the filter, thus diluting it and causing an additional diffusion process to occur.

Buffer

Whichever technique is employed, vast quantities of fluid are required for the process to take place. One of the many small molecules that are cleared is bicarbonate. Bicarbonate is central to the acid–base balance of the human body, and its steady removal in renal-replacement therapy and without replacement would lead to increasing acidosis and ultimately to the patient's death.

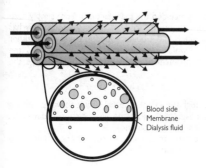

Fig. 16.13 Haemodialysis

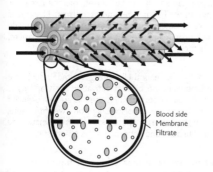

Fig. 16.14 Haemofiltration

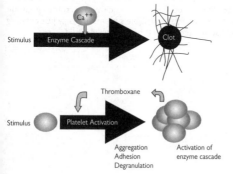

Fig. 16.15 Activation of clotting cascade

Initial stability difficulties precluded the manufacturer from simply adding bicarbonate to the dialysis or replacement fluids (although this has now been overcome). So fluids had a buffer added in the form of either lactate or acetate, both of which are converted to bicarbonate by the patient. This can become problematic if the patient cannot utilize the buffer.

Anticoagulation

The passage of blood through the extracorporeal circuit activates clotting pathways. The resulting coagulation clogs the filter circuit, reducing its efficiency and ultimately destroying its patency.

Anticoagulants are employed to maintain circuit patency, unless the patient is particularly coagulopathic.

Heparin

Heparin has long been used to maintain filter patency through its inhibitory effects on the enzyme cascade. It can be infused into the circuit or the patient, to maintain an APTT of 1.5–2 times normal. Heparin is poorly cleared by renal-replacement therapy. Attempts have been made to neutralize heparin with protamine before it is returned to the patient, although the technique is tricky and not widely used.

Epoprostenol

Prostaglandins produced by the endothelial lining of the vasculature inhibit the effect of thromboxane on platelet activation. This activity is lost in an extracorporeal circuit. Epoprostenol is used as an anticoagulant and is infused into the circuit at 1–5 nanograms/kg body weight/minute, and occasionally at even higher doses. Hypotension is a problematic side effect. The combination of heparin and epoprostenol is synergistic.

Citrate

Citrate has been used to bind up ionised calcium in the circuit, thus inhibiting several calcium dependant steps in the clotting cascade and inhibiting calcium influx into platelets, preventing platelet activation. Large quantities of citrate are needed and this results in a large solute load and metabolic alkalosis. Specialized fluids are required and sourcing citrate can be problematic. Commercially available systems are only just entering the UK market and so the technique is not yet widely used.

Stress-ulcer prophylaxis

Over three-quarters of intensive-care unit patients have endoscopic evidence of mucosal damage within one or two days of admission to intensive care, although in most cases the damage is superficial and will heal quickly. Clinical evidence for gastric bleeding occurs in up to one-quarter of patients ('coffee grounds' or malaena) and up to 6% of patients suffer clinically important bleeding that results in haemodynamic instability or a requirement for blood transfusions. The incidence of stress ulceration seems to be falling, probably because of general advances in the management of critically ill patients, in addition to specific prophylactic measures for stress ulceration.

Pathophysiology

It is thought that mucosal damage is brought about by a number of factors, such as disturbances in mucosal blood flow caused by cardiovascular instability and hypoperfusion, leading to a relative mucosal ischaemia, the presence of ↓ gastric luminal pH and altered mucosal protective mechanisms. At pH<4, the proteolytic enzyme pepsin destroys clots forming on damaged gastric mucosa, increasing the probability of bleeding and the extent of gastric damage.

Risk factors

There are a large number of risk factors identified for stress ulceration, although the two most important risk factors are mechanical ventilation for >48h and coagulopathy (Table 16.46).

Aim of therapy

An ↑ in the gastric pH to >4 is thought to be sufficient to prevent superficial stress ulceration progressing to a more serious pathological state, which is much more difficult to treat. The aim of therapy is to prevent further attack on already injured mucosa by ↓ acidity and/or preventing proteolytic enzymes from attacking unprotected gastric mucosa. This can be differentiated from the aim of therapy for nonvariceal upper GI bleeding, where a higher pH is required (pH>6)

Methods of stress ulcer prophylaxis

- Several large randomized, placebo-controlled studies have been conducted, with conflicting results arising from each. The therapy of choice has changed a number of times over the years.
- Histamine H2-receptor antagonists are usually used as first-line therapy; ranitidine, 50mg bolus injection three times daily is common.
- Proton-pump inhibitor use is growing, although there is at present no defining study that places this agent at the heart of stress-ulcer-prophylaxis therapy. Once daily injections of omeprazole or pantoprazole have been used, and some centres use an extemporaneously prepared enteral formulation of omeprazole (simplified omeprazole suspension).

- The use of sucralfate has almost disappeared, and antacids are no longer used. It is common practice to cease stress-ulcer prophylaxis when nasogastric feeding is established, although the limited evidence available suggests that feed is not an effective form of stress-ulcer prophylaxis.
- Some surgical procedures can result in a ↓ acid-secretory function through denervation of the stomach (such as in oesophagectomy), but the effect this has on stress-ulcer formation has not been studied.
- Pharmacological stress-ulcer prophylaxis is so routine in critical care that the prescribing of prophylaxis becomes an almost reflex response. Stopping acid-suppression therapy in patients with a total gastrectomy can be a common pharmacist's intervention. Partial gastrectomy might still require stress-ulcer prophylaxis if the acid-secretory function remains in tact (ie where the antrum of the stomach remains).

Unwanted effects of stress ulcer prophylaxis.

- One large study found an ↑ incidence of nosocomial pneumonia in the ranitidine arm. This has largely been ignored because it was not found in subsequent studies, although an ↑ incidence of pneumonia in an ambulatory population taking acid-suppressant therapy has also been reported.
- The incidence of *Clostidium difficile* is greater in patients who take acid suppressants (higher for PPIs when compared with H_2 antagonists).
- The use of pH-testing strips to confirm the correct placement of enteral tubes is unreliable if acid-suppressant therapy is used.
- Ranitidine is associated with a number of side effects, including cardiac rhythm disturbance, but the evidence that it causes thrombocytopenia is very poor.

Table 16.46 Risk factors for stress ulceration

- >48h mechanical ventilation
- Coagulopathy
- Acute renal failure
- Acute liver failure
- Sepsis
- Hypotension
- Severe head injury
- History of GI bleeding
- Burns covering >35% of body surface
- Major surgery

Vasoactive agents

A variety of agents can be used to manipulate the cardiovascular system in critical care. These agents should only be used after the patient has been adequately fluid resuscitated. Terminology is often used incorrectly and interchangeably—the following; terminology should be used:

- Inotropes—affect the force of contraction of the heart.
- Chronotropes—affect the heart rate.
- Vasopressors—↑ BP.

Charts of receptor activity are widely available; however, they can be tricky to use because different activities predominate at different infusion rates.

Adrenaline (epinephrine) (α_1^{+++}, β_1^{+++}, β_2^{++}, $D_1^{°}$, $D_2^{°}$)

Dose range effects

- Low doses (<0.01mcg/kg body weight/min):
  - Predominant β_2-adrenoceptor stimulation leads to dilatation of skeletal vasculature, resulting in a fall in BP.
- Medium doses (0.04–0.1mcg/kg body weight/min):
  - Predominant β_1-adrenoceptor stimulation leads to an ↑ in heart rate, stroke volume and cardiac output.
- Large doses (0.1–0.3 mcg/kg body weight/min):
  - α_1-adrenoceptor stimulation predominates, leading to vasoconstriction, which ↑ systemic vascular resistance and ∴, ↑ BP.
- Larger doses (>0.3mcg/kg body weight/min):
  - Increased α_1-adrenoceptor stimulation causes ↓ renal blood flow and ↓ splanchnic vascular bed perfusion. GI motility and pyloric tone are also ↓

Uses

Anaphylactic shock, severe congestive cardiac failure, septic shock and status asthmaticus.

Other effects

Infusions of adrenaline can lead to arrhythmias, hyperglycaemia and metabolic acidosis.

Noradrenaline (norepinephrine) (α_1^{+++}, β_1^{+}, $\beta_2^{°}$, $D_1^{°}$, $D_2^{°}$)

Dose range effects

- Low doses (<2mcg/min):
  - Predominant β_1-adrenoceptor stimulation leads to an ↑ in heart rate, stroke volume and cardiac output.
- Higher doses (>4mcg/min):
  - Predominant α_1-adrenoceptor stimulation leads to vasoconstriction. Baroreceptor-mediated bradycardia is possible.

Uses

Septic shock and to ↑ mean arterial pressure in severe head injury.

Other effects

Infusions of noradrenaline can lead to arrhythmias, hyperglycaemia, and metabolic acidosis. Not useful for cardiogenic shock because of increased afterload.

Dopamine (α_1^{++}, β_1^{++}, β_2^{++}, D_1^{+++}, D_2^{+++})

Dose range effects

- Low doses (<2mcg/kg body weight/min):
  - Predominant D_1-receptor stimulation leads to ↑ renal, mesenteric and coronary perfusion.
- Medium doses (2–5mcg/kg body weight/min):
  - Predominant β_1-adrenoceptor stimulation leads to an ↑ in heart rate, stroke volume and cardiac output.
- Large doses (>6mcg/kg body weight/min):
  - α_1-adrenoceptor stimulation predominates, leading to vasoconstriction, which ↑ systemic vascular resistance and, ∴, ↑ BP.

Uses

Cardiogenic shock. Should not be used as a 'renoprotective' agent, except occasionally where it is used as a vasopressor on general wards to support BP (and hence improves renal perfusion).

Dobutamine (α_1^{+}, β_1^{++}, β_2^{+}, D_1°, D_2°)

Dose range effects

- Usual dose (2.5–10mcg/kg body weight/min):
  - Predominant β_1-adrenoceptor stimulation leads to ↑ cardiac output.

Uses

Cardiogenic shock.

Other effects

BP can fall in hypovolaemic patients.

Dopexamine (α_1°, β_1^{+}, β_2^{+++}, D_1^{++}, D_2^{++})

Dose range effects

- Usual dose (0.5–6mcg/kg body weight/min):
  - Strong β_2-adrenoceptor stimulation leads to vasodilatation. D_1 receptor leads to ↑ renal perfusion. Splanchnic perfusion might also be ↑.

Uses

Can be useful to improve splanchnic perfusion.

Other effects

Heart rate ↑ in a dose-dependent manner.

Phosphodiesterase inhibitors (nonreceptor-mediated effect)

Pharmacology

Inhibits phosphodiesterase, causing an intracellular excess of cAMP and consequent calcium ion influx. This causes ↑ myocardial contractility and smooth-muscle relaxation.

Uses

Cardiac failure.

Other effects

Hypotension caused by vasodilatation.

Treatment of alcohol withdrawal

Alcohol withdrawal syndrome is characterized by a range of symptoms, including tremor, paroxysmal sweats, nausea and vomiting, anxiety, agitation, headache and perceptual disturbances. Seizures are occasionally observed. Half of patients who experience a seizure only suffer a single fit. Some patients with severe withdrawal will progress to delirium tremens. Symptoms usually appear within 6–24h of the last consumption of alcohol and typically persist for 72h, but can last for several weeks.

Many alcohol-dependent people require no medication when withdrawing from alcohol. Supportive care, including information on the withdrawal syndrome, monitoring, reassurance and a low-stimulus environment, are effective in ↓ withdrawal severity.

Many alcohol-dependent patients might not be obvious 'alcoholics'.

If medication is required, a benzodiazepine loading-dose technique is usually employed. The patient is given repeated doses until symptoms have diminished to an acceptable level. Chlordiazepoxide or diazepam are effective in the prevention and treatment of acute alcohol-withdrawal seizures. Because of the relatively large doses usually given, and the long half-lives, it might not be necessary to give any further medication for withdrawal relief. If symptoms reappear, however, further doses should be administered, with doses titrated according to symptom severity.

Suggested withdrawal regimen

Therapy should be started as soon as the patient can tolerate oral medication. Patients should be sedated on admission, with chlordiazepoxide, 20mg four times daily for 1–2 days, followed by rapid tailing-off over the subsequent 3–4 days.

- Day 1—20mg four times daily—10mg when required, up to a maximum of 200mg daily.
- Day 2—20mg four times daily—10mg when required, up to a maximum of 200mg daily.
- Day 3—20mg three times daily.
- Day 4—20mg twice daily.
- Day 5—10mg twice daily.
- Day 6—STOP.

Review dose daily and titrate on individual patient basis

There is a clinical opinion that patients given the recommended maximum dose and still suffering symptoms of withdrawal should be given further doses every 2h until symptoms are controlled or are obviously too drowsy to swallow any more!

Cautions

- Patients might experience seizures as the dose of benzodiazepine is tailed-off.
- Patients who are sedated for too long might develop a chest infection.
- The dose should be adjusted to provide effective sedative and anticonvulsant end points while preventing oversedation, respiratory depression and hypotension.

- Doses of benzodiazepine should be reduced in severe liver dysfunction. Alternatively, a shorter-acting benzodiazepine, eg lorazepam, can be used (seek specialist advice). Patients with chronic liver disease should have their dose assessed twice daily to avoid oversedation.
- A maximum 24h dose (10mg twice daily) should only be prescribed on discharge from hospitals if necessary.
- Clomethiazole, although historically used for the treatment in alcohol withdrawal of in-patients, has the potential for life-threatening respiratory depression if the patient continues to drink alcohol, which precludes its use.

Thiamine and vitamin supplements

Poor nutrition is common in patients who drink for the following reasons:
- Inadequate intake of food.
- Associated chronic liver disease.
- Chronic pancreatitis.
- Malabsorption (water-soluble and fat-soluble vitamins should be replaced and severely malnourished patients should be considered for enteral feeding).

Thiamine

Thiamine deficiency leads to polyneuritis with motor and sensory defects. Ophthalmoplegia (paralysis of the eye muscles), nystagmus and ataxia are associated with Wernick's encephalopathy, in which learning and memory are impaired; there is an estimated 10–20% mortality. Korsakoffi's psychosis is characterized by confabulations (the patient invents material to fill memory blanks) and is less likely to be reversible once established.

IV thiamine replacement

There is no licensed IV thiamine preparation in the UK. one pair of pabrinex® IV high-potency (vitamin B and C injection BPC) ampoules contain 250mg of thiamine.

IV Pabrinex® should be given initially to those with severe withdrawal symptoms.

Dose:

One pair of ampoules should be added to 100mL/sodium chloride 0.9% solution or glucose 5% solution and administered intravenously over at least 10mins once daily for 3 days or until the patient can take oral thiamine. In established Wernicke's encephalopathy higher doses are needed (consult product literature).

Oral thiamine replacement

If symptoms of withdrawal are not severe the following regimen is the recommended:
- Oral thiamine, 100mg four times daily should be given until withdrawal is complete, and reduce the dose to 100mg twice daily.

Other vitamins
- Forceval® (or locally approved multivitamin product), one capsule daily.
- Folic acid, 5mg once daily (if folate deficient).

At discharge

Oral supplements should be continued at discharge in patients who are malnourished or have inadequate diets. Thiamine should be continued long term if there is cognitive impairment or peripheral neuropathy (100mg twice daily).

Consideration should also be given to the setting in which withdrawal occurs. In all cases, careful monitoring of withdrawal severity is essential, while more severe withdrawal requires inpatient care. Specialist alcohol treatment services and most hospitals can provide charts to be used in the monitoring of symptom severity.

Dealing with poisoning enquiries

Poisoning incidents can be caused by the following means:
- Accidental poisoning—eg small children eating tablets or berries.
- Nonaccidental—eg Munchausen's syndrome by proxy (in this syndrome one person creates symptoms in another by, for example, administering drugs).
- Deliberate self-poisoning—eg tablets or chemicals are ingested intentionally, sometimes to manipulate family or friends and, rarely, with the intention of (successful) suicide.

Any enquiry regarding a possible acute poisoning incident should be treated as potentially serious and urgent. Questioning can quickly establish if there is little possibility of harm, but if there is any doubt the patient should be referred to the nearest A&E department and/or a poisons information centre should be contacted for advice.

Some misconceptions

Members of the public might not be aware of the following:
- Alcohol poisoning can be potentially fatal, especially in children and adolescents. In children, if there are any signs of intoxication the patient should be referred to an A&E department.
- Some forms of poisoning might not cause symptoms initially, eg paracetamol overdose, ingestion of sustained-release tablets and capsules. This can create the impression that there is no intoxication. Referral to an A&E department should be made if sufficient tablets have been taken, even in the absence of symptoms.

Be aware that some over-the-counter preparations might have similar brand names, eg Piriton® and Piriteze® and, Anadin® and Anadin®-paracetamol. Ensure that you and other healthcare professionals are clear what product is involved.

Sources of information

TICTAC is a computerized tablet and capsule identification system used by the medicines information and poisons information centres. Information required to identify a tablet or capsule using TICTAC includes the following:
- Shape—straight, rounded or bevelled edge for tablets.
- Colour—cap, body and contents for capsules.
- Markings—including whether one-half or one-quarter scored.
- Coating—film, sugar or uncoated.
- Length and width (in millimetres)—at longest/widest point.
- Weight.

Toxbase[1] is an online poisons information database that covers drugs (including over-the-counter medication), plants, household, industrial and agricultural chemicals, and snake and insect bites[1]. Details of probable toxic effects and appropriate management are provided. Toxbase is password-protected. Medicines Information and poisons information centres have access to Toxbase and NHS pharmacy departments can apply for a password through the website.

1 www.spib.axl.co.uk

Poisons information centres provide 24h telephone advice. If there is any cause for concern in an acute-poisoning incident, a poisons information centre should be contacted immediately. It is inappropriate to cause unnecessary delay in what might be a life-threatening situation by looking elsewhere for information. The doctor dealing with an acute incident should contact the poisons information centre direct so that first-hand information is given and received. Advise the doctor of the sort of information the poisons information centre might require. For a nonacute or general enquiry, it is appropriate for a pharmacist to contact the centre.

Information required to deal with a poisoning enquiry

Eliciting as much information as possible about a poisoning incident can facilitate speedy management. It is especially important to have the relevant information available when contacting a poisons information centre:

- Identity—brand name and active ingredients.
- Timing—when did the incident occur relative to the time of the enquiry.
- Quantity—number of tablets and volume of liquid. An estimate is better than no information. Checking the quantity left in a container versus its full volume at least gives an estimate of maximum quantity ingested.
- If tablets or capsules—are these sustained-release?
- Age and weight of the patient—especially if a child.
- Any signs and symptoms observed.
- If the patient has vomited—any sign of the poison, eg coloured liquid, undigested plant material or tablet fragments.
- Any treatments or first aid already administered and the outcome.

If attendance at an A&E department is recommended, the enquirer should be advised to take any containers or plant material with them that could help with identification (taking suitable precautions to avoid skin or clothing contamination with the poison).

First aid for poisoning incidents

- Do not induce vomiting.
- If fully conscious, give sips of water or milk.
- If unconscious, check ABC. As needed, perform the following:
  - Perform CPR but not mouth-to-mouth resuscitation, except with a face shield (because of the risk of contaminating first aider).
  - Place patient in the recovery position.
- Take the patient to an A&E department or phone the emergency services.

Drug desensitization

Patients with drug hypersensitivity can usually be treated with an alternative agent. However, on rare occasions if there is no suitable alternative, drug desensitization might be appropriate. Drug desensitization is potentially hazardous and should never be attempted in patients who have had a severe allergic reaction, such as bronchospasm, facial swelling or anaphylaxis. However, it can be attempted in those who have had a rash—provided this was not a severe skin reaction, such as Stevens–Johnson syndrome.

Desensitization schedules using both oral and parenteral administration have been developed for a variety of drugs but mostly for antibacterials (notably penicillins) and some chemotherapy drugs. Examples of these are listed at the end of this topic as further reading.

Drug desensitization is potentially hazardous because there is always a risk of anaphylaxis. Thus, when attempting the procedure, the following precautions should be observed:
- The patient is informed of the potential risks (it is advisable that they give written consent to the procedure).
- The patient must be reasonably well (ie no active disease other than the current infection).
- The patient's drug history should be reviewed and any drugs known to exacerbate allergic reactions stopped—notably β-blockers and NSAIDs.
- Desensitization should be carried out as an in-patient or closely monitored day-case procedure.
- A doctor or appropriately trained nurse with authority to administer emergency drugs should be present throughout.
- Drugs and equipment required for treatment of anaphylaxis should be available.
- The patient should have an IV cannula placed for administration of emergency drugs before starting the procedure.
- Prophylactic antihistamines, adrenaline or steroids should not usually be given as these can mask a reaction:
- Patient monitoring should be carried out before each dose and every 30min (if the dose interval is longer), including
  - temperature, pulse and BP.
  - respiratory signs, including peak-flow measurement.
  - observation and direct questioning of the patient for signs and symptoms of allergic reaction, eg skin flushing, rash, itching, wheeze, shortness of breath and tingling lips or tongue.
- Patients should continue to be monitored for at least 1h after the final dose of the desensitization schedule.
- Observations and details of drug administration should be documented in the patients medical notes.

It is important to ensure that the desensitization schedule is followed as rigorously as possible:
- Measure doses accurately, eg using an oral syringe.
- The patient should rinse their mouth with water and swallow after oral doses.
- Doses should be administered at exactly the specified time intervals.

Because of the requirement for direct medical observation throughout the procedure, most schedules involve rapid desensitization. However, some longer schedules have been used, in which case the procedure is carried out on an out-patient basis. The patient's GP should be informed that out-patient desensitization is planned.

It is important that patients doing drug desensitization at home are carefully selected and that the patient agrees to the following:

- Undertakes never to be on their own throughout the procedure.
- Understands the risks and what action to take if a reaction occurs. Ideally, another responsible person in the home should also be informed.
- Should have access to a telephone and contact numbers for the physician supervising the procedure.
- Has access to suitable transport so that they can attend the hospital in the event of a minor reaction (the patient should call emergency services if a major reaction).
- Lives reasonably close to the hospital and certainly not in a remote area with difficult access.

After the schedule is complete and treatment doses of the drug are being administered without adverse effects, a treatment course of the drug can be given. Desensitization is usually lost within 1–2 days of stopping the drug. If it is probable that further courses of the drug will be needed, low doses should be administered until the next course is required. It is important that patients understand that drug desensitization is only temporary.

Further reading

Examples of drug desensitization schedules

Sullivan TJ et al. (1982). Desensitisation of patients allergic to penicillin using orally administered beta-lactam antibiotics. *Journal of Allergy and Immunology* **69**(3): 275–82.

Kalanadhabhatta V et al. (2004). Successful oral desensitisation to trimethoprim-sulphamethoxazole in acquired immune deficiency syndrome. *Annals of Allergy, Asthma and Immunology*, **92**(4): 409–13.

Confino-Cohen R et al. (2005). Successful carboplatin desensitisation in patients with proven carboplatin allergy. *Cancer* **104**(3): 640–3.

Eapen SS et al. (2005). A successful rapid desensitisation protocol in a loop diuretic allergic patient. *Journal of Cardiac Failure* **11**(6): 481.

Pathology ranges and interpretation

Table A1

	Levels ↑ by	Levels ↓ by	Comments
Sodium (Na⁺) 135–145mmol/L	Water depletion, nephrogenic diabetes insipidus, (eg lithium toxicity), mineralocorticoid excess (eg Cushing's syndrome), corticosteroids, 2° aldosteronism (eg CCF), nephritic syndrome, hepatic cirrhosis and uraemia *Symptoms: dry skin, postural hypotension, oliguria. Cerebral dehydration → thirst, confusion and eventually coma*	Water excess, mineralocorticoid deficiency (eg Addison's, thyroid deficiency), thiazide and loop diuretics, burns, SIADH, excess sweating, diarrhoea, vomiting, aspiration, atypical pneumonia, haemodilution caused by cardiac, hepatic or renal failure, oedema, infection and carcinoma *Symptoms: headache, nausea, hypertension, cardiac failure, cramps, confusion convulsions and overhydration*	Regulated by aldosterone (ADH)
Potassium (K⁺) 3.5–5.0mmol/L	Mineralocorticoid deficiency (eg Addison's thyroid deficiency) ACE inhibitors, K⁺: sparing diuretics, renal failure, severe tissue damage (eg burns), hypoaldosteronism, diabetic ketoacidosis, excess K⁺ therapy, NSAIDs, β-blockers, heparin infusions and sodium depletion (very rare) *Symptoms: muscle weakness and abnormal cardiac conduction (eg ventricular fibrillation, and asystole)*	Thiazide and loop diuretics, vomiting, diarrhoea, ileostomy, fistula, steroids, glucose and insulin therapy, mineralocorticoid excess (eg Cushing's syndrome), β-agonists, aspiration and metabolic alkalosis *Symptoms: hypotonia, cardiac arrhythmias, muscle weakness and paralytic ileus*	Regulated by aldosterone, insulin/glucose For hypokalaemia, if on diuretics, then ↑ bicarbonate is the best indication that hypokalaemia is likely to be long-standing. Magnesium might be low and hypokalaemia is often difficult to correct until magnesium normalized

Table A1 (*Contd.*)

	Levels ↑ by	Levels ↓ by	Comments
Chloride (Cl^-) 95–105mmol/L	Excess ingestion and dehydration *Symptoms: nonspecific*	Vomiting, diarrhoea, diuretics, dehydration and nephropathy *Symptoms: nonspecific*	Cl^- follows Na^+ movement
Bicarbonate (HCO_3^-) 24–30mmol/L	Excessive antacid use, thiazide and loop diuretics, metabolic alkalosis, bicarb, hypokalaemia, vomiting and Cushing's syndrome *Symptoms: vomiting*	Diarrhoea, renal failure, diabetes mellitus, metabolic acidosis, respiratory alkalosis and hyperventilation *Symptoms: headache, drowsiness and coma in severe acidosis*	Reflects renal, metabolic and respiratory functions
Glucose 3.0–8.0mmol/L	Diabetes mellitus, severe stress, occasionally after CVA, corticosteroids, thiazides and relative insulin deficiency caused by ↑ growth hormone, ↑ glucocorticoids or placental lactogen during pregnancy (glucagonaemia) *Symptoms: polyuria, polydipsia and ketoacidosis*	Insulin overdose, sulphonylureas especially in the elderly, insulinoma, alcohol and hepatic failure *Symptoms: dizziness, lethargy, sweating, tachycardia, agitation and coma*	
Magnesium (Mg^{2+}) 0.70–1.10mmol/L	Renal failure and excessive antacids *Symptoms: loss of muscle tone, lethargy and respiratory depression*	Severe diarrhoea, fistula, alcohol abuse, diuretics, diabetes mellitus, TPN, hyperaldosteronism, hepatic cirrhosis and malabsorption *Symptoms: tetany, parathesiae, cramps, arrhythmias, neuromuscular excitability and hypoparathyroidism*	Deficiency can exacerbate digitalis toxicity and Mg^{2+} is excreted by the kidneys

Table A1 (Contd.)

	Levels ↑ by	Levels ↓ by	Comments
Zinc (Zn^{2+}) 11–24µ	Zinc therapy	Cirrhosis, diarrhoea, alcoholism, drugs, parenteral nutrition, inadequate diet, steroids, diuretics, malabsorption syndrome and rarely genetic *Symptoms: poor wound healing and growth, alopecia, infertility and poor resistance to infection*	
Calcium (Ca^{2+}) 2.20–2.60mmol/L (Beware to determine correct calcium level in hypoalbuminaemia and hyperalbuminaemia)	Paget's disease, vitamin A overdose, hyperparathyroidism, vitamin D overdose, thiazides, oestrogen, lithium, tamoxifen, excess milk ingestion, excess calcium absorption, Hodgkin's disease and myeloma *Symptoms: nausea, vomiting, constipation, abdominal pain, renal stones, cardiac arrhythmias, headache, depression, mental fatigue and psychosis*	Thyroid surgery, hypoparathyroidism, alkalosis, renal failure, osteomalacia, vitamin D deficiency and acute pancreatitis *Symptoms: ↑ nervous excitability, tetany, convulsions, muscle cramps, spasms, tingling, numbness of fingers, and ECG changes*	Apparent hypocalcaemia might be caused by hypoalbuminaemia. Regulated by parathyroid hormone calcitonin (1,25-dihydroxycholecalciferol)
Phosphate (PO_4^{3-}) 0.8–1.4mmol/L	Renal failure, hypoparathyroidism, diabetic ketoacidosis and ↑ vitamin D	Osteomalacia (starvation) Hyperparathyroidism, alcohol abuse, ↓ vitamin D Al(OH)$_3$ therapy and septicaemia	Ca^{2+} and PO_4^{3-} metabolism closely linked
Urea 2.5–7.0mmol/L	Renal failure, elderly (caused by ↓ renal function), urinary tract obstruction, CCF, dehydration, corticosteroids, high-protein diet, ↑ catabolism (eg starvation), sepsis and GI bleed	↑ GFR, pregnancy, excessive IV infusion, low protein intake, anabolic states or synthesis, liver failure, diabetes insipidus, diuresis and overhydration.	Derived from amino-acid metabolism in the liver; indicator of kidney function

Table A1 (*Contd.*)

	Levels ↑ by	Levels ↓ by	Comments
Creatinine 20–110μmol/L (Cr/Cl) 80–139ml/min (not considered impaired unless <50ml/min)	Dehydration, renal failure ↓ GFR, urinary tract obstruction and ↑ meat/vitamin C	Pregnancy and chronic muscle wasting	Derived from muscle mass, determined by lean body mass and indication of glomerular insufficiency
Alkaline phosphatase <125IU/L	Renal failure, cholestasis, liver cell damage, osteomalacia and bone disease, hyperparathyroidism (eg Paget's disease) and metastases. Also during third trimester of pregnancy, postmenopause, carcinoma of liver/prostrate and drug-induced (eg chlorpromazine)	Hypothyroidism and growth retardation	~50% bone-related, ~50% hepatic fraction and ~2–3% intestinal fraction
Creatine kinase 32–184IU/L	MI, skeletal muscle damage even IM injection, muscular dystrophy, acute psychotic episodes, head injury, surgery, hypothyroidism, alcoholism and neonates		Found in heart, skeletal and smooth muscle, and brain
Haemoglobin ♂: 13.5–18g/dL ♀: 11.5–16g/dL	Polycythaemia, and dehydration	Sickle cell disease, thalassaemia, GI bleed, haemorrhage, (acute/chronic) deficient RBC production, iron deficiency, marrow depression, renal failure, ↑ haemolysis and chronic liver disease	

Table A1 (*Contd.*)

	Levels ↑ by	Levels ↓ by	Comments
White cell count 4.0–11.0×10⁹/L	Drugs, infection, septicaemia, malignancy, drugs (eg steroids), sulphonamides bacterial infection, alcohol hepatitis and cholecystitis	Drugs, bacterial infections, HIV, hypersensitivity reactions, surgery, trauma, burns, haemorrhage, leukaemia, radiation, cytotoxics, ↓ vitamin B_{12} and ↓ folate	Produced in bone marrow and stimulated by GSF
Haematocrit or packed cell volume ♂: 0.4–5.0 ♀: 0.37–0.47	Addison's thyroid deficiency, dehydration, polycythaemia and pregnancy	Anaemia and haemorrhage	Relative measure of cells in blood and packed cell volume
Platelets 150–400×10⁹/L	Inflammatory disorders, bleeding, malignancy, splenectomy and polycythaemia	↓ production: bone-marrow failure/suppression, leukaemia, drugs (notably cytotoxic drugs), megaloblastic anaemia, SLE. Heparin. ↑ consumption: DIC, splenomegaly, furosemide, gold, idiopathic thrombocytopaenia. and HIV drugs.	Derived from megakaryocytes in bone marrow and destroyed in spleen
Prothrombin time 10–14s INR — 0.8-1.2	Severe liver damage, cholestasis causing malabsorption of vitamin K and warfarin		Used to monitor anticoagulant therapy and assess liver function
Thrombin time 12–15s	Heparin and DIC		
APPT	Heparin, haemophilia and liver failure		Used to monitor heparin therapy
Fibrinogen 1.7–4.1g/L	Nephrotic syndrome, Hodgkins and PE	DIC and massive blood transfusion	
Total protein 60–80g/L	Mineralocorticoid deficiency (eg Addison's thyroid deficiency) and myeloma	Catabolic states (eg septicaemia)	

Table A1 (Contd.)

	Levels ↑ by	Levels ↓ by	Comments
Albumin 35–50g/L $t_{\frac{1}{2}}$=20–26days	Dehydration and shock	Lost through skin (eg burns and psoriasis) liver disease, malnutrition, septicaemia, nephrotic syndrome and late pregnancy *Symptoms: oedema and toxic effects of drugs normally bound to albumin (eg calcium, bilirubin and phenytoin)*	
Bilirubin—total <17μmol/L Bilirubin-conjugated (bound to albumin) <4μmol/L	Hepatocellular damage (eg viral hepatitis–inability to conjugate bilirubin), cholestasis (eg by phenothiazines and flucloxacillin) gallstones, inflammation, malignancy, Gilbert's syndrome, haemolysis, methyldopa, GI bleed, extensive bruising and sulphonamides (displace bilirubin from albumin) *Symptoms: Jaundice*		Derives from breakdown of red blood cells by monocyte macrophage system
γ-Glutamyl transpeptidase ♂: 11–51IU/L ♀: 7–33IU/L	Cholestasis (eg carcinoma of pancreas or biliary tract), liver cell damage (eg hepatitis and cirrhosis). Enzyme inducers (eg alcohol, phenytoin, and phenobarbitone) and alcoholism		Found in liver, kidneys, pancreas and prostrate; released by tissue damage
Aspartate transaminase 5–35IU/L	Hepatocellular damage, cirrhosis, viral hepatitis, severe haemolytic anaemia, myocardial injury (eg MI), cholestasis, trauma or surgery	Renal failure and vitamin B deficiency	Found in liver, heart, kidneys, skeletal muscle and erythrocytes

Table A1 (Contd.)

	Levels ↑ by	Levels ↓ by	Comments
Amylase <180U/dL random urine <650IU/L	Acute pancreatitis, abdominal trauma, diabetic ketoacidosis, chronic renal failure, cholecystitis, intestinal obstruction, mumps, ruptured ectopic pregnancy, post-MI ruptured DU and morphine	Hepatitis and pancreatic insufficiency	Found in paratoid glands and pancreas. Smaller amounts in ovaries, intestine and skeletal muscle
Fibrin degradation products <10μg/mL	DIC and adult respiratory distress syndrome		
Cholesterol 3.9–6mmol/L	Diabetes mellitus, familial hypercholesterolaemia excess alcohol, hypothyroidism and hepatic and renal diseases	Severe illness, severe weight loss and MI (during first 2wks)	Treatment will depend on other risk factors
pH 7.35–7.45	Vomiting, K^+ loss, burns, hyperventilation, stroke, SAH, anxiety, hyperthyroidism, excess antacids, aspirin overdose, fever and uncompensated alkalosis	Respiratory failure, hypoventilation, diarrhoea, renal failure, ketoacidosis trauma, shock, high plasma lactate (eg liver failure), hypoxia, anaemia and uncompensated acidosis	Reflects ratio of acid to base and not absolute concentration. It might, ∴, mask a defect for which the body has compensated
PaO_2 >10.6kPa	Artificial overventilation with O_2	COAD, respiratory failure, ARDS, and cardiogenic pulmonary oedema	
$PaCO_2$ 4.7–6.0kPa Total CO_2 24–30mmol	COAD, hypoventilation respiratory acidosis and ARDS-compensated metabolic alkalosis	Hyperventilation, respiratory alkalosis, CVA, anxiety, aspirin overdose, compensated metabolic acidosis, pulmonary embolism and non-cardiogenic ARDS	Indicator of respiratory function

Normal ranges

Table A2

Sodium	135–145mmol/L	White cell count	$4.0–11\times10^9$/L
Potassium	3.5–5.0mmol/L	PCV/haematocrit	♂=0.4–0.54
Chloride	95–105mmol/L	PCV/haematocrit	♀=0.37–0.47
Bicarbonate	24–30mmol/L	Platelets	$150–400\times10^9$/L
Glucose (fasting)	3.5–5.5mmol/L	INR	0.8–1.2
Magnesium	0.75–1.05mmol/L	KCR	0.8–1.2
Phosphate	0.8–1.4mmol/L	Thrombin time	Ratio <1.2
Zinc	11–24µmol/L	Fibrinogen	1.7–4.1g/L
Calcium	2.12–2.65mmol/L	Albumin	35–50g/L
FDP	<10µg/ml	Total protein	60–80g/L
Urea	2.5–6.7mmol/L	Bilirubin(total)	3–17µmol/L
Creatinine	70–150µmol/L	Bilirubin-(conjugated)	<4µmol/L
Cr/Cl	80–139mL/min	GGT	♂: 11–40IU/L :7–33IU/L
Alk. phos	<150IU/L	AST	5–35IU/L
Creatine kinase	♂: 25–195IU/L ♀: 25–170IU/L		
Haemoglobin	♂=13.5–18g/dL	Amylase	<180IU/L
Haemoglobin	♀=11.5–16g/dL	Amylase (random urine)	<650IU/L
Cholesterol	3.9–6mmol/L	PaO_2	>10.6kPa
pH	7.35–7.45	$PaCO_2$	4.7–6.0kPa

Paediatric normal laboratory values

These values are a guide; local laboratories may differ. Check normal values with the laboratory you use.

Table A3 Biochemistry

Alanine aminotransferase	Newborn–1 month		≤70IU/L
	Infants and children		15–55IU/L
Albumin	Preterm		25–45g/L
	Newborn (term)		25–50g/L
	1–3 months		30–42g/L
	3–12 months		27–50g/L
	1–15yrs		32–50g/L
Alkaline phosphatase	Newborn		150–600U/L
	6 months to 9yrs		250–800U/L
Amylase			70–300IU/L
Aspartate aminotransferase			<45IU/L
Bilirubin	Full term	day 1	<65µmol/L
		day 2	<115µmol/L
		day 3–5	<155µmol/L
		>1 month	<10µmol/L
Calcium	Preterm		1.5–2.5mmol/L
	Infants		2.25–2.75mmol/L
	>1yr		2.25–2.6mmol/L
Chloride			95–105mmol/L
Creatine kinase	Newborn		<600IU/L
	1month		<400IU/L
	1yr		<30IU/L
	Children:	♂	<190IU/L
		♀	<130IU/L
Creatinine	0–2yrs		20–50µmol/L
	2–6yrs		25–60µmol/L
	6–12yrs		30–80µmol/L
	>12yrs	♂	65–120µmol/L
		♀	50–110µmol/L
Creatinine clearance	<37wks' gestation		<15mL/min/m^2
	Neonate		10–20mL/min/m^2
	1–2wks		20–35mL/min/m^2
	2–4 months		35–45mL/min/m^2
	6–125 months		45–60mL/min/m^2
	12 months to adult		50–85mL/min/m^2

Table A3 (*Contd*)

C-reactive protein		<20mg/L
γ-glutaryl	Newborn	<200IU/L
transferase	1 month to 1yr	<150IU/L
	>1yr	<30IU/L
Glucose	Newborn to 3 days	2–5mmol/L
	>1wk	2.5–5mmol/L
Lactate		0.7–1.8mmol/L
Magnesium	Newborn	0.7–1.2mmol/L
	Child	0.7–1mmol/L
Phosphate	Preterm first month	1.4–3.4mmol/L
	Full term newborn	1.2–2.9mmol/L
	1yr	1.2–2.2mmol/L
	2–10yrs	1–1.8mmol/L
	>10yrs	0.7–1.6mmol/L
Potassium	0–2wks	3.7–6mmol/L
	2wks to 3 months	3.7–5.7mmol/L
	>3 months	3.5–5mmol/L
Protein (total)	1 month	50–70g/L
	1yr	60–80g/L
	1–9yrs	60–81g/L
Sodium		135–145mmol/L
Urea	0–1yr	2.5–7.5mmol/L
	1–7yrs	3.3–6.5mmol/L
	7–16yrs ♂	2.6–6.7mmol/L
	♀	2.5–6mmol/L

Table A4 Haematology

Age	Hb (g/dL) Mean (range)		MCV (fl) Mean (range)		WBC (x10⁹/L) range	Reticulo-cyte (%) range
Birth	18.5	(14.5–21.5)	108	(95–116)	5–26	3–7
1 month	14	(10–16.5)	104	(85–108)	6–15	0–1
6 months	11	(8.5–13.5)	88	(80–96)	6–15	0–1
1yr	12	(10.5–13.5)	78	(70–86)	6–15	0–1
6yrs	12.5	(11.5–14)	81	(75–88)	6–15	0–1
12yrs	13.5	(11.5–14.5)	86	(77–94)	5–15	0–1

Note: an artefactual high neonate WBC may be reported because automatic cell counters may wrongly include in the WBC the many normoblasts (red cell precursors) in the neonate.

Table A5 Respiratory rate

Newborn	30–60 breaths/min	Heart rate is usually four times the respiratory rate
6months	30–45 breaths/min	
1–2yrs	25–35 breaths/min	
3–6yrs	20–30 breaths/min	
>7yrs	20–25 breaths/min	

Table A6 Blood pressure

	Mean (mmHg)	
	Systolic BP	Diastolic BP
Newborn to 2yrs	95	55
3–6yrs	100	65
7–100yrs	105	70
11–15yrs	115	70

Table A7 Urinary output

	mL/day
Infant	250–600
Child	500–1000
Adolescents	500–1500
Adult	500–2000

Table A8 Hypoglycaemia

	Serum glucose
Pre-term	<1.4mmol/L
Term	<2.0mmol/L
Child	<2.5mmol/L

Table A9 Electrolyte requirements

Na^+	2–4mmol/kg body weight/24h
K^+	1–3mmol/kg body weight/24h
Cl^-	3–5mmol/kg body weight/24h
Ca^{2+}	1mmol/kg body weight/24h
Mg^{2+}	0.15mmol/kg body weight/24h

Drug interference with laboratory tests

Drugs interfere with laboratory diagnostics, which can lead to wrong diagnoses or treatments and unnecessary further tests.

Table A10 Drug–laboratory interferences are usually overlooked

Drug	Laboratory test	↑/↓	Mechanism of action
Acetazolamide		Leads of spurious ↑ of theophylline levels	Interferes with certain HPLC assays for theophylline
Amiloride	Creatinine	Leads of falsely high measurements of serum creatinine and ↓ creatinine clearance	Doesn't alter renal function, but blocks tubular secretion of creatinine
Amiodarone	T4		Amiodarone inhibits peripheral conversion to T3
Ascorbic acid	Urine sugar	(false + and −)	Clinitest
Oestrogens	Dexamethasone suppression	(false +)	Caused by ↑ corticosteriod binding globulin
Ketamine	Alkaline phosphatase, GGT, ALT		Mechanism unknown
Levodopa	Urinary glucose Urinary ketones	False + False +	
Lithium	Serum lithium levels		Inadvertent use of lithium–heparin collection tube leads to spuriously high serum lithium determination
Oral contraceptives	Glucose		Alters glucose tolerance test
Spironolactone	Digoxin assay	↓ of true level, ie can mask test confirmation of digoxin toxicity	Interferes with certain specific digoxin assays. Refer to Biochemistry department for type of assay used locally
	Plasma cortisol levels (synacthen test)	Erroneously ↑ cortisol levels	Metabolites of spironolactone fluoresce, which interferes when fluorometric analysis is used for tests

Therapeutic drug monitoring (TDM) in adults

The aim of TDM is to provide an assessment of the drug concentration that will assist in achieving rapid, safe and optimum treatment.

TDM is generally of value in the following situations:

- Good correlation between blood concentration and effect.
- Wide variations in metabolism.
- High risk of side effects.

Routine measurements might be warranted, for example, in determining adequate concentrations postorgan transplantation or more commonly ordered to add evidence to a specific clinical problem, eg investigate handling by a patient with concurrent disease or confirm excessive dosing correlating to signs of toxicity.

Table A11 covers common drugs, but other drugs might also benefit from TDM, such as drugs used to treat HIV.

Table A11 Common drugs

Drug	Therapeutic range— standard units	Ideal sampling time	Comments and SI units	Type of sample required
Carbamazepine	4–12mg/L	Trough measurement before dose.	Therapeutic ranges: adults, 34–51. Units: mmol/L ranges desired from predose specimens.	Serum or plasma—SST (orange) or PST heparin (green).
Ciclosporin	Varies with indication.	Trough measurement before dose.	Therapeutic range depends on the disorder/ clinical situation being treated.	Whole blood–EDTA (lavender).
Digoxin	0.8–2mcg/L. The reference range is valid for specimens taken 6–8h postdose.	Sampling 8–24h after last dose.	Adults, 1.0–2.0. Units: nmol/L.	Serum or plasma–SST (orange) or PST heparin (green).
Lithium	Minimum effective concentration in mania prophylaxis is 0.5–1.2mmol/L. Toxic concentration >1.5mmol/L.	12h post dose.	Therapeutic range: 0.5–0.8. Toxicity: >1.0. Units: mmol/L. Not in lithium Heparin tube Please measure Maintenance range 12h after last dose.	Serum–SST (orange).
Phenytoin	10–20mg/L	Trough Measurement before dose.	Therapeutic levels (predose Specimen): 40–80. Units: mmol/L	Serum or plasma—SST (orange) or PST heparin (green).

Table A11 (*Contd.*)

Phenobarbitone	15–40mg/L	Trough Measurement before dose.	Therapeutic range desired from predose. Specimens: adults, 65–170. Units: µmol/L	Serum or plasma —SST (orange) or PST heparin (green).
Theophylline /aminophylline	10–20mg/L	1) During a continuous infusion, preferably at 6h. and 18h. 2) SR preparation – predose.	55–110. Units: µmol/L.	Serum or plasma—SST (orange) or PST heparin (green).
Tacrolimus	5–15ng/mL	Trough measurement before dose	N/a	Blood—EDTA (lavender).

Table A12 Antibiotics

Drug	Therapeutic range mg/l	Ideal sampling time	Comments	Type of sample required
Gentamicin, Once daily	5–10mg/L	Trough level 18–24h after the first dose (ideal <1.0mg/L).	Not necessary to do a post-dose level	Blood SST (orange).
Gentamicin, conventional dosing	Trough <2 Peak 5–10	Trough Peak–1h postdose. dose.	Peak for endocardititis if having synergistic therapy 3–5mg/L	Blood SST (orange).
Amikacin	Trough <10 Peak 20–30	Trough Peark–1h postadministration.	Further usually twice weekly predose levels if no dose changes and normal renal function.	Blood SST
Vancomycin	Trough 5–10	Predose before fourth dose.	Further monitoring usually twice weekly.	Blood SST (orange).
Teicoplanin	Trough 10–20	Trough	>20mg/L (<60mg/L) for deep seated infection.	Blood SST (orange).
Tobramcyin	Trough <2 Peak 5–10	Trough 1h post-administration	Samples should to the fourth dose, depending on renal function.	Blood SST

- For antibiotic assays, doses should ideally be timed for convenience, eg 10.00am. For predose levels, a sample should be taken and the dose administered.
- For dosage adjustment, sampling at steady state is essential, except for suspicion of toxic concentrations.
- Sampling is taken at an appropriate time during a dose interval. You must co-ordinate when, or if, your pathology department can undertake the test or co-ordinate from another centre.
- Concentrations can be affected by various factors, such as age, drug interactions, protein binding, metabolism and organ dysfunction.
- The pharmacist has a very important role in interpreting results from TDM:
  - Advice on what to do if unexpectedly high/low result, eg check that dose was given, timing of sample in relation to dose or sampling technique.
  - Advice on whether or not another dose should be given if a waiting result.
  - Dose adjustment—most drugs follow linear kinetics ie doubling the dose will double the level, but certain drugs, eg phenytoin, exhibit non-liner kinetics and require small, incremental dose adjustments.
  - Timing of sampling if there is a suspicion of drug interaction from the introduction of new therapies.

Useful websites

Useful websites

Description	Web address (URL)
Americal Society of Clinical Oncology (ASCO)	www.asco.org
American Society of Haematology (ASH)	www.hematology.org
American Society of Health-System Pharmacists	www.ashp.org
Annals of Internal Medicine	www.annals.org
Australian therapeutic goods administration	www.tga.gov.au
Bandolier 'Evidence-based thinking about healthcare'	www.jr2.ox.ac.uk/bandolier
BNF	www.bnf.org
British Committee for Standards in Haematology (BCSH) guideliness	www.bcshguidelines.com
British medical Journal (BMJ)	www.bmj.bmjjournals.com
British Oncology Pharmacy Association (BOPA)	www.bopa-web.org
British Society for Haematology (BSH)	www.b-s-h.org.uk
Canadian Health Technology Assessment Programme	www.ccohta.ca
Cancer services Collaborative	www.modern.nhs.uk
CancerlineUK	www.cancerlineuk.net
COREC	www.corec.org.uk
Counterfeit drugs	www.pharmacistscombatcounterfeiting.org
Cytotoxic guidelines	www.marcguidelines.com
Department of Health	www.doh.gov.uk
Drug information	www.druginfozone.nhs.uk
Drugs in breast milk	www.ukmcentral.nhs.uk
Drugs of porcine origin-downloadable booklet	www.medicines-paternship.org/ourpublications/drugs-of-porcine-origin
Electronic medicines compendium	www.medicines.org
European Society for Medical Oncology (ESMO)	www.esmo.org
Extemporaneous formulations	www.ghp.org.uk/cig
Foreign medicines, identification of	www.pharmj.com/noticeboard/info/pip/foreignmedicines.html
Free full-text journals online	www.freemedicaljournals
Gene Therapy Advisory Committee (GTAC)	www.advisorybodies.doh.gov.uk/genetic/gtac
Health and Safety Executive (HSE)	www.hse.gov.uk
Herbal medicines—includes evidence for efficacy, ADRs and drug interactions	www.herbmed.org

International Society of Oncology Pharmacy Practitioners (ISOPP)	www.isopp.org
Journal of Clinical Oncology (JCO)	www.jco.org
Malaria advice (no prophylaxis advice)	www.malariahotspots.co.uk
MHRA	www.mhra.gov.uk
Medicines management and pharmaceutical care	www.pharmalife.co.uk
Merck manual full-text online	www.merck.com/pubs/mmanual
MI network	www.ukmi.nhs.uk
MI tutorials and extemporaneous formulations	www.phaminfotech.co.nz
National electronic library for health	www.helh.nhs.uk
National Institute for Clinical Excellence (NICE)	www.nice.org.uk
National prescribing centre	www.npc.co.uk
National Translational Research Centre (NTRAC)	www.ntrac.org.uk
National treatment centre for substance misuse	www.nta.nhs.uk
Oxford Handbook of Clinical Medicine	www.oup.co.uk/ohcm
Palliative care	www.palliativedrugs.com
Paracetamol information centre (includes guidelines on treatment of overdose)	www.pharmweb.net/ paracetamol.html
Patient-group directins	www.groupprotocols.org.uk
RPSGB	www.rpsgb.org.uk
Scottish Intercollegiate Guideline Network (SIGN)	www.sign.ac.uk
TB information in various languages	www.immunisation.nhs.uk
The Journal of the American Medical Association (JAMA)	www.jama.ama-assn.org
The Lancet	www.thelancet.com
The New England Journal of Medicine	www.content.nejm.org
The Pharmaceutical Journal	www.pharmj.com
Travel advice, specific to destination—includes vaccinations and malaria prop	www.fitfortravel.scot.nhs.uk
Travel—health information (subscription required, free NHS Scotland)	www.travax.scot.nhs.uk
Travel shop, includes travel health information and medical supplies	www.nomadtravel.co.uk
WHO action programme on essential drugs	www.who.int/dap

Index

Reference intervals—biochemistry

Drugs (and other substances) may interfere with any chemical method; as these effects may be method dependent, it is difficult for the clinician to be aware of all the possibilities. If in doubt, discuss with the lab.

Substance	Specimen	Reference interval (labs vary, so a guide only)	Your hospital
Adrenocorticotrophic hormone	P	<80ng/L	
Alanine aminotransferase (ALT)	P	5–35IU/L	
Albumin	P[1]	35–50g/L	
Aldosterone	P[2]	100–500pmol/L	
Alkaline phosphatase	P	30–150U/L (adults)	
α-amylase	P	0–180 Somogyi U/dL	
α-fetoprotein	S	<10ku/L	
Angiotensin II	P[2]	5–35pmol/L	
Antidiuretic hormone (ADH)	P	0.9–4.6pmol/L	
Aspartate transaminase	P	5–35IU/L	
Bicarbonate	P[1]	24–30mmol/L	
Bilirubin	P	3–17µmol/L	
bnp	P	<50ng/L	
Calcitonin	P	<0.1µg/L	
Calcium (ionized)	P	1.0–1.25mmol/L	
Calcium (total)	P[1]	2.12–2.65mmol/L	
Chloride	P	95–105mmol/L	
[3]Cholesterol	P	3.9–6mmol/L	
VLDL	P	0.128–0.645mmol/L	
LDL	P	1.55–4.4mmol/L	
HDL	P	0.9–1.93mmol/L	
Cortisol	P	a.m. 450–700nmol/L midnight 80–280nmol/L	
Creatine kinase (CK)	P	♂ 25–195IU/L ♀ 25–170IU/L	
Creatinine (∝ to lean body mass)	P[1]	70–≤150µmol/L	
Ferritin	P	12–200µg/L	
Folate	S	2.1µg/L	
Follicle-stimulating hormone (FSH)	P/S	2–8U/L in ♀ (luteal); >25U/L in menopause	
Gamma-glutamyl transpeptidase	P	♂ 11–51IU/L ♀ 7–33IU/L	
Glucose (fasting)	P	3.5–5.5mmol/L	
Glycated (glycosylated) Hb	B	2.3–6.5%	
Growth hormone	P	<20mu/L	
HbA1c (= glycosylated Hb)	B	2.3–6.5%	
Iron	S	♀ 14–31µmol/L ♂ 11–30µmol/L	
Lactate dehydrogenase (ldh)	P	70–250IU/L	
Lead	B	<1.8mmol/L	
Luteinizing hormone (lh) (premenopausal)	P	3–16U/L (luteal)	
Magnesium	P	0.75–1.05mmol/L	

1 See *OHCS* p81 for reference intervals in pregnancy.
2 The sample requires special handling: contact the laboratory.
3 Desired upper limit of cholesterol would be ~ 6mmol/L. In some populations, 7.8mmol/L is the top end of the distribution.

P = plasma (eg heparin bottle); S = serum (clotted; no anticoagulent); B = whole blood (edetic acid EDTA bottle)

Reproduced with permission from Longmore ML, Wilkinson IB, Rajagopalan S (2004). *Oxford Handbook of Clinical Medicine*, 6th edn. Oxford: Oxford University Press.